THE
COMPLETE
PROSTATE BOOK

"This is indeed the single most complete source of information on the prostate gland. All of your questions and concerns about prostate health are fully addressed in an unbiased, honest, and reassuring manner. The chapters on prostate cancer are outstanding. This reference will eliminate most if not all of your confusion and anxiety surrounding the complexities of prostate cancer."

Christopher S. Ng, MD
Director of Laparoscopic Urologic Oncology
Minimally Invasive Urology Institute
Cedars-Sinai Medical Center (Los Angeles)

"All men should have a doctor as wise, witty, and straightforward as Dr. Jones. His book avoids boring chapters filled with confusing medical jargon and instead presents an accessible, informative, and entertaining guide to a man's most vexing gland. If you have a prostate (or love someone who does) read this book."

Kate Dailey
Associate Editor, *Men's Health Magazine*

"This extraordinary book from a respected colleague offers a uniquely informative review of the entire spectrum of prostate disorders in language that everyone can understand."

Andrew C. Novick, MD
Chairman, Glickman Urological Institute, Cleveland Clinic Foundation, and
Associate Dean for Faculty Affairs and Professor of Surgery
Cleveland Clinic Lerner College of Medicine of Case Western Reserve University

"This is an excellent book that thoroughly covers the evaluation and treatment of both benign and malignant diseases of the prostate. Dr. Jones has done a tremendous job of critically summarizing and reviewing the data on all prostate conditions and has produced a clear, concise synopsis for the public."

Joseph Presti Jr., MD
Director, Urologic Oncology Program
Stanford University School of Medicine

"This book provides helpful, straightforward guidance for the majority of men who know little about the prostate gland and the common medical conditions surrounding it. Dr. Jones excels at providing a wealth of information in clear, easy-to-read language."

Richard R. Kerr
Editor-in-Chief, *Urology Times*

"Dr. Stephen Jones has created a very user-friendly guide to prostate health. The book is written in an easy-to-understand style that is filled with the most up-to-date information on 'what every man needs to know' to live a healthy life. As a urologist specializing in prostate cancer, I enjoyed reading his clear explanations of the causes and treatments of prostate problems that many men will face in their lifetime. I will definitely recommend this book to my patients who want the best information on these important issues in men's health."

Leonard G. Gomella, MD, FACS
The Bernard W. Godwin Jr. Professor of Prostate Cancer
Chairman, Department of Urology, Jefferson Medical College (Philadelphia)

"This interesting and easy-to-read book supplies essential information to enable men to make an educated decision about their treatment. Every aspect of prostate cancer is covered, and I enjoyed reading it. I believe it is required reading for any member of the public interested in this condition."

John M. Fitzpatrick
Professor and Chairman, Department of Urology
University College—Dublin

"Stephen Jones's *Complete Prostate Book* is an easy, yet accurate and detailed read that allows the men and their significant others to be informed prior to as well as after seeking medical attention."

Mark S. Soloway, MD
Professor and Chairman, Department of Urology
University of Miami School of Medicine

"This is a remarkably comprehensive yet easily readable text. All of the facts and myths are presented in a very practical manner to help men who are faced with sometimes difficult treatment decisions about prostate problems."

Joseph A. Smith Jr., MD
Professor and Chairman of Urologic Surgery
Vanderbilt University Medical Center (Nashville)

"*The Complete Prostate Book* addresses a very complex organ and its diseases in a comprehensive yet succinct manner. Jones has not only targeted the lay public effectively, but there are pearls of clinical practice for the medical professional as well. What is truly remarkable is the seamless incorporation of new surgical technology and molecular medicine in prostate disease such that it is easily comprehended. This manual for men may be the 'tipping point' for education in prostate health."

Louis S. Liou, MD, PhD
Boston Medical Center
Boston University School of Medicine

THE COMPLETE PROSTATE BOOK

WHAT EVERY MAN NEEDS TO KNOW

BENIGN PROSTATE PROBLEMS

PROSTATE ENLARGEMENT

REDUCING YOUR RISK OF CANCER

SEXUAL HEALTH

LATEST TREATMENTS FOR PROSTATE CANCER

J. STEPHEN JONES, MD

A LEADING UROLOGIST AT GLICKMAN UROLOGICAL INSTITUTE,
CLEVELAND CLINIC FOUNDATION

Foreword by COACH RICK PITINO

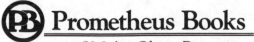 Prometheus Books
59 John Glenn Drive
Amherst, New York 14228-2197

Published 2005 by Prometheus Books

Inquiries should be addressed to
Prometheus Books
59 John Glenn Drive
Amherst, New York 14228–2197
VOICE: 716–691–0133, ext. 207
FAX: 716–564–2711
WWW.PROMETHEUSBOOKS.COM

09 08 07 06 05   5 4 3 2 1

Library of Congress Cataloging-in-Publication Data

Jones, J. Stephen, 1960–
    The complete prostate book / J. Stephen Jones.
        p. cm.
    Includes bibliographical references and index.
    ISBN 1–59102–304–1 (pbk. : alk. paper)
    1. Prostate—Diseases—Popular works. I. Title.

RC899.J66 2005
616.6'5—dc22

2005012247

Printed in the United States of America on acid-free paper

To Jared, Katie, and Kathryn—
the reasons I wake up each morning.

CONTENTS

2: THE BOTHERSOME PROSTATE

3: THE DANGEROUS PROSTATE

ACKNOWLEDGMENTS

A book with the word "complete" in the title requires a monumental effort on the part of many people, only one of whom has the privilege of being featured on the cover. The work of a number of other critical players turned an idea into reality.

Linda Greenspan Regan at Prometheus Books sprung her trap at my most vulnerable moment—during the delight as my previous book was going to print. She envisaged the book she felt needed to be written, and knew we could create it together. Despite my weariness, I could only withstand the first two times she said, "Please." The third one broke me, and I remain grateful. Chris Kramer and the entire production staff at Prometheus can be thanked for perfecting the little details that make a difference.

Coach Rick Pitino is a true leader of men both on and off the basketball court, with his consistent focus being a drive to help others. I appreciate his support for this project and for the men we hope to help with this book.

As I sat writing early drafts of this book, I observed the hundredth anniversary of Dr. Hugh Hampton Young's first radical prostatectomy in 1904. The occasion made me acutely aware that the work of my forebears and colleagues is a legacy I proudly embrace. Through the vision and support of Dr. Andrew C. Novick, the environment of the Glickman Urological Institute of the Cleveland Clinic Foundation allows talented people to reach their potential. The urologists around me are the top of our profession; to work in their presence is humbling. Contributions to prostate disease care by my colleagues whose work is referenced in this book, such as (alphabetically!) Dr. Ken Angermeier, Dr. Jay Ciezki, Dr. Rob Dreicer, Dr. Inderbir Gill, Dr. Jihad

25

26   ACKNOWLEDGMENTS

Kaouk, Dr. Eric Klein, Dr. Cristina Magi-Galluzzi, Dr. Drogo K. Montague, Dr. Raymond Rackley, Dr. Lynn Schoenfeld, Dr. Jim Ulchaker, Dr. Sandip Vasavada, Dr. Ming Zhou, Dr. Craig Zippe, and many others have made me a better urologist and brought this book closer to fulfilling its title. Work of many more colleagues from around the world is referenced herein; they are too numerous to count, but their input and discoveries were crucial to the process.

Jeff Loerch and his team of medical illustrators have redefined urological artwork, and I am pleased to feature a small representation of their portfolio. Joe Pangrace, Ross Papalardo, Joe Kanasz, and Beth Halasz have an uncanny ability to create medical art that bridges a divide; physicians can learn complex principles while the lay public can easily comprehend the needed perspective from their beautiful work.

The staff members at the Glickman Urological Institute are a vital part of my world and key to the many successes we have achieved. Sticking with us through the years have been Nancy Mart, Shelley Angie, Shelly Kovacevic, Renée Kitay, Samaria Sanders, Lisa Iafelice, and Sandy Ausmundsen. Marge O'Malley makes these things happen before I can finish asking, and always does everything with excellence.

My mother, Mary Jones, taught me the value of education and the written word. More significantly, she taught me important values. Her fingerprints are indelibly on my work. My grandmother, Betty Young, was the greatest fan of my previous book. I hope this one survives the absence of her advocacy. I know she has already told Saint Peter that he must have a copy. Since prostate cancer can be a hereditary disease, I had originally planned to thank my grandfather, Howard Jones, and my father, Gene Jones, for *not* having prostate cancer. Dad took that line away halfway through the manuscript when he was diagnosed with early stage, low-grade (read: curable) prostate cancer. I am confident that the courage and common sense he used in dealing with it will assure a successful outcome, although he unfortunately made me begin prostate cancer screening six years earlier than I had intended because of my newly revealed family history. Thanks for nothing!

My children are the source of immeasurable pride, fulfillment, and inspiration. Jared, the award-winning humanitarian leader, has now assured us that his parents are the least gifted writers in the family. Katie is the award-winning wordsmith whose creations frequently bring tears to her mother's eyes, though I try to maintain dignity while holding in my pride.

Most important, Kathryn is the real key to each of my successes, professionally or otherwise. She suffered the writing of yet another book and the costs it brings. Nevertheless, she edited every word and told me all the things I needed to take out to make it readable for a broader audience—that is, anyone not related to me. While doing so, she often revealed a wonderful clarity, further confirming my absolute faith in her wisdom. I hope she will someday grant me the honor of returning the favor.

—J. Stephen Jones

FOREWORD

Rick Pitino
Head Coach, Louisville Cardinals

Most men worry about prostate problems at some point. After all, a majority will experience at least some symptoms during their lifetimes, and prostate cancer is by far the most common malignancy in men. My concerns were simply more public than most because I had to take a couple of days off in order to get help—and taking days off makes headlines in my business. Fortunately, in doing so I found that my symptoms were not only significant, but also common and correctable. Following a successful outcome, I also learned that many men I knew or encountered had similar concerns ranging from pain to urinary difficulty to cancer. In introducing this book, I hope to help you learn that such problems are nothing to be embarrassed about, and that almost all are manageable if you simply seek help.

For the last ten years, between ages of forty-two and fifty-two, I have experienced symptoms of prostatitis and urinary difficulties. After several examinations, doctors said that my prostate felt "boggy." This was concerning to them, so a biopsy was performed in Boston with negative results and my PSA remained below one, which is completely normal. Medication was prescribed throughout the years ranging from Flomax to Cipro. None ever caused relief of my symptoms or made a significant difference. In January 2004, I started having pain in my groin area. A "sports hernia" was a possible diagnosis. An ultrasound revealed a mass, which was possibly malignant. Another biopsy was performed, as well as a cystoscopy. Both proved negative. I decided at that point to get a more definitive answer once and for all. Unlike correcting a poor foul shot, there were too many different viewpoints and methods of attack.

A few years back, I had given a motivational speech to a group of doctors and administrators at the Cleveland Clinic. Physicians gathered from there and the Mayo Clinic. The doctors were kind enough to offer to reciprocate if they ever could be of assistance. I now needed an answer quickly as we were making our stretch run toward March Madness. After a battery of tests under the supervision of Dr. J. Stephen Jones and the Cleveland Clinic, I realized that my problems were being experienced by thousands of other men my age. This is not a solution, but it does help in understanding the problem.

Pelvic pain, prostatitis, cystitis, and sports hernia have all been possible diagnoses in the past. It is crucial to appreciate that those problems must be correctly diagnosed and then treated. Dr. Jones helped me understand that as we get older, these problems can be controlled with the right treatments.

Dr. Jones and the Cleveland Clinic allowed me to return to work within forty-eight hours. Prostate and bladder problems in men must be diagnosed correctly to help relieve the stress of feeling ill. This book will help you recognize that you are not alone. It will help you understand the role of a healthy prostate as part of the larger, overall health of its owner. This includes advice on a healthy diet, exercise, and sex life. It also includes advice on smoking and stress, as well as helpful information on how to become an active participant in, and to get the most out of, your healthcare experiences.

Prostate problems and urinary difficulties are common and here to stay. Our understanding and optimistic way of dealing with these problems will aid us on a path of recovery. Upon my return from Cleveland, my twelve-year-old daughter, Jacqueline, asked me why the word "urological" was used in the press release that described my illness. I laughed and explained to her that urological was a perfectly normal way of describing the problem. This book will help you recognize the role of a man's family in his experiences, decisions, and outcomes.

I've witnessed many friends and associates deal with prostate cancer in the last couple of years. When we see that it affects sports leaders such as Joe Torre, Jim Boeheim, and Jim Calhoun, we recognize how close to home prostate difficulties are for men. Dr. Jones points out prevention strategies for prostate cancer and helps manage those who may need prostate surgery.

The focus of this book is clearly illustrated by the three main section titles: "The Basic Prostate," "The Bothersome Prostate," and "The Dangerous Prostate." The author is a surgeon who openly acknowledges that nonsurgical treatment, delayed treatment, or—in some instances—no treatment at all, are all acceptable approaches to many problems, including those of many men with conditions as serious as cancer. However, when surgery is indicated, this book guides you through what to expect and how to optimize your outcome.

Many of us need to know the true cause of urinary symptoms and pain of the abdomen and pelvis—whether the real cause is related to the prostate, bladder, or any other connections to the prostate area.

This book is written in direct and honest language. It's easy to understand and follow correctly.

In recommending it, I know that you will discover a clearer picture of how the prostate works, how to avoid its problems, and what options are available.

1.

The Basic Prostate

1.

INTRODUCTION TO THE PROSTATE: WHAT IS IT GOOD FOR?

A man spends the first fifty years of his life trying to make money—the rest of his life trying to make water.
—Henry M. Weyrauch, MD, *Life after Fifty: The Prostatic Age*

The prostate seems to be a gland that materializes on a man's fiftieth birthday. Most men become aware of it only around that time, either because of urinary difficulties or when a doctor puts on a glove to begin checking for cancer. Before then, many have heard that it may be somehow responsible for sexual activity, although they don't know exactly how.

In actuality, the prostate is a secondary sex organ that has nothing to do with sexual performance. The primary sex organ—the penis—has that job. In contrast, the prostate sits silently in the pelvis doing all its work during the brief period in which men procreate (make babies).

The prostate has one simple but crucial function: preservation of the species. By that, I mean that it produces the fluid that allows normal sperm function. The majority of this fluid is a sugar-based substance that gives sperm cells energy for their journey to the egg. The potential result is fertilization, enabling procreation. Therefore, the prostate is responsible for preventing extinction of the species—not quite the titillating role most people believe.

Although extreme exceptions exist (tabloid reports of young boys fathering children, or real reports of elderly senators doing so), most men use the prostate for reproduction only during early adulthood. Therefore, the prostate has completed its useful life span before most men ever become aware that it exists.

After fulfilling its role of enabling paternity, the prostate simply sits in the pelvis occupying space—a setup for mischief. It often begins to grow until its size becomes a nuisance (making urination difficult) or until it develops cancer and becomes dangerous.

The prostate's location—deep in a man's pelvis—plays a role in most of the problems it can cause. Side effects associated with treating prostatic conditions are also related primarily to where it sits. This book will help you understand the prostate in sickness and in health.

THE "PRIVATE GLAND"

Unlike other male sex organs, the prostate is almost always spoken of in negative terms. No one brags about his prostate or how well it works. Have you ever heard anyone say he had the prostate of a thirty-year-old? Few men brag about its size.

Few men know where the prostate is (although after their first prostate examination they get a pretty good idea it is located somewhere they wish it weren't). In contrast to the reality, many men believe that the prostate is at least partially responsible for an erection. This is not so, but the assumptions are understandable because of a couple of facts. First is that the age at which men develop prostate ailments or cancer is around the same age when erectile dysfunction becomes common. These problems arrive in each other's company, so they seem related. In addition, men treated for prostate problems may experience damage to erections (as discussed later in this book). Such damage is certainly not inevitable, so don't stop reading here! Moreover, such damage is often readily correctable.

This book is intended to clarify and delineate the facts surrounding prostate issues. Since women are often known to be the seekers of truth regarding medical information, it may be of as much use to the women who intend to keep prostates (and the men who own those prostates) healthy.

WHAT'S IN A NAME?

The word "prostate" comes from the sixteenth-century French anatomist and surgeon Ambrose Pare, who named it for the Greek term meaning "guardian." He chose this name based on its strategic location surrounding the lower urinary tract, which he apparently thought helped it guard against any possible enemies that might work their way upstream. Its vital location makes it essentially the Panama Canal of human anatomy—the gatekeeper to urinary tract transportation.

However, instead of guarding the bladder from foreign invaders, it may serve more as an embedded enemy if it goes bad. If it obstructs urinary out-flow or develops cancer, it may harm the bladder and the man as much as an external enemy. Fortunately, although such damage is common, it is usually manageable.

The name seems to stump some people. It is a pros*tate*—not a pros*trate*. Urological purists may end up lying pros*trate* if they hear enough people mispronounce pros*tate* (the gland). They may also shake their heads when they hear men discuss their pros*tates*, since not one man in the history of medicine has ever been found to have more than one prostate. The coup de grâce for urological purists occurs when they hear men discuss their *pros-trates*—a combination of the wrong word with the wrong number.

WHAT'S THE PROBLEM?

Men become fixated on the prostate for a multitude of reasons. First, its loca-tion deep in the pelvis lends itself to a sense of hidden mystery. Many of us fear the unknown. Since we can't see it, it may take on a mythic life of its own, and it's blamed for an unlimited number of ailments. Second, women don't have one, so there must be something very mystical and masculine about it. Finally, it really does cause a number of ailments, usually associated with aging. From the annoying (prostatitis), to the harmful (enlargement), to the dangerous (cancer), the gland sits there finding new ways to cause havoc. As we age, few men escape some form of trouble from the gland. (A gland, by the way, is a group of cells that secretes something the body needs—in this case, fluids necessary for reproduction.)

Indeed, the specialty of urology originally arose in large part due to the frequency of prostate problems. Ounce for ounce, it may be the source of more ills than any other structure in man.

In the following chapters we will explore normal prostatic anatomy and function in detail. We will find out how neighboring organs are related to many problems caused by an abnormal prostate, as well as the ill effects that it can cause. We will also focus on the full array of treatments for these disorders. After completing this book, you will have an understanding of the prostate that will prepare you to handle essentially any issues that arise.

WARNING FOR CONCRETE THINKERS

You will find that there are many points of controversy in this material. The goal of this book is to bring some sense to them. There are many alternatives available for management of prostate issues. Since controversy abounds, it might be tempting to interpret this to mean that we don't completely understand the prostate or know exactly what to do if things go wrong. There is a little truth to that. However, it should really be interpreted as meaning that the prostate—like every organ in the human body—is a wonderfully, albeit frustratingly, complex entity. Nature didn't make the organ or its dysfunctions simple, so evaluation and management may not be straightforward.

Therefore, you will note that I refer at many points to controversies or various alternatives that might be used by different physicians. Your urologist might approach you differently than I would. He and I may approach your best friend differently than we approach you. That doesn't mean either approach is wrong. Our mission should include helping you understand that more than one approach has merit. If we believe one approach is best for your situation, we should be able to help you understand why. This book is designed to help you to be knowledgeable in consultation with your physician.

As you read this book, please note that any term in **bold** is defined at the end of the book in the glossary. This will avoid my redefining the terms repeatedly, so you may want to refer to this section at various points. Please note that I describe the experiences of several men dealing with prostate problems. Although their names and other features of their lives have been changed, their stories are the experiences of real patients. I have taken liberties when appropriate to clarify issues that are common to many.

Finally, in order to avoid confusing attempts to remove gender from the language, I have chosen to use the male pronoun in reference both to prostate patients (who are ALL male) and their urologists (who are usually, but certainly not always, male). This should not be misinterpreted in any way to disregard the wonderful reality that women have gone from a curiosity in urology a few decades ago to now comprising a growing, *vital*, part of our specialty, strengthening our profession. This is purely for simplicity, and not to offend.

WHAT THIS BOOK WILL NOT DO FOR YOU

It will not tell you what to do—or make decisions for you. The purpose of many health books is to advocate one treatment—turning them into sales pamphlets. This is not one of them.

My intent is to give you information in the clearest manner possible. Removing all bias is impossible, of course. However, I will try to make my viewpoint known and try to minimize its impact on your decision making when there are legitimate alternatives.

Knowledge is power. Arm yourself with the following information no matter what your prostate problem. Do so even if you don't have prostate problems yet. This book will help prepare you for now and the future.

2.

IN THE NEIGHBORHOOD: UNDERSTANDING THE ANATOMY

*Anatomy is the only solid foundation of medicine; it is to the
physician and surgeon what geometry is to the astronomer.*
—William Hunter

Everything that happens to the prostate is affected by its location deep
in the male pelvis. Its "neighbors" are all organs that can be affected
by problems occurring in the prostate, or that can be injured by treatments administered to the prostate. Therefore, understanding the anatomical
area allows us to understand many aspects that will be covered in this book.
Medical students learn anatomy before anything else. Likewise, let's consider the anatomy, as it explains so many issues involving the prostate.

Imagine the prostate as the ground floor of an apartment building, with
several nearby organs as its neighbors (see figure 2-1). This chapter will
explain why the geographical (i.e., anatomical) relationships are so important
to understanding functions, abnormalities, and treatments of the prostate.

INSIDE THE PROSTATE

Before considering the neighboring organs, you should be aware of the inner
makeup of the prostate. Prostatic anatomy is really very simple. It is primarily composed of gland tissue that is about the firmness of a rubber ball.
Counterintuitively, the base is actually the top of the gland at the site where
it attaches to the bladder. From there it tapers slowly before narrowing below

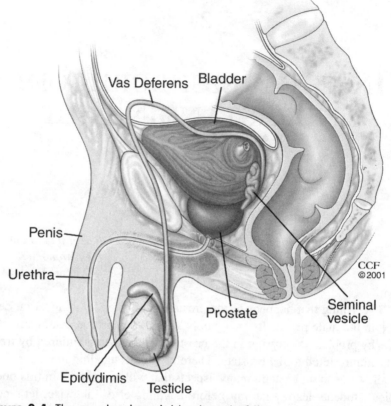

Figure 2-1: The anatomic neighborhood of the prostate.

the **apex**—a conical-shaped opening located where the urethra exits the prostate on its way to traverse the length of the penis. Due to its size and shape, it is often described as "walnut-shaped."

There are many different approaches used to describe prostatic anatomy. I recommend the simplest—the prostate is basically composed of an outer layer called the peripheral zone and an inner layer called the **central** or **transition zone.** The most important distinction is that benign enlargement (as discussed later) is more likely to affect the central/transition zone, whereas cancer is more likely to form in the peripheral zone. The front or anterior portion is an area that is actually part of the peripheral zone. Its importance relates to the frequency that difficult-to-diagnose cancers are often located there.

UPSTAIRS NEIGHBORS

The prostate sits just under the urinary bladder. As a result, urine can escape only from the base of the bladder (**bladder neck**) by traversing a tube running through the middle of the prostate. This tube, called the **urethra**, is a flexible conduit leading to the outside of the body.

Once urine enters the urethra, it flows through based on simple fluid dynamics. In other words, it runs just like water through a fire hose. The urethra doesn't contract or otherwise push urine along, so sometimes drops get caught inside. This leads to *dribbling* later on when the remaining drops work their way outside at a less convenient time.

When the prostate grows upward, it can lift the bladder. A portion might actually grow inside the bladder. This *intravesical* (inside the bladder or *vesical*) growth will occasionally act like a benign tumor and take up some of the bladder's capacity.

Surgery of the prostate inevitably ends up being surgery of the bladder due to their proximity. Realistically, it is often difficult to tell where the prostate ends and the bladder begins, similar to determining the spot in midstream where a river ends and the ocean begins. We will thus cover many bladder and urination issues in this book. The merging of bladder and prostate is so entwined that at least a little portion of bladder is inevitably removed if any (or all) of the prostate is removed.

Several flights up in our anatomical apartment building are the kidneys. These urine factories are responsible for filtering all unwanted substances out of the bloodstream, thereby cleaning the entire body. The product of this removal is urine (urological nectar). The kidneys send this unwanted urine down the ureters, their drainage route to the bladder. Most people have one ureter draining each kidney to the bladder, although about 1 percent of people have two ureters per side, which is known as *duplication*. This duplication may reach all the way to the bladder, or the two duplicated portions may join somewhere downstream before reaching the bladder.

The kidneys are far enough away that the prostate doesn't directly affect them. However, the ureters pass through the base of the bladder wall where the bladder and prostate merge. As noted above, that makes them pass within millimeters of the prostate. Therefore, if the prostate pushes on them, one or both ureters can become elevated or *obstructed*. This type of direct compression is rare with benign enlargement, but it is not uncommon for prostate cancer to grow into the bladder base and obstruct the ureters.

Another problem occurs when the bladder muscle thickens as a result of working too hard to push urine through the obstructing prostate. Like any muscle, use and exercise cause it to become larger. This thickening can block the ureters as they pass through the muscle. The ureters can become blocked up if the bladder outlet is obstructed. Urine pressure builds and pushes back up the ureters. Any of these situations, if unnoticed or untreated, may lead to kidney failure.

Finally, the intestines are located immediately above the bladder and prostate, but are rarely affected by activities at the level of the prostate.

NEIGHBORS TO THE NORTH, SOUTH, EAST, AND WEST

Determining direction is a little tricky (and all relative) in the human body, but we can describe structures at the same level as the prostate in these terms. The most obvious structure at that level is southerly behind the building—the rectum. Its proximity allows access to examine the prostate. Moreover, visualization of the prostate is possible using an ultrasound probe placed into the rectum. This enables investigation and biopsy to determine if cancer is present, as well as measurement of its size.

Also at the level of the prostate and slightly above are the *seminal vesicles*, small sacs attached to the prostate that sit behind the bladder. Over half of the *ejaculate* is produced by these hidden secondary sex glands. Each *vas deferens* joins the tube from a seminal vesicle in a joint structure called the *ejaculatory duct*. During ejaculation, muscle contractions push semen down the ejaculatory duct, through the prostate, and out to do its work if things are working properly.

The seminal vesicles and *vasi deferentia* (the plural of vas deferens) may be the most boring organs in the body. However, because they attach to the prostate, they inevitably are affected by prostate treatments. The owner rarely notices these boring structures unless he undergoes a vasectomy for sterilization.

The only important east-west neighbors are a key set of nerves that pass along each side, as described below.

DOWNSTAIRS: THE PELVIC FLOOR

The pelvic floor is a like a muscular hammock that holds everything in place. The *levator ani* are muscles that originate on either the bony pelvis or its ligaments. In a circular manner they secure the pelvic floor as if it were a sagging trampoline.

The hammock has two openings in men. (Toward the back, the rectum must pass through, while the urethra exits through a much smaller opening in the front.) Between these openings is the point at which all the muscles come together in the middle of the hammock, which is called the **perineal body**. It is a small fibrous tendon that the muscles pull against to maintain support. It sits between the base of the scrotum and the rectum, and is easily strained due to its central location in the pelvic-floor muscle. This entire area is called the **perineum**.

Most men never even know they have a perineal body unless they have pain in this sensitive area and an astute physician notes that this tendon has been pulled or irritated. This can occur during a sneeze, straining, or even a bowel movement. Just like other pulled tendons, it is treated with heat, rest (difficult to do), and sometimes medication. This problem is often mistaken for prostatitis.

URINARY RHABDOSPHINCTER: THE DOORMAN

A tiny, horseshoe-shaped muscle sits over the urethra just below its exit from the prostatic apex. This muscle is called the *rhabdosphincter*, named such because it is a skeletal muscle under voluntary control (*rhabdo*) that closes the urethra (**sphincter**). Its function is to enable a man to keep the urethra closed so that urine doesn't escape. It is sometimes referred to as the *external urinary sphincter* to differentiate it from the muscle of the bladder neck, known as the *internal urinary sphincter.* When a man has both sphincters intact, urinary control is usually very good. Even if he loses one of the two to surgery or injury the other can do an adequate job. However, if he loses one to surgery, as often occurs as a normal and expected outcome during prostate surgery, the other has to be intact or he will not have adequate bladder control.

IN THE YARD: THE NOT-SO-GREAT SANTORINI

Surrounding most of the surface of the prostate is a network of veins called *Santorini's plexus*. This group of veins carries blood primarily from the penis—a major area of blood flow activity if there ever was one. The veins draining the penis traverse the pelvic floor in a grouping called the **dorsal vein complex**—named such because of their location on the dorsal or back side of the penis. (This terminology is interesting because the dorsal or back side is the top, so that the official anatomical position of the penis for descriptive purposes is straight up!).

Soon after coming through the pelvic floor, the dorsal vein complex divides into three main (and many minor) branches. These branches, which are varied in every man, similar to the variations of snowflakes, comprise Santorini's plexus.

This complex serves its purpose well except when confronted with prostatic surgery. Due to the large size, immense variability, and significant amount of blood flow through these thin-walled veins, prostatic surgery involves the risk of substantial blood loss. Until the anatomy was more clearly defined by Dr. Patrick Walsh, prostate surgery almost always involved severe blood loss and transfusions. Now that we understand this anatomy and how to control the vessels, major blood loss is rare and patients do not commonly need transfusion with prostate surgery.

NORTHERN NEIGHBOR: THE PENIS

This is the big one. Few men can name all the organs in the neighborhood of the prostate, but all of them know the penis is right out the front door. Not only does this make men nervous about treating prostate problems, but it also makes some erroneously assume that problems with the penis must have started in the prostate. With that thought in mind, some men will complain that they are having prostate troubles when they experience impotence, premature ejaculation, or other sexual difficulties.

Just like the power lines supplying a nearby building, the *penile nerves* reach their destination by going through the prostate neighborhood (i.e., passing east and west). Therefore, radiation and surgery involving the prostate could injure these microscopic wires.

The penile nerves weren't fully understood until recently. These tiny strands of tissue are hard to see, so they're often overlooked by surgeons and anatomists alike. In 1981 Dr. Patrick Walsh was in the Netherlands to address a medical meeting. Since it was Dr. Walsh's birthday, his hosts reserved a free afternoon for any leisure activity he desired. Most people could think of dozens of things to do for a birthday party in the Netherlands; he chose to spend the afternoon in the anatomic dissection lab on campus exploring the exact route that the nerves took through the pelvis en route to the penis. This discovery completely changed our understanding of these nerves. Since we know where the nerves are located, we can usually preserve them during prostate and other urological surgery.

Males clearly fixate on their penis, but most don't really know what one consists of. The main bulk of the penis is composed of three tubes running lengthwise. On top are two side-by-side cylinders, each of which is called a *corpus cavernosum* (the plural of which is *corpora cavernosae*). During erection they fill with blood under pressure, kind of like airing up a tire or an inflatable raft.

Immediately below the corpora cavernosae runs the third tube, called the *corpus spongiosum*. The *urethra* exits the prostatic apex and carries urine and semen through the spongiosum to the tip of the penis. The spongiosum spreads out at the end of the penis to form the helmet-shaped *glans penis* or "head." The glans penis holds the nerve fibers that give the penis its sensitivity.

AROUND THE PERIMETER

Surrounding much of the neighborhood is the bony pelvis, a solid ring that protects its contents from harm like the rock wall of a gated community. The downside is that the pelvis limits expansion of its contents. The result is that if the prostate grows the bones don't move aside. Therefore, if it needs more room it will likely push on the other structures. The only saving grace is that all these contents are flexible, so this doesn't always result in harm.

NEIGHBORS DOWN THE STREET

As vital organs go, the testicles are greatly underappreciated. They may be relatively unnoticeable, but they carry inside them the future of the species. All mammalian life relies on a male animal producing sperm to fertilize the female's eggs. This whole process originates in the testicles.

The inside of each testis is packed tightly with tiny tubes that do nothing but crank out sperm all day. These tubes, called seminiferous tubules, are coils that can stretch out to about a yard long. One hundred of these tubules could stretch the length of a football field, and all of them from one testis might stretch for miles. Between the spaces in these coils are the *Leydig cells*—little cellular testosterone factories. Based on its control of these Leydig cells, the only male sexual organ under predictable regulation of the brain is the testis; testosterone production of these Leydig cells is turned on and off by the brain's tiny *pituitary gland.*

Right behind (and sometimes on top of) each testicle is the epididymis. This structure holds maturing sperm preparing for their journey. Their final launch from the epididymis is only an intermediate stage, however, as the sperm must then travel into the pelvis for final preparations.

The testicles are suspended precariously from each side of the abdomen by the *spermatic cords*—woven ropes of arteries, veins, muscles, nerves, and other tissues. The most important and strongest structure in the spermatic cord is the *vas deferens*, the hard structure in the upper scrotum that feels like a matchstick. This structure carries sperm on the first part if its journey from the epididymis. It enters the abdomen through the *inguinal canal* (*groin*) and heads toward the prostate. There it joins the duct to the seminal vesicle to form the *ejaculatory duct* as described above.

The testicles' need for the cooler environment outside the main body cavity is puzzling. This is the only body process that requires a temperature different from standard body temperature. The enigmatic part is that this makes it necessary for the testes, truly vital organs from the standpoint of preservation of the species, to be the only vital organs so exposed in their location.

DISTANT NEIGHBORS: LYMPH NODES AND BONES

Although lymph nodes and bones are not neighbors in the sense that prostate problems affect them directly, these are the areas where prostate cancer spreads most commonly, so an understanding of these distant neighbors is in order.

Lymph nodes are small nodules of tissue throughout the body where lymphatic vessels deposit and cleanse their fluid. Lymphatic vessels work in concert with blood vessels to drain body areas, primarily as a front line in the body's defense system. If something harmful (such as a virus or a grain of dirt) enters the body, the lymphatic vessel's job is to carry it to a lymph node, where it can be isolated and neutralized. This is similar to an antivirus program on a computer, which whisks up the software virus and isolates it. If it can't be fixed, it is either destroyed or isolated in a place where it can't hurt the rest of the system.

The body recognizes cancer cells in a similar manner to the way it recognizes other "foreign" invaders. Therefore, a lymph node will often capture cancer cells. The only problem is that the cancer cells sometimes develope the ability to defeat the body's defense system, so they simply set up a satellite location as a second cancer in the lymph node. Eventually, multiple lymph nodes end up overburdened and the cancer proceeds to spread to vital organs. Like the antivirus computer program, the lymph node may not always be able to defeat the intruder.

The other common site of spread is to the bones. Certain types of cancer go to certain areas preferentially. Prostate cancer's preferred site is into the bones, especially those of the spine, pelvis, and femurs (upper leg bones). Why this pattern occurs is a matter of controversy, but recall that Santorini's plexus surrounds the prostate and carries blood (and potentially cancer cells) away. Interestingly, it proceeds to drain into a similar group of veins in the spinal canal called *Batson's plexus*. Although unproven, it is possible that this allows cancer cells access to the spine.

WHY DOES THE NEIGHBORHOOD MATTER?

Now let's talk about why these anatomical relationships in the prostate's neighborhood matter. First, a change in any of these organs can affect any of the others. Enlargement of one pushes the others away. Worse, it may cause blockage of some of these structures.

Targeted medical treatment isn't always as accurate as the "smart bombs" on the news. Although accuracy improves all the time, radiation treatments aimed at the prostate must pass through the other neighbors. The closer the structure is, the more likely it is to be affected. This can cause scarring or other damage, and this damage can build over the years. That means that the true amount of damage may not be evident when treatment is completed, but may cause problems several years down the line. By that time it's too late to change it, which can be a particularly frustrating occurrence.

Prostate surgery also risks injury to the neighbors. Even in the hands of the most skilled surgeon, a surgical instrument may inadvertently injure adjacent structures. The most obvious occurrence of this is when the fragile penile nerves are damaged. Moreover, swelling and scarring in the surgical area can also damage these nerves even if they are unharmed by the operation itself. Without understanding these relationships, it might appear that the removal of the prostate can cause impotence. On the contrary, losing the prostate does nothing. Instead, damage to neighboring nerves is the problem. Likewise, damage to the external urinary **sphincter** (the muscle that maintains urine control) can have problematic consequences. Keeping in mind all these relationships of the prostate neighborhood will allow you to better understand such issues throughout this book.

KEY POINTS

- The prostate is hidden deep in the male pelvis. This leaves it well protected, but means that anything affecting the prostate may cause harm to its important neighbors.

- The simplest way to think of prostatic anatomy is to regard the gland as having an inner transition/central zone and an outer peripheral zone.

- Specific issues of the anatomy are discussed throughout this book, so please refer back to this chapter to aid your understanding.

3.

SYMPTOMS:
THE PROSTATE AND ITS
IMPERSONATORS

The bladder often proves to be an unreliable witness, claiming for instance to be full when empty and empty when overfull.
—Patrick Bates

Dan came to the office complaining of "prostate troubles." He sought a second opinion because the antibiotics he had taken for years no longer brought relief. "I have prostatitis," he declared. "But antibiotics don't work anymore."

Prostatitis is an easy—but frequently wrong—self-diagnosis. If a man has symptoms anywhere between collarbone and knees, there is the real possibility he may call it prostatitis. Taking antibiotics is usually the next step, often from the flouroquinolone drug class. The Cipro Dan took was one such drug.

"What do you mean by 'prostatitis'?" I questioned. He looked at me like I was daft.

"You're a urologist and you don't know what prostatitis is?" he jeered. "My prostate gets swollen and tender. It burns when I urinate unless I stay on antibiotics."

I clearly had disappointed him already. I wasn't done. "What do you mean by your 'prostate'?"

His derision could not be concealed. He didn't even ask how I could be unaware of its location. Only when he decided to educate me on pelvic anatomy did we begin to make progress. "My prostate," he said with increasing frustration, "is right here," he showed with his fingertip. How-

ever, instead of pointing somewhere behind the pubic bone, his finger was higher and to the left. I wasn't sure yet what was going on, but was confident that his symptoms were not from prostatitis—unless his prostate was in a location never previously identified.

After I convinced Dan that I wasn't clueless, we proceeded to investigate. Digital rectal examination (DRE) confirmed his prostate was neither swollen nor tender. It was normal. His colon, however, was not. Dan suffered from diverticulitis, a condition where small sacs (diverticulae) dilate and expand like little balloons from a chronically constipated colon. Years of poor dietary habits and straining during bowel movements had finally reached a critical point. One of the diverticulae had ruptured into the dome of his bladder, causing urinary infections from small amounts of stool bacteria that leaked through the opening. Antibiotics initially controlled the infections, but eventually the amount of stool coming through overwhelmed both the drugs and his system.

I recommended cystoscopy (as described in detail in the next chapter), which allowed me to visualize his bladder from the inside. A small opening made the diagnosis obvious. He didn't need more antibiotics; he needed surgery to correct the problem.

The prostate was exonerated.

***

Patients and some physicians both tend to blame a plethora of symptoms on the prostate or bladder. The tendency is based on the concepts discussed in the introduction of this book. Because the prostate is hidden and mysterious, it is easy to ascribe evildoing to it whenever there is a problem.

There is no one symptom exclusively related to the prostate or bladder. Indeed, the prostate is capable of causing a number of problems. However, many of its neighbors can create the same havoc, as evidenced by the quote above. If it is accurate that the bladder is an "unreliable witness," the prostate is even more so. These symptoms are divided into three main categories: irritative (frequency, urgency, nighttime frequency), obstructive (slow stream, hesitancy, intermittency, incomplete emptying), and painful.

We will describe here the most common symptoms and distinguish them. Since this can be difficult, all but the most straightforward—and self-limiting—will probably lead you to the doctor's office for further investigation. However, some simple guidelines within your control are offered here.

URINARY FREQUENCY: TOO LITTLE, TOO OFTEN

Urinary **frequency** simply means you void frequently. Although the term is clear, its full definition is not. There is no such thing as a normal voiding frequency. Frequent to me might be more than three or four times a day whereas to you it might mean twice an hour.

Frequency can be due to a number of things. It may occur when the bladder doesn't empty completely, and remains partly or mostly full when the person leaves the restroom. Incomplete emptying will obviously lead to the need to void again soon. A sensation of incomplete emptying may suggest this possibility but by no means assures the diagnosis. Sensations can mislead. An absence of such sensation means little as well, as many people with incomplete emptying either have diminished sensation as the cause, or develop it as bladder damage insidiously develops. Diabetics are particularly vulnerable to this because of nerve damage known as *diabetic neuropathy*.

Frequency also occurs when the bladder cannot hold normal volumes of urine. Sometimes this is due to bladder irritation from an infection or a stone. Most neurological conditions such as multiple sclerosis, stroke, and Parkinson's disease can cause frequency. Bladder cancer also can, but this is uncommon.

It is also important to be sure frequency is not simply the result of excessive fluid intake. It suggests something amiss if you void small amounts frequently. By small amounts, I mean only an ounce or two at a time. However, if you drink a lot and void large amounts frequently it simply suggests the bladder is doing what it was intended to do—fill and empty. It doesn't matter what you drink; what goes in must come out, so drinking a large volume will make you void a large volume no matter what it is you drink.

Sometimes people think they have frequency when they actually have a normal voiding pattern. It is common that people tell me they "go to the bathroom all the time," but when we review a voiding diary (as described below) they find they go to the restroom every few hours—a normal pattern.

Finally, frequency can occur simply from a condition known as **overactive bladder** (**OAB**). This occurs from the sensation of mild bladder contractions, often the result of urinary obstruction overworking the bladder. This obstruction might come from prostate problems (as discussed in chapter 7). As the bladder muscle works harder because of prostatic obstruction, the muscle becomes stronger and more active, similar to a bicep when worked hard in the gym. This bladder strengthening helps overcome obstruction for awhile, but eventually leads to symptoms if untreated.

URGENCY: "GOTTA GO"

An abnormal—usually sudden—urge to void is simply called **urgency**. It occurs mainly because of the sensation of a bladder contraction. This may be due to anything described above that causes frequency, but it is often a symptom complex on its own.

My friend and ski buddy Professor Paul Abrams, from the United Kingdom, was the president of the International Continence Society a few years ago when this organization adopted the term overactive bladder as a way to describe the condition. This means exactly what it sounds like—the bladder is overactive. The confusing part is that it might be overactive as a result of a bladder or prostate abnormality—including the problems listed above—but commonly occurs spontaneously.

Patients with OAB often recognize themselves in pharmaceutical advertisements. The most recognizable is the "I gotta go" line that summarizes the condition and their chief complaint.

The most severe stage of OAB occurs when you get a sensation to void and cannot make it to the restroom in time. When an accident occurs, it is called **urge incontinence** (or OAB-wet, as opposed to OAB-dry). Aggressive intervention including medications or surgery is needed at that point, so you should see a urologist if you haven't already.

NOCTURIA: FREQUENCY AT NIGHT

Frequent urination during hours normally reserved for sleep is called **nocturia**. The source can again be any of the problems listed above, but additional factors may come into play. Whether you actually get up or simply lie there trying not to, nocturia leads to tiredness, potential marital difficulties (if you awaken a spouse who doesn't return to sleep easily), or frustration. It is often the symptom that leads to the first doctor's appointment for men with prostate problems.

Initially, some people simply get up to go to the restroom because they awaken and assume they should void so they won't need to later. Others use a trip to the restroom to get things off their minds. Habit plays a substantial role. When symptoms are mild, the prostate may be blamed for a simple case of chronic insomnia.

A bladder that empties incompletely will inevitably lead to nocturia because it is already partially filled the minute you leave the restroom. In this situation the bladder will obviously become too full to make it through a full night's sleep.

The final issue with nocturia involves the body's normal night-day cycle, called *diurnal rhythm*. We normally produce more urine in the daytime than at night based on hormonal factors. The evolutionary advantage of a full night's sleep is obvious.

This cycle can be overwhelmed by several things. First, we may simply lose this hormonal effect for unrelated medical reasons. Second, drugs such as caffeine, alcohol, Lasix (furosemide), or other diuretics ("water pills") taken late in the day can force fluids out at night. The first two are especially likely to awaken you. Both come with their own fluid supply, plus they make you sleep more lightly.

Finally, fluid buildup during the daytime from *congestive heart failure* (weakness of the heart muscle leading to poor circulation) or other unrelated medical conditions settles in the legs because of gravity. Lying down at night allows this fluid to become absorbed back into the body in large amounts. This is similar to drinking several glasses of water (or having an infusion of several liters of IV fluids) while sleeping. The bladder will obviously detect this amount of fluid soon, which may lead to nocturia. Excessive *volume* or amount of urinary output at night, as opposed to excessive *frequency* at night, is called *nycturia*.

MANAGING IRRITATIVE SYMPTOMS

Irritative symptoms—urgency and frequency—usually respond to a group of medications known as *anticholinergics*. They temporarily block muscle contractions that cause such sensations. That doesn't mean that beginning a prescription commits you to lifetime use. However, the pills work only while present in the person's system, so those who respond with acceptable side effects usually continue their use in order to avoid the symptoms.

There are some nonmedical options to manage irritative symptoms as well. First, you should become aware of your actions that may be affecting bladder function. You should know whether you drink so much fluid that your bladder simply voids often because it is full. The easiest way to determine this is to complete a "voiding diary" or "intake and output" diary. This involves recording exactly what you would expect—your intake and output. Measure both in ounces (or metrics if you prefer), and write them on a piece of paper, noting the times each occurs.

Intake is easy to measure by determining the size of your glasses and cups. Pour a glass full of water and then transfer it to a measuring cup. Thereafter simply estimate. If you consume drinks outside the home, the volume is usually provided. If not, make a good guess.

Measuring output is a little trickier. The easiest way is to use a large measuring cup. Take it into the restroom with you and void into it instead of the toilet. Note (and write down on the diary) the amount prior to emptying it into the toilet. Throw it away when you have completed the voiding diary— it is inexpensive at the local discount retailer and (definitely) not worth trying to wash. Alternatively, the urologist can give you a "hat" that sits in the toilet to catch urine. (Women find this easier, but the measuring cup works better for men.)

If you find your bladder held at least six to eight ounces each time you voided, you can conclude it was doing what it should—holding a normal amount of urine and emptying when full. You might find that your fluid intake is excessive. That observation can save the trouble and cost of a clinic visit, since the cure is obvious. If you drink less and the problem continues, then you should see your physician. Frequent voiding of small amounts indicates the problem is a true bladder problem, possibly including OAB. Seeing the urologist can help.

LIMITING FLUIDS

Most people with frequency naturally decrease their fluid intake based on common sense. If the diary reveals excessive intake to be the problem, this is a logical step.

However, if you already void small amounts this strategy can become a losing game. As you decrease fluid intake the urine becomes more concentrated. This may make it even more irritating and (counterintuitively) cause even more urgency and frequency.

In fact, this principle can sometimes be used to correct irritative symptoms. Some people get in the habit of voiding frequently and actually seem to train the bladder to signal urgency at low volumes. Breaking this cycle sometimes involves simply holding it longer.

When I instruct people with irritative symptoms to try this they typically react with incredulity: "I came to you because I go to the bathroom too often and you tell me to not go to the bathroom so often?" Only with weeks (or more) of retraining do they begin to believe the bladder can sometimes be retrained. Medications such as those listed in chapter 8 can help in the transition.

SLOW STREAM

A slow stream, otherwise known as "decreased force of stream," suggests a likelihood of obstruction or blockage. It often occurs due to compression of the urethra, similar to the effect of someone stepping on a garden hose. In contrast to irritative symptoms (urgency, frequency, and nocturia), it is the classic **obstructive symptom**.

Sometimes compression is the result of an enlarged prostate, but it can also occur at the bladder outlet because of contraction of muscle fibers, which is called a **primary bladder neck obstruction**. This poorly understood entity is uncommon but usually requires surgery.

A **urethral stricture** or **bladder neck contracture** also causes obstructive symptoms by narrowing the urethra with a fibrous waistband at either of their respective locations. Although they can occur spontaneously, they are usually due to scarring from previous surgery or instrumentation, such as catheter placement or injury.

Finally, a decreased force of stream or other obstructive symptoms may occur in the complete absence of obstruction. A weak bladder barely able to generate enough pressure to void will mimic obstruction. Differentiating obstruction from a weak bladder is obviously important if considering surgery.

HESITANCY, INTERMITTENCY, AND STRANGURY

Hesitancy is a delay prior to beginning the stream. After the bladder finally generates enough pressure to overcome the resistance, the stream begins. Erratically, the prostate may slam shut for a moment, leading to **intermittency**. This is the classic spurt-spurt as a man tries to completely empty his bladder.

The penultimate obstructive symptom is *strangury*, which means what it sounds like. The urinary stream is almost strangulated. Straining and other attempts to maintain voiding are the final countermeasures before you can no longer void at all. This complete inability to void is called **urinary retention**.

DRIBBLING

Competing with nocturia, *dribbling* may be the most common symptom in men with prostatic obstruction. It is usually due to incomplete emptying of the urethra, but can also occasionally be due to bladder contractions that occur after emptying if you rush to return the penis to its usual place. However, dribbling really isn't a disease and is mainly a nuisance resulting in an embarrassing spot on your pants.

The ditty about "the last drop will never fall" is true, but there are ways to manage the annoyance. First, beware that the urethra is like any other tissue—it loses elasticity with aging. In the child or young man, its natural contractility is enough to compress all urine out quickly. Increasingly with age, it is common for a few drops to become trapped in little "pockets" of less elastic urethra. This tendency would not cause a problem except that the little pockets eventually work their way out and dribble into the shorts. This is especially common following prostate surgery.

The best way to avoid this happening is to not allow such pockets to form. The best strategy is to wait a few seconds after voiding is complete. Make sure the penis is directed downward throughout its length so that drainage is straight down. This allows wayward drops time to come out while aimed at the toilet instead of the shorts. Some men simply pull the penis out through a minimal opening so that it drapes up over the shorts. This essentially creates a trap like the one under your sink. As soon as the urethra is directed downward into the shorts, any urine trapped in the "S" will dribble out at a most inconvenient location and time.

Another maneuver involves "stripping" the urethra like a tube of toothpaste. With the penis pointed down, use the thumb and forefinger several times to milk residual urine out. Waiting a few seconds allows more to reach the penile urethra, when a second or third stripping can empty most of it. Stripping directed at the very base of the penis also helps remove the rogue drops.

A final maneuver used successfully is to reach for a piece of toilet tissue. Wadding up enough to absorb the offending drops and placing it over the urethral opening as the penis is replaced into the shorts will usually catch the stragglers. It can then be tossed and flushed. If you use these maneuvers a drier pair of shorts should brighten your day.

UROLOGICAL BLEEDING

No man likes to see his own blood, especially coming from the penis. Its presence may or may not be significant. The most common occurrence of bleeding from the penis occurs during ejaculation. Blood in the semen is called **hematospermia**, usually the result of prostatic veins bursting during or before ejaculation. It is usually not indicative of any problem, although men who experience hematospermia should have prostate cancer ruled out prior to assuming anything. As long as the doctor has confirmed that the DRE and a PSA are normal, he will probably reassure you and recommend observation. Hematospermia also normally occurs following prostate biopsy in a majority of men.

Blood in the urine is another matter. Its presence, called **hematuria**, is suspicious for the possibility of something serious and warrants urological investigation. You should seek specialty consultation immediately if you experience visible hematuria.

A PAIN IN THE BACKSIDE—OR FRONT SIDE

Lower abdominal and pelvic pains are often blamed on the prostate, but it is usually not the culprit. Acute **prostatitis** is one of the rare causes of severe pain in these locations. Although an easy diagnosis to make, it is often wrong. More often, men like Dan at the beginning of this chapter have an "ache" somewhere in the area and assume it originates in the prostate.

Some physicians perpetuate this myth by incorrectly diagnosing "prostatitis" for abdominal or urinary symptoms they cannot explain. Multiple courses of antibiotics or other medications often follow. Failure to respond sometimes simply instigates further inappropriate treatment. Far more often, pain in these locations is due to musculoskeletal or gastrointestinal conditions.

PAINFUL EJACULATION

One symptom that actually is often related to the prostate is *painful ejaculation*. Men with symptoms suggestive of chronic prostatitis may complain of this. They are more likely to respond to antibiotics than are men with vague pelvic pains, suggesting that they actually do have bacterial prostatitis.

IMPOTENCE

I am always amazed at how many men blame impotence on the prostate. Although it may result from almost any treatment for prostate problems, *impotence is never due to the prostate*. Regardless, since many men with prostate problems experience impotence, this problem is covered in detail in its own chapter.

SYMPTOMS OF PROSTATE CANCER

Prostate cancer usually causes no symptoms. This becomes significant in two ways—that is, the presence of symptoms should not worry you about cancer and the absence of symptoms should not make you believe cancer is impossible.

Urinary symptoms are usually due to benign conditions of the bladder or prostate, while prostate cancer usually causes symptoms only when severely advanced. Bone pain, weight loss, and other end-stage symptoms of malignancy are part of the discussion only in advanced prostate cancer.

KEY POINTS

- Urinary symptoms usually relate to benign conditions—not cancer.
- Urinary symptoms are divided into **irritative** and **obstructive**. The former include urgency, frequency, and nocturia. The latter include hesitancy, intermittency, and decreased force of stream.
- An intake and output diary is an easy way to determine if you have a normal voiding pattern. If you drink large amounts of fluid and void large volumes, the problem is likely not in the urinary tract. If you drink normal amounts of fluids but void small amounts frequently, you may have a problem to discuss with your physician.

4.

GETTING THE MOST FROM A TRIP TO THE UROLOGY OFFICE

A urologist is another personality type altogether. There's a civility and seriousness to urologists, but also a strange wryness. You have to tell them things you'd just as soon not tell yourself, and so the patients tend to speak in euphemisms: "Doc, I got a thing with my thing."

People who know doctors swear they can always spot the urologist. It's the lack of pomposity, but also the surety of ego. Stern, unfazed, methodical, frequently German, as if for effect.
—Hank Stuever, *Washington Post*

Urologists tend to be class clowns who may seem to take everything lightly, but somehow end up winning a competitive spot in one of medicine's "hot" specialties. Combining the academic standing required to make the cut with the personality suited to deal with peoples' most private issues, we are known as a unique, perhaps quirky, group.

Whereas neurosurgeons are asked intriguing questions about the origin of human thought or the neurobiological implications of the soul, urologists are more likely to be asked: "Why would anyone want to do that for a living?"

Urologists are admittedly a different breed. We spend our days doing things that would mortify our mothers. "Take your daughter to work day" is never an option. Most patients we meet drop their pants at some point in the conversation. That takes a little getting used to.

Since you are reading this book, it is likely you could end up in a urology office at some point. The following pages are designed to prepare you for that interaction.

GETTING READY FOR THE UROLOGY APPOINTMENT

Prior to seeing the doctor, you will probably be asked to fill out a detailed medical history form. The information requested will address two needs. The first is to find out why you are there and what your problem is. The second need is to fulfill requirements placed on physicians by Medicare and other insurers. These regulations require the collection and documentation of a great deal of information that may seem like overkill but must be charted in order to remain within federal guidelines.

The first question asks for your *chief complaint*. Literally, this means, Why are you here? Next, some general medical information will be gathered. The *past medical history* (PMH) and *past surgical history* (PSH) list illnesses, hospitalizations, and operations that have affected your present physical state. *Medications* and *allergies* are listed and flagged for future reference, to be checked before writing a prescription. An abbreviated *social history* asks about marital status, occupation, and tobacco and/or alcohol use. Finally, a *review of systems* will ask some simple questions about all organ systems, from the neurological to the urological. This information is pertinent whether you have a bad heart, a bad knee, or a bad prostate.

CHECKING IN: BE PREPARED

Gordon arrived for his consultation with Dr. Brown for urinary difficulties ten minutes after his scheduled appointment. He didn't have an insurance card or any information on how the visit was financially covered. He said that he took some medications prescribed by an internist, but didn't know anything except their color and that they "cost too damned much." He was "deathly allergic" to some pill "that a quack doctor made me take," but had no idea what it was, or even why he had taken it. For that matter, he didn't recall what side effect it caused—just that he was sure he was allergic to it. Despite his inability and unwillingness to supply any information except the fact that his primary care physician thought he should see a urologist because he couldn't help him, he was ready for a diagnosis to be dished out and a prescription to be written within seconds of sitting down in the office. He was certain that more important things waited back at his office.

***

When people go to the movies, they go prepared. They know why they are there and which movie they want tickets for. They have money ready. If hungry, they go straight to the concession stand and order exactly what they want. They knowingly empty their bladder if they think the movie will be long or if they suffer from prostate ailments. My wife always remembers to bring a sweater, even in summer, because the theater may be too cool.

If only people came to the doctor's office so well prepared. Many, like Gordon, come without having their necessary medical information available. They expect the doctor to make recommendations on their health care without providing the necessary information to do so.

***

The pill to which Gordon was "deathly allergic" was *prazosin*, which had been prescribed for severely elevated blood pressure. The reason he had vomited the time he took it was that his blood pressure was out of control, almost high enough to have a stroke. He wasn't allergic—just clueless. He was no longer taking it, but was taking a similar drug, **doxazocin** (**Cardura**). The prescription he now demanded without an examination or gathering of any history was for yet another drug from the same class, **tamsulosin** (**Flomax**). A friend was taking it successfully to treat urinary difficulties. Had Gordon received that prescription as requested, he would have been taking two drugs that did essentially the same thing. A drug interaction was possible. Fortunately for Gordon, Dr. Brown did his homework before agreeing to his demand.

***

An inadequate medical history can yield disastrous results. If Dr. Brown had not figured out that Gordon took Cardura, its interaction with other medications that he considered prescribing could have caused significant problems. Fortunately, the doctor was able to make a determination once the patient finally slowed down enough to clarify his medications.

Before checking into any doctor's office these days you should know your insurance status. Some people take the approach that it is someone else's responsibility. Those are the people likely to be left responsible for the bill. Your insurance may not pay for any of the visit or tests obtained unless preapproved. Ignorance of this policy won't remove your financial responsibility, so be prepared. Moreover, your insurance policy may favor certain medications over similar ones, and may only pay for limited quantities. If your insurance covers one drug instead of another equivalent drug, you'll want to let the doctor know so he can decide if the suggested drug is an acceptable alternative. If it would pay for a ninety-day supply of medications, you should know that before paying the same amount (*copay*) for a thirty-day supply.

Upon check-in, provide the necessary information to the office staff. Have your medical history information available and ready. If any tests have been previously performed that are related to this visit, be certain to ask the staff to assure that the results are on your chart instead of waiting until you are face-to-face with the doctor. Although your referring physician may have asked his staff to fax or mail pertinent information, don't assume it is on your chart until you confirm it.

The General Examination

Although an examination below the belt might be the only thing expected, remember that no prostate is an island. The doctor will begin the examination before you probably even realize it. He will note your weight, build, and general health, and will be especially interested in the organs around the prostate "neighborhood." An abdominal examination to check for tumors or hernias (more common in men with prostate problems) is part of a routine physical examination, in addition to checking for an overdistended bladder.

The Genital Examination

Men love dropping their pants—except in the urologist's office. Suddenly, modesty abounds. Try to get over it. The most important thing you can do to improve the genital examination is to drop your pants adequately while standing for the examination. Let the doctor do his work so you can move on to treatment.

The genitals are checked for abnormalities, especially involving the **urethra** because of its role in urination. The testicles are examined mainly for size and tumors. If they appear large, it is usually due to fluid around them. This fluid might be a small collection of sperm (*spermatocele*) or routine body fluid (*hydrocele*), neither of which should be considered problematic unless it becomes large enough to bother you or get in the way. A collection of *varicose veins* in the scrotum is called a *varicocele*.

The Rectal Exam: DRE

This is the biggie, the part of the urology appointment men dread the most. "I hate this," is the comment most often heard. Well, from the urologist's standpoint, "It ain't the high point of my day, either."

The digital rectal exam is often abbreviated DRE. Digital doesn't suggest a technological or computerized assessment. Quite the opposite, it is the most low-tech prostate test. A digit is a finger (or toe, but not in this case). The DRE is performed by placing a gloved finger into the rectum in order to feel the prostate.

Despite bias to avoid it, the rectal examination should be performed annually on all men old enough to have significant disease that could be detected by doing so. That usually means rectal or prostate cancer, so the recommendation is to usually begin having a rectal examination after the age of fifty. Black men and men with a family history of prostate cancer should begin a year earlier because they have an increased risk of developing cancer. Mayo Clinic researchers have predicted that at least half of all prostate cancer deaths could be prevented by annual DRE.[1]

There are a couple of things that help make the rectal examination more tolerable. First, you should try to get over any anxiety or embarrassment. Face it, the urologist sees essentially every patient's backside at some point, and yours isn't substantially different. The reason to get over the anxiety is that nervousness makes the pelvic floor muscles tighten and lowers the pain threshold. That means the doctor has to push harder to get a gloved finger into the rectum, and more discomfort sensations will consequently be sent to the brain.

Some men complain about the amount of lubrication used on the gloved finger. Don't. Lubrication does more to lessen discomfort than anything else the doctor can do (except being gentle, which should be a given). The lubricating jelly is water soluble, so it washes or wipes off easily. Encourage him to use as much as needed.

Finally, your body position makes a big difference. The best position for a rectal examination is standing with the legs slightly apart. Leaning over an examining table with the knees slightly bent and your elbows placed at the *edge* of the examining table is optimal. This position puts maximum bend into the waist, shortening the distance that the doctor must reach inside to be able to check the prostate. The shorter distance means that he pushes less— which is obviously in everyone's best interest. In obese men, this offers the best hope for the urologist to reach the entire prostate.

What Does DRE Check For?

The prostate is a smooth gland can be felt when palpated through the rectal wall. Any irregularity could be prostate cancer, so assessment of anything that feels "different" is the focus of the examination. To visualize the prostate, imagine a clenched fist. Normal consistency is about the same as that of the tissue between thumb and forefinger that rises to form a thick hump when the fist is clenched tightly. In contrast, cancer might feel like an irregular bump, but will classically feel like a knuckle of that same clenched fist (see figure 4-1).

Sometimes the differences are subtle—and subjective. It is not uncommon that a good physician refers a patient whose findings are not at first evident to a urologist. Sometimes it is only after several passes of the finger, applying varying degrees of pressure, that I can feel the area of concern. Sometimes I can't feel anything. It may be disconcerting to the patient if the doctors disagree on their assessment of DRE, but this is not necessary. Because the DRE is subjective, I sometimes recommend waiting a few weeks before reassessing the examination if I am not certain.

By the same token, if the DRE detects a definite abnormality, don't become overly concerned, since the PSA (prostate-specific antigen) helps us know how likely it is that you have cancer. Prior to our recent knowledge of PSA, an abnormal DRE indicated that prostate cancer was present in about half of men. Now that we have the additional information provided by PSA, an abnormal DRE combined with a completely normal PSA suggests a chance of cancer well below that. Therefore, the DRE is an adjunct for prostate cancer diagnosis, but it is not the definitive test. A biopsy is, as described later. Finally, DRE also detects rectal cancers, another major cause of death in men of the same age at risk of prostate cancer.

URINALYSIS

The word *urologist* begins with "uro," as in *urine*. That means that this specialty involves diseases that often exhibit findings in the urine. It also means that you shouldn't empty your bladder before coming into the office. You will most certainly be asked to give a specimen. If you start with an empty bladder you will need to drink several paper cups of water in order to give at the office. If you want to avoid the delay, save a donation until you check in.

Urosocopists were ancient physicians who made diagnoses by holding the patient's urine up to the light. They supposedly could see abnormalities

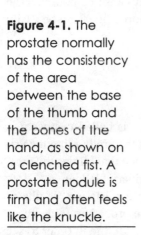

Figure 4-1. The prostate normally has the consistency of the area between the base of the thumb and the bones of the hand, as shown on a clenched fist. A prostate nodule is firm and often feels like the knuckle.

that provided a view into the patient's constitution. So significant is the role of uroscopy in *uromythology* that the traditional logo of the *Journal of Urology* is a drawing of a urosocopist performing his craft. (The *Journal of Urology* is one of the most prestigious journals in our field, but true to the mischievous nature of urologists, it was designated as "the *official organ* of the American Urological Association" for more than fifty years. The journal retained its whimsical moniker until 1972, when some predictable ribbing by *Playboy* magazine made the editors relinquish the inside joke. The Europeans retain their sense of humor to this day and still call *European Urology* and the *Scandinavian Journal of Urology and Nephrology* "official organs.")

PSA AFTER DRE?

Some physicians will not order a PSA blood test to be drawn immediately after DRE, believing the DRE will cause a misleading elevation in its level. This is an interesting holdover from the days of an older blood test, PAP, which could be elevated simply by performing DRE. The older test should not be drawn following DRE.

In contrast, we know that routine DRE will not cause PSA to become abnormal (although it might go up an insignificant fraction). Therefore, there is no reason to wait or to make a man wait for results or return on another day for lab work. Like many old habits, this one has taken a while to go away. Many physicians still follow the habits they formed during an earlier era.

No one today looks at urine held up to the light to make a diagnosis, but its appearance under the light of a microscope yields crucial information. Red or white blood cells indicate abnormalities of the urinary tract. Chemical tests for sugar indicate diabetes, which is a frequent cause of both erectile dysfunction and urinary problems. Several other abnormalities can be easily detected through the urinalysis.

CYSTOSCOPY

One specialized test performed in the urology office is called **cystoscopy**. This involves the placement of a small scope through the urethra into the urinary bladder. The scope is a relatively soft, flexible tube that allows the urologist to see the inside of the urethra, prostate, and urinary bladder.

A gel containing *lidocaine* (the same anesthetic dentists use) is placed into the urethra and bladder a few minutes before the procedure to decrease sensation. The cystoscope is then inserted through the urethra in order to see the lower urinary tract. In our office, the patient can actually watch the same image that the urologist sees on a television screen. Photographs can be taken if anything abnormal is identified.

These scopes were traditionally composed of fiber optic bundles, but we now use a new generation with digital chips embedded at the end that allow us to visualize the bladder with magnification and clarity better than can be seen with the naked eye. One such image of a normal bladder lining is seen in figure 4-2.

Cystoscopy is not part of the routine workup for prostate problems, but may help evaluate suspected abnormalities of the lower urinary tract. The most important use is to rule out bladder cancer in someone who has blood in the urine. (Stones, benign prostate enlargement, and some uncommon kidney disorders might cause blood in the urine. In addition, obstruction, infections, incontinence, and other concerns might also indicate the need for cystoscopy on occasion.) Planning for prostate surgery sometimes involves cystoscopy as well.

The procedure is usually not painful, although most men describe mild discomfort or a "funny" sensation inside the urethra. The flexible scopes used today are small enough to be well tolerated. The most common comment I hear when completing the procedure is, "So that's what I worried about?" Don't worry. Cystoscopy is completed in minutes and the urologist can immediately tell you the results.

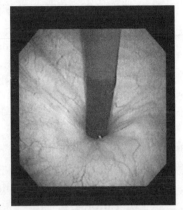

Figure 4-2. View inside normal bladder showing a flexible cystoscope coming through the prostate, emerging out of the bladder neck, and looking back onto itself (the black tube).

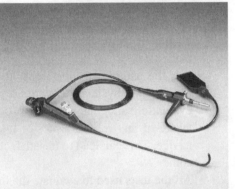

Figure 4-3. The flexible cystoscope is usually used in men because of its low profile and small size. It can be placed comfortably, enabling the urologist to evaluate the urethra, prostate, and bladder in the office under local anesthesia. (Courtesy of Olympus, USA)

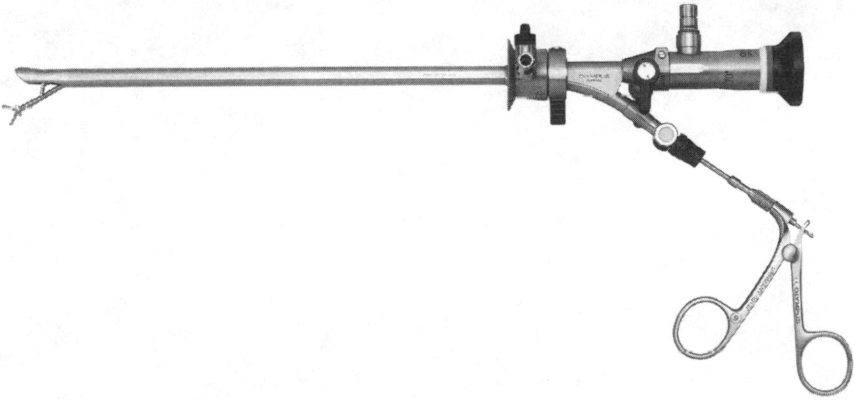

Figure 4-4. The rigid cystoscope is used mainly in the operating room, when the urologist needs to perform a bladder biopsy or other procedure under spinal or general anesthesia. (Courtesy of Olympus, USA)

BIOPSY AND OTHER TESTS

The most specific test regarding the prostate is the transrectal ultrasound, or TRUS. Most of chapter 12 is devoted to this procedure. Urodynamics and other tests to evaluate the prostate are covered in chapter 7.

KEY POINTS

- A doctor's appointment is for *your* good—not the doctor's. Therefore, make sure you communicate all your related history and symptoms to your urologist.
- It is the doctor's responsibility to attempt to find out what your needs are from an examination. Then he should determine the appropriate diagnostic evaluation and therapeutic options to assure these needs are met.
- It is the patient's responsibility to communicate all relevant information to the physician. If you ask the physician to give advice on the evaluation and management of your problem without making him aware of any related issues or history, you should expect inadequate advice. This can lead to unsatisfactory, or occasionally dangerous, outcomes.
- All the tests used to evaluate the urinary tract are, in general, tolerated well and certainly are much easier to take than most people expect.

5.
A Tomato a Day Keeps the Urologist Away: Maintaining Prostate Health

Still I would trade it all for a good pee.
—William Henry Devereaux Jr.
in Richard Russo, *Straight Man*

A cottage industry has arisen based on prostate health. You can buy vitamins, supplements, and other substances of unclear origin, many promising to provide the prostatic fountain of youth.

The "natural" trend began primarily in Europe in the late twentieth century. The widespread appeal was bolstered by the costs of supplements and "neutraceuticals" often being reimbursed in the same manner as prescription medications. Though not reimbursed, Americans followed by embracing "natural" remedies as a result of aggressive marketing and public awareness of prostate disease. These elements created a huge industry, which topped sales of $1 billion a year.[1] Here we will discuss the limited information known about these and other issues related to prostate health.

THE PROSTATE AS PART OF THE WHOLE: NO PROSTATE IS AN ISLAND

It amazes me that men obsess over their prostatic health while letting the remainder of their bodies fall apart. While taking supplements by the handful at the urging of advertisers with unproven claims, many neglect exercise, eat a diet of fast food and processed dishes, and smoke and drink to excess.

71

This makes no sense. First, it will do you no good to prevent prostate disease if you simply die of a heart attack before you have time to develop cancer. Second, avoiding side effects from prostate treatments won't help if you develop impotence or other problems from deterioration in overall health.

Therefore, before you invest too much time in tuning up your prostate, look around it first. If it is inside a healthy body, you can do some things to keep the prostate from threatening your health. If it is inside a body in need of major rehabilitation, then this is a good time to take a fresh look at your overall health. This means you should exercise for at least thirty minutes three times a week. You should eat a diet based on real foods (beer and chips don't count). You should drink no more than two alcoholic beverages a day and you should never smoke again. Until you have made a serious effort at those goals, your prostate may not play a major role in your future.

Once you have decided to maintain your overall health, then your desire to take care of your prostate is worth the effort. This chapter will provide you with our current understanding of what can be done to preserve prostatic health. Most of the following are designed to protect from prostate cancer, but some may help prevent benign prostate problems as well.

SMOKING

> *A custom loathsome to the eye, hateful to the nose, harmful to the brain, dangerous to the lungs, and in the black stinking fume therof, nearest resembling the horrible Stygian smoke of the pit that is bottomless.*
>
> —King James I, 1604

Everyone knows smoking hardens arteries. As a result, vital organs don't receive enough oxygen, which leads to heart attack, stroke, and other life-threatening diseases. Although the surgeon general warned us decades ago, the threat of illness or death still doesn't stop enough people from smoking.

Although smoking causes many forms of cancer, it probably plays a minor role at most in developing prostate cancer. Some studies have indicated a small increased risk, but most have not. Smokers with prostate cancer have a worse prognosis despite treatment, though this may simply be due to their risk of dying from smoking-related risks.

If you are still asking the question, Is smoking really that bad? you have been brainwashed by tobacco company propaganda. Don't listen! Cigarette smoking kills about a half million Americans a year—more than AIDS, automobile accidents, murders, suicides, drug overdoses, and fires combined. Studies estimate the chance of a man reaching normal life expectancy is almost twice as good for a nonsmoker. Quitting early, before too much permanent damage is done, adds almost ten years to a man's life.[2]

Americans spend more than $50 billion each year on smoking-related health costs, on top of the billions spent on cigarettes themselves. Cigarettes emit uncountable poisonous chemicals, including cyanide, benzene, methanol, acetylene (think blowtorches), carbon monoxide, and ammonia. Another gas emitted is formaldehyde, which is the pathologists' chemical you'll end up bathed in if you don't quit.

Secondhand smoke also affects those around you, especially children. Spouses of smokers are at increased risk of the above diseases. Children of smokers have many times more lung problems, including asthma and pneumonia. Sudden infant death (SIDS) is increased in babies of smokers. Most important, smoking around children teaches them that smoking is acceptable to the people whose approval they most need, so they are likely to carry on this tragic family tradition. Finally, smokers have worse outcomes following radiation therapy for prostate cancer (as discussed in chapter 16).

Therefore, if you are worried about dying of prostate cancer but continue to smoke, you are being shortsighted. For most men with that combination, the risk of early death is greater from smoking than it is from prostate cancer.

NO EASY ANSWERS

This and chapter 10 ("Causes of Prostate Cancer") were the hardest to write, because the information available on causes and dietary or other factors that might affect the risk of prostate cancer is inconclusive. As you read these two chapters, you must keep in mind that some studies support the role of issues that other studies contradict. I have tried to clarify when a majority of urologists have concluded that a preponderance of evidence supports an approach. Although a majority may share certain views, it is rare in such topics that there is universal agreement.

Recall the warning for concrete thinkers. The role of the topics covered in these two chapters will remain controversial and under investigation for years to come. You should consider the information with this understanding, and decide with your doctor whether you believe any approach herein is in your best interest. Thereafter, you must keep up with developments in research that may affect interpretation of these factors and adjust accordingly.

DIET FOR A HEALTHY PROSTATE

You Say Tomato—I Say Lycopene

Antioxidants are chemicals that seem to block destructive *free radicals* and protect from cancer. One of the best natural sources appears to be *lycopene*. Its presence in tomatoes is credited for an approximately one-third lower risk of prostate cancer in men who consume large amounts of tomato sauce.[3]

It appears that cooking releases the active ingredient, because men who consumed similarly large amounts of tomato juice (uncooked) don't have the same protection.[4] An even greater benefit may relate to the ability of cooked tomatoes to prevent more severe forms of prostate cancer by as much as 50 percent.

Some studies question whether this is due to lycopene or to some unidentified substance in tomatoes. In addition to lycopene, other *phytonutrients* (substances found naturally in food that are believed to have a possible protective effect) include vitamin C, vitamin E, selenium, carotenoids (the orange-red pigments in fruits and vegetables), bioflavonoids (including soy isoflavones, proanthocyanidins, Quercetin, and ginkgo biloba), alpha-lipoic acid, and coenzyme Q10. Although marketed widely, there is no good proof any of these except soy and vitamin E have an impact.

Soy

Isoflavone is thought to be the active ingredient in soy products such as tofu, tempeh, and soy milk. Soy products have become popular with women to treat conditions as varied as hot flashes, decreased libido, and cancer. Their use is based on a belief that they increase estrogen levels.

This effect on estrogen levels would theoretically protect against prostate problems in men, because estrogen slows the development of prostate enlargement and cancer. Soy is now available in a number of new processed foods—from ice cream to meat substitutes—although it is found in greatest concentration with intact soybeans. This has also led to an explosion of supplements and products promoted to save lives by their isoflavone content.

Soy supplements aren't well regulated and most have less isoflavone than a half cup of soybeans. Content labeling can also be misleading, as the dose listed often refers to the size of the pill and not the active ingredients. Therefore, like other natural products, soy isoflavone should probably be obtained through natural foods. Whether it is helpful for prostate cancer prevention remains questionable. Despite this, some studies suggest that intake of natural soy foods might reduce prostate cancer risk, so most urologists believe soy is a reasonable dietary weapon.[5]

Because soy might increase estrogen, it has also been advocated as a possible (but unproven) treatment for hot flashes in men undergoing hormonal ablation (as described in chapter 22).

Other Possible Sources of Dietary Protection

Flaxseeds, pumpkin seeds, shark cartilage, a macrobiotic diet (whatever that is), garlic, vitamin C, and a number of other sources have been advocated. None of these has been proven to have a positive effect on prostate health or on prostate cancer prevention.

Fat

A fatty diet, especially one high in animal fats, has been implicated as increasing the risk of a number of malignancies, including prostate cancer.[6] However, a summary of the studies has failed to clarify the importance of this.[7] Thus, at this time most authorities still recommend a low-fat diet, but this will continue to be a source of controversy for some time.

Green Tea

All true teas come from the *Camellia sinensis* tree, which is really more of a bush. The difference between classic black tea most familiar to Americans and green tea is the processing. Green tea is unfermented, whereas black tea is fermented. Theoretically, this leaves antioxidants in green tea that help prevent innumerable diseases, including prostate cancer. Studies have suggested it may play a role, but no definitive proof exists.

VITAMINS, MINERALS, AND SUPPLEMENTS FOR A HEALTHY PROSTATE

What's Inside?

One problem with nutritional supplements is that there is no standardization regarding content. It is legal to claim a supplement contains a certain dosage of the presumed active ingredient even if that is not true. For example, one study looked at the levels of active ingredients in "natural" products. They found that fewer than half actually contained what their labels claimed.[8]

Similarly, some "natural" supplements for erectile dysfunction work because they contain substantial amounts of unnatural ingredients. One example is the reputed potency miracle, "Super X." Its miracle appears to come not from nature, but rather from the laboratories of major pharmaceutical companies. Samples tested were found to contain twenty-seven to thirty-one milligrams of sildenafil, better known as Viagra. Such amounts are within the range prescribed for impotence. Another such agent is named with the manly and impressive, "Stamina Rx." It contains eighteen to twenty-two milligrams of *tadalafil*. That is the active ingredient in the longer-acting impotence prescription medication Cialis. The dosage is impressive considering the maximum dose that I—as a board certified urologist—can prescribe for the same medication is twenty milligrams![9]

This all points out that "natural" isn't synonymous with healthy. Remember that tobacco—the biggest killer of them all—comes straight from Mother Nature.

Saw Palmetto

The most popular supplement for prostate problems is **saw palmetto**, made from the bark of the small palm tree, *Serenoa repens*. In the past two decades it has became popular as a prostate cure-all. It is touted for urinary difficulties, prostate cancer prevention, and prostate cancer treatment. With a mixture of traditional Native American medicine and the marketing machine of the complementary medicine industry, it has become perhaps the most widely used agent for prostate problems—prescription or not—in the world.

It seems that saw palmetto may block *5-alpha reductase*, the enzyme that converts **testosterone** to its active form, *dihydrotestosterone* (DHT). The prescription medications *finasteride* (Proscar) and *dutasteride* (Avodart) work by doing so. Studies regarding this effect are contradictory, with some showing saw palmetto effective in this way and others not. Most studies are of poor design and not believable because of their unscientific approach, which seem designed to generate marketing data instead of real evidence.

One effect of blocking DHT is a decrease in PSA of 40 to 50 percent and a reduction in prostate size of up to one-third. In comparison, saw palmetto has minimal if any impact on PSA, and at best reduces size by 6 percent.[10]

The problem with most studies that have looked for an effect of saw palmetto is that they are not *placebo controlled*. When we investigate a prescription medication we always give some people the drug and approximately the same number a placebo. This is because people who believe they will get better because they are taking a drug usually will experience some improvement in symptoms simply by wishing it so. As a result, we see a response rate (the placebo effect) of approximately 25 percent even in the placebo group. This finding has disproven a multitude of proposed prescription medications and kept most of the ineffective ones from ever reaching the marketplace. When the makers of these agents advertise charts showing a response rate but do not have a placebo group, we must be aware that the placebo effect may be responsible.

Other proposed mechanisms for saw palmetto (all unproven) include anti-inflammatory effects, estrogen-like activity, interference with growth factors, and free radical scavenging. A host of other unproven effects is bounced around, but at least some of these effects appear to be placebo related. Regardless, side effects with saw palmetto appear to be limited, but you should discuss it with your physician before taking this or any supplement.

Selenium

An antioxidant that appears likely to have an effect on prostate cancer prevention is selenium. This trace mineral is not naturally a major part of the American diet. A number of plants and some animal products contain selenium, but its presence is highly dependent on soil content. Therefore, men from areas with high levels in the soil receive greater levels in locally grown foods. The soils of the high plains of the American heartland are reportedly selenium rich, whereas the soils of Russia and China are deplete.

The role of selenium in preventing prostate cancer was found serendipitously when researchers were investigating its ability to prevent skin cancer. It failed to do so, but the investigators noticed that 63 percent fewer men developed prostate cancer while on selenium supplementation.[11] Others found that men with the highest levels of selenium in toenail clippings (an interesting but objectionable way to detect selenium levels) developed prostate cancer half as often.[12]

Although the above studies provide only indirect evidence, selenium seems to be a promising preventive agent. Since most foods consumed in modern society don't grow in local soil, geography isn't vital to receiving adequate selenium. We know that oral supplementation with selenium can compensate for deficiencies, if toenails are any guide. Men with low levels who begin supplements catch up in a matter of months.

The USDA (United States Department of Agriculture) recommends intake of only fifty-five micrograms—a minuscule amount. Recommendations for cancer prevention usually involve two hundred micrograms (one millionth of a gram) per day—still small, but enough to warrant its own tablets or capsules. This is a safe dose for most people, but overdosing can cause side effects or even poisoning, so consult your physician before beginning its use.

Catching up on selenium purely through diet is tricky, with most foods having only a few micrograms per serving. However, beef liver and cod each have over half the daily requirement in a single serving. A can of tuna has more than a day's supply. The big one is the Brazil nut. One ounce (unblanched, so none is washed away) has twelve times the daily requirement.

Although we don't know for sure the effect of selenium once prostate cancer develops, we do know that in laboratory studies, it slows the growth of hormone refractory prostate cancer cell lines.[13] Its role in men who have already developed prostate cancer remains unclear at this point.

Vitamin E

Vitamin E is an antioxidant that slows the growth of or kills prostate cancer cells in laboratory dishes. Studies in Finland attempting to prevent lung cancer with vitamin E failed to do so, but men taking the vitamin had a one-third lower incidence of prostate cancer and a 41 percent lower risk of dying from prostate cancer.[14] Studies comparing vitamin E levels with prostate cancer risk have been contradictory, with some finding a protective effect and others showing none.

Alpha-tocopherol is the natural form of vitamin E, found in highest amounts in vegetable oils, nuts, and green leafy vegetables. Supplemental forms found in the capsules familiar to most consumers are slightly less active, but can compensate for a diet short of the desired amount. Preventive doses used in most studies are 400 to 800 IU daily.

The main risk with vitamin E is bleeding. It serves as a blood thinner similar to aspirin. Therefore, it should be discontinued prior to surgery or biopsy in order to minimize bleeding risk. In addition, there is one report showing increased risk of death from cardiovascular or other unrelated causes in men who take doses of 400 IU or larger.[15] Always consult with your doctor before taking any drugs or supplements.

A large multi-institutional trial is currently under way to find out whether men who take vitamin E and selenium will have less incidence of prostate cancer down the road. This trial is creatively named SELECT, meaning the **SEL**enium and Vitamin **E** Cancer Prevention Trial. This study, led by Dr. Eric Klein of the Cleveland Clinic and involving thousands of men, is designed to determine whether this combination truly protects from the development of prostate cancer.

MEDICATIONS FOR A HEALTHY PROSTATE

Finasteride: The Prostate Cancer Prevention Trial

Finasteride is marketed as two different prescription drugs. The first is the stronger, five-milligram size called Proscar, which is used to shrink an enlarged prostate. The one-milligram size of the identical chemical is marketed as *Propecia*, familiar as the once-a-day pill prescribed for male pattern baldness.

The active ingredient selectively blocks 5-alpha reductase, one of the two enzymes that convert **testosterone** into its active form, *dihydrotestosterone* (DHT). Since DHT is responsible for prostate growth, this blockade shrinks the prostate and can effectively treat symptoms of prostate enlargement in some men. DHT also causes prostate cancer to grow, so blocking it has obvious promise for prostate cancer prevention.

HOW ARE DOSES CHOSEN?

You might be interested to know how doses are usually determined. Most commonly, they are made up. This is especially true of supplements such as vitamin E and selenium. Because vitamins and supplements are unregulated, a manufacturer basically picks a dose. Once the tablets or capsules are so designated, any study that follows will use that dose. If successful, the die is cast.

This principle also sometimes applies to designated doses of prescription medications. Dr. A. Morales of Ontario was the first to introduce the use of the biological therapy BCG for the treatment of bladder cancer in 1976. He administered six weekly treatments of this drug and reduced cancer recurrence significantly. When asked why he chose six treatments instead of some other regimen, he readily conceded that the drug came in a "six-pack," so that seemed to be the amount to try. Once a week made sense from a scheduling standpoint. "This regimen is arbitrary, and may be modified in the future as additional data become available," he wrote in a reply to an editorial comment.[16]

Dr. Morales's arbitrary dosing of BCG is the same one we still use today—quite successfully, I might add.

The Prostate Cancer Prevention Trial (PCPT) used finasteride in an attempt to prevent the development of prostate cancer. In the study, 18,882 men were given either finasteride or a placebo for seven years and then underwent prostate biopsy to determine whether the drug had lowered the risk of cancer. This was a double-blind study, meaning neither the men nor their doctors knew whether they were taking the drug or a placebo.

This important study yielded some contradictory findings that created confusion. Indeed, in 2003 it was closed early because it reached the primary goal of creating a 25 percent reduction in the incidence of prostate cancer in men who took finasteride. However, a troubling caveat emerged. Although men were overall less likely to develop prostate cancer, those who did appeared to have higher-grade (potentially more serious) tumors. Those who took finasteride had a 6.4 percent chance of having high-grade prostate cancer, whereas those who didn't had a 5.1 percent chance. Although this was a small difference, the size of the study assured that it was statistically significant and was unlikely to be due to chance.[17]

As discussed in the following chapters, cancer of a higher grade is more dangerous than a lower-grade cancer, so this finding is potentially alarming. Moreover, finasteride reduces PSA by approximately 50 percent, so it may mask prostate cancer if this effect goes unrecognized.

Therefore, you could interpret this information in either direction. If you wanted to believe in its value, you could say that finasteride reduced prostate cancer by about 25 percent. But you could also say that 1.3 percent more men who took finasteride developed high-grade cancer. What you can't say is which is best, because we don't know how many men in each group eventually will have serious problems or die from their disease. Only time will tell, and with prostate cancer that might be a long time. Recall that prostate cancer can progress very slowly, so it may be a decade or two before we can make any bold proclamations.

A final issue with the PCPT involves the concept of "burden of cure." This is based on the concern that most men with prostate cancer will have to consider curative therapy. If cancer is prevented, they will avoid not only the stress of this diagnosis, but also the burden of whichever treatment is ultimately chosen. Whether preventing the disease saves lives remains unclear, but if one-fourth fewer men will have to undergo treatment as a result of prevention, they will have received benefit.

The PCPT has been debated widely. Authorities can't agree on whether to be pleased that 25 percent of cancer cases were prevented, or to be concerned that cancer was higher grade in some of those that did develop the disease. We honestly can't yet determine which finding is more important, and may not be able to until we see how these men do in long-term follow-up. The ultimate test will be when we see how many men in each group ultimately die of prostate cancer. Therefore, I currently advise men that the verdict is still out on this question. I tell them the evidence that it might make things worse is weak enough that they should not automatically discontinue using finasteride if it is helping their urinary symptoms. Alternatively, the evidence that it will help prevent cancer is not overwhelming enough to automatically recommend its use for this purpose until further evidence becomes available. This is something for you to discuss with your physician.

The Prevention Bandwagon

A couple of other trials are underway that are using medications in an attempt to prevent prostate cancer. The first is the REDUCE (**RE**duction by **DU**tasteride in Prostate **C**ancer **E**vents) trial using dutasteride, a drug similar to finasteride that blocks the same enzyme as finasteride, plus a sister enzyme. Whether the additional blockage is significant is debatable, and will potentially be clarified by this study.

Nonsteroidal Anti-Inflammatory Drugs

Nonsteroidal anti-inflammatory drugs such as aspirin and ibuprofen may slow cancer growth. If this effect is proven, such agents might be used to both prevent and treat prostate cancer.[18] The major problem with these medications is side effects, including bleeding abnormalities, ulcers, and kidney damage.

These risks can potentially be overcome by a new generation of such medications called COX-2 inhibitors.[19] Unfortunately, these drugs have their own downside. One member of the group, Vioxx, was withdrawn from the market in 2004 because of an increased risk of heart attack in patients taking it. This risk could occur with other similar medications, and must be weighed against the possible benefit of prostate cancer prevention.

ACTIVITIES FOR A HEALTHY PROSTATE

Sex Is Good—and Good for You

Sex is good for health. Men who are sexually active and pleased with their sex lives are healthier, happier, and live longer.[20] In addition, at least two studies have found that increased ejaculation frequency was related to lower risk of prostate cancer.[21] Do not miss out on the most appealing opportunity to reduce your risk of cancer or early death.

Many urologists believe prostatitis can occur with extremes of sexual activity. Ejaculation on an excessive basis (as if that were truly definable, but generally believed to be more than twice daily) might irritate the prostatic ducts. Going prolonged periods without ejaculation (similarly impossible to define, but probably a matter of months) might lead to congestion. Either might create the irritation synonymous with prostatitis, although this remains unproven.

Of course, the other responsibilities of sexual activity still apply. Unless you are in a monogamous relationship and desiring paternity, you should use condoms or whatever means necessary to protect from pregnancy or sexually transmitted diseases, including HIV.

Other Activities

Some men may develop prostatitis as a result of trauma to the perineum. The classic occurrence is among bicycle riders, whose seats press against the gland during riding. Excessive bicycle riding can also cause erectile dysfunction. Similarly, truck and tractor driving or other forms of driving for long periods is sometimes blamed on prostate problems. There is no clear causative effect.

President Bill Clinton was infamously asked whether he wore boxers or briefs. Although some men believe briefs cause excessive heat accumulation, leading to a decreased sperm count and prostate problems, there is no evidence of this.

KEY POINTS

- The Prostate Cancer Prevention Trial showed that finasteride could reduce cancer incidence by 25 percent. However, if cancer did develop, it was more likely to be high grade.
- Natural prevention techniques remain the source of controversy as studies have not been absolutely clear of the role of many strategies. However, many urologists have concluded that five things may reduce your risk of prostate cancer. You should discuss these with your physician:

    1. Vitamin E, 400 IU (the most common tablet), daily
    2. Selenium, 200 micrograms (the most common tablet), daily
    3. A diet high in soy products
    4. A diet high in cooked tomatoes
    5. A low-fat diet

- Any prevention strategy requires you to weigh the potential risks versus the potential benefits.

2.

The Bothersome Prostate

6.

PROSTATITIS: THE IRRITATED AND IRRITATING PROSTATE

The diagnosis of "prostatitis" is often made by the physician, but rarely is substantiated in the laboratory.
—E. M. Meares Jr. and Tom Stamey, 1972

Prostatitis—inflammation of the prostate—is one of the most frequent diagnoses in urology. Although the most common form is only a mild inflammation, its acute or most severe form can be a serious illness. Unfortunately, the term is applied incorrectly far more often than accurately. It has become a catchall phrase used to describe many otherwise vague or inexplicable symptoms. Here we will clarify the difference between the infectious and noninfectious types, and discuss management in both cases.

ACUTE PROSTATITIS

Diffuse muscle aches and pelvic pain had annoyed Jim for two days. He had cancelled a business trip because he couldn't sit long enough to make it through the flight. Hot baths and Tylenol helped temporarily.

A temperature of 101.6° finally brought him to the emergency room. Though he looked ill, most of the examination was unremarkable. He had some mild abdominal tenderness and was sweaty and red from the fever, but otherwise it looked like another case of influenza. He was ready for discharge with a prescription for influenza medication. He had a sudden urge to urinate and asked for the restroom.

Fifteen minutes and two degrees later, Jim called for the nurse. He was unable to urinate. The urology resident physician on call was paged.

***

Acute is the term used to describe a sudden illness. Acute prostatitis is a serious bacterial infection arising suddenly when microorganisms that are normally relegated to other body areas infect the prostate. Their presence elicits a serious inflammatory reaction similar to that occurring anywhere in the body when bacteria reach areas where they don't belong. The body's immune system sends chemicals to the area, which causes fluid accumulation and swelling. White blood cells arrive en masse to perform their duty of attacking the foreign invader. The area becomes red, hot, and tender.

Fever is common in this "true" form of prostatitis, sometimes due to bacteria circulating through the bloodstream. This also leads to muscle aches and signs of a widespread systemic infection.

Bacteria usually reach the prostate either through the bloodstream or through its ducts (tiny tubes that drain secretions). These ducts also serve as a potential backdoor access for bacteria. They are especially likely to allow bacterial invasion if voiding pressure pushes urine containing bacteria into the ducts during voiding. A final route for bacteria into the prostate involves instrumentation such as cystoscopy or prostate biopsy. Regardless of the route, once bacteria reach places they don't belong, the immune system recognizes the attack and begins its counteroffensive.

This is similar to any inflammatory reaction. A similar response can occur under the skin. Bacteria are often *on* the skin, but never normally burrow *inside* the skin. Only when they reach through a crack, cut, or duct do they cause problems. The redness, pain, swelling, and warmth you experience with skin inflammation also occur in response to prostatic inflammation.

Additional problems arise when the location is prostatic because of its anatomic neighborhood. Swelling obstructs urination and can lead to strangury and other obstructive symptoms.

***

The resident covering the hospital that weekend ordered a urine specimen to check for infection, but Jim's inability to urinate presented a barrier. He reached for an examination glove. Jim was too sick to argue, but almost came off the table because of severe pain as soon as the examination started.

"Just as I thought," the doctor stated. "You have prostatitis." He reached for a catheter tray. Jim simply moaned.

TREATING ACUTE PROSTATITIS

Antibiotics to destroy offending bacteria are the key to treating acute prostatitis. They usually work within a few days. Unless the infection is very serious, most people can be treated with oral therapy. However, severe cases or those not responding to oral medications may require hospitalization for IV antibiotics.

The most common antibiotics used are those from the *flouroquinolone* class. Common examples include *Ciprofloxaxin* (Cipro, of anthrax scare fame) or *levofloxacin* (Levaquin). This class is favored because these drugs concentrate in prostatic tissue better than most antibiotics, and they are *broad spectrum* enough to kill most bacteria. Combination sulfa pills such as Bactrim and Septra, as well as doxycycline and tetracycline, also work in the absence of drug allergies. They are markedly less expensive but bacteria are sometimes resistant to them.

The required duration of antibiotic treatment is complex. Though most infections clear in a matter of days, the prostate is prone to having protected pockets of bacteria that refuse to die, so prolonged regimens are usually used. I recommend a minimum of ten to fourteen days, and usually prescribe the more expensive flouroquinolones for that duration and then another two to four weeks of *sulfa* or *doxycycline* to assure that the infection is eradicated.

Urinary difficulties are usually managed by taking medications such as *Hytrin, Cardura, Flomax,* or *Uroxatrol.* These can be taken with antibiotics without fear of drug interactions. If urinary retention occurs, a catheter can be placed temporarily to allow urine to pass until the swelling resolves. Acetaminophen (found in Tylenol) reduces fever and helps with pain and muscle aches.

It is reassuring to know that acute prostatitis completes its course and goes away. Once bacteria are dead, they no longer cause a problem. Their attack becomes a memory, but doesn't cause repeated returns to the doctor unless a completely new infection arises in the future, which is very uncommon. Some residual inflammation may persist, but is usually asymptomatic.

***

Although Jim assumed it would be torture, the catheter actually made him feel better almost immediately. Well over a liter of cloudy urine drained within minutes. A sample was sent to the lab, which confirmed a bacterial infection.

I was called and admitted him to the hospital for IV antibiotics because of the severity of the illness. A urine culture returned two days later identifying a common bacterial infection as the cause. It also proved that Cipro was active against this type of bacteria, so he was switched to a daily pill. His fever spiked several times, reaching over 104° twice, but for three days his temperature stayed below 100. Given his progress, the catheter was removed and he urinated without difficulty. He was tired, but able to go back to work within days. Since he had been so ill, I kept him on antibiotics for a month. I saw him a few days later in the office and confirmed the problem had resolved. Since then he has had no further problems.

CHRONIC PROSTATITIS

Unlike the acute or episodic form, chronic prostatitis implies a long-standing or repeat condition. This would be similar to chronic sinusitis. They both manifest by repeated or sometimes constant irritation in their respective locations. Neither becomes severe (and in fact might be present without being noticed at all), but can be frustrating in their perseverance.

The source of prostatic inflammation is not always obvious, but it is sometimes caused by a low-grade bacterial infection. However, irritation can also occur due to *sterile* (uninfected) urine backing up into the prostatic ducts, causing an intense inflammatory response that mimics an infection.

Men with chronic prostatitis have low-grade inflammation (sometimes caused by *infection* and sometimes simply caused by *irritation*) that can cause urinary difficulties, as well as pain and discomfort in the prostate. It might be felt as lower abdominal, back, penile, or perineal pain.

Note that these are vague symptoms that most people have at one time or another, so it is easy to find an excuse to blame chronic prostatitis for a multitude of otherwise unexplained symptoms. This leads to its inaccurate and overused diagnosis for pain anywhere from the waist to the knees, almost any urinary symptom, and even sexual difficulties.

Therein lies the problem—since all men experience one or more of these symptoms at some point, it is feasible that almost anyone could be diagnosed with chronic prostatitis.

PROSTADYNIA

There is a third category of prostatitis which most urologists call **prostadynia**, meaning "painful prostate." This is the term for prostatic inflammation in the absence of infection, and may be the source of most cases diagnosed as "prostatitis." In the past this was also called *nonbacterial prostatitis*.

The old way to determine the difference between bacterial and nonbacterial prostatitis was to perform *prostatic massage*, which was exactly as appealing as it sounds. The gloved finger used for DRE "milked" fluid from the prostate into the penis through the urethra by pressing so hard that the prostatic fluid had nowhere else to go. This fluid, *expressed prostatic secretions*, was checked under the microscope and was presumed to indicate inflammation if white blood cells were present. If they were seen, antibiotics were prescribed. The problem with this method is that it had only a limited basis in scientific fact. White blood cells might be present in normal seminal fluid or might not escape into the semen even in the presence of infection. Either one would lead to misdiagnosis. Moreover, men didn't like having prostatic massage in the presence of a tender prostate.

HOW CAN YOU TELL?

Doctors use a couple of indicators to determine whether the diagnosis should be related to the prostate. The first is obvious—the prostate should be tender. *It is almost impossible to*

Many people confuse inflammation with infection and have a hard time accepting that bacteria are not the source of symptoms, whether in the prostate, upper urinary tract, or other places in the body. They usually want antibiotics to treat their ailments whether the physician feels they are appropriate or not.

I find an easy way to understand the difference is in the joints. When a joint such as the knee or shoulder hurts people usually assume arthritis or irritation as the source. They don't require antibiotics, but rather seek medications to relieve the inflammation. As it turns out, anti-inflammatory drugs such as ibuprofen, aspirin, etc., are designed to relieve not only inflammation, but also associated pain or discomfort.

The source of joint pain and swelling is rarely a bacterial infection that warrants antibiotics, but usually is simply due to inflammation. The same situation exists in the prostate and should be managed accordingly.

diagnose prostatitis accurately without examining the prostate. If the prostate is not tender, the diagnosis is unlikely.

I find that DRE can be misleading to many patients and nonurologists. Either might make the mistake of assuming a case of prostatitis whenever DRE is painful. But that overlooks the fact that the tenderness may not be in the prostate. DRE should reveal tenderness *in*, not near, the prostate. Tenderness in the anatomic neighborhood of pelvic floor, lower back, groins, or scrotum doesn't count. If those are the areas of tenderness, then the problem is irritation of something else, not the prostate. Other areas of concern should be addressed.

In order to determine the difference, I press against the prostate first when performing DRE looking for symptoms of prostatitis. If it is not tender I know that the diagnosis is apparently not prostatitis and seek a better explanation for the symptoms. If it is tender, I then try to determine if it is truly the prostate or simply the rectal wall or pelvic floor muscles by pressing on these areas separately. If there is more pain with a firm push against the pelvic floor muscles near the prostate, I know that we are dealing with a muscular issue and can treat it as I would a sore muscle anywhere else in the body.

The second issue that appears commonly with a true prostatitis is painful ejaculation. Men with symptoms suggestive of chronic prostatitis who also complain of painful ejaculation are more likely to respond to antibiotics, suggesting they actually do have bacterial prostatitis. Unfortunately, they are also more likely to experience longer, more significant symptoms on a recurrent basis.

TRADITIONAL DIAGNOSTIC METHODS

Many older urologists (and a few younger ones) continue to differentiate the various conditions using urinary tests performed before and after *prostate massage*. The idea is that a massage might press out bacteria, white blood cells, or other evidence of infection.

Because of the expense and discomfort of doing so, a majority of urologists have abandoned these techniques. Even superspecialists in prostatitis have greatly simplified them. However, for especially complex cases this method still occasionally plays a role, particularly if you see a urologist who specializes in prostatitis and chronic pelvic pain syndromes.

PROSTATITIS ON PROSTATE BIOPSY

Signs of inflammation are often found through a prostate biopsy. The presence of white blood cells and other signs of irritation determine the diagnosis. This irritation is sometimes the cause of an elevated PSA, but may be a coincidental finding.

Most of these men have *no symptoms,* suggesting inflammation is an insignificant finding. It is unclear whether anything should be done about it. For one thing, it is unrewarding to treat symptoms that do not exist. Doing so risks side effects and costs. For these reasons, if prostatitis is identified through prostate biopsy, most doctors will not recommend intervention.

One reason to treat might be an attempt to reduce the PSA if you believe inflammation is the reason for its elevation. This might avoid further concern of cancer in the future if the PSA returns to normal as a result. In my experience this is rarely successful.

I usually do not recommend antibiotics in this circumstance. However, sometimes the biopsy causes symptoms of prostatitis and reveals that bacterial prostatitis triggered the PSA elevation. This is the most significant complication of prostate biopsy and should be treated with antibiotics as is *acute prostatitis.*

HOW COMMON IS PROSTATITIS?

About 15 percent of men who see a physician for urinary complaints are diagnosed with prostatitis.[1] Many additional men with pelvic, back, or abdominal pain also receive the diagnosis. With the vague nature of many of the symptoms, it is easy to use the diagnosis of prostatitis when we don't know for certain what the real problem is.

This leads to significant inappropriate treatment. The economic impact of treatment for men with the presumed diagnosis of prostatitis is huge, costing almost $4,000 per case yearly. The indirect cost, such as missed days of work or lost productivity in 79 percent of these men, is more than $2,000 a year for each.[2]

Fortunately, most men with such symptoms have either mild urinary difficulties or pain from muscular problems of the back or pelvic floor that will resolve no matter what—so misdiagnosis in this case may not be harmful. However, many men receive countless doses of antibiotics or prostate medications on a repeated basis. Such is the case of Dan at the beginning of chapter 3. He had been treated with almost every antibiotic known to man. His failure to respond was predictable since the treatment was for a condition he did not have. Moreover, overuse and inappropriate use of antibiotics renders many of them ineffective as bacterial resistance develops.

Many such men too often receive prostate massage intended to remove the bad humors, in addition to prescription medications. I have known countless men over the years who were probably psychologically dependent on these medications not because they helped, but because they hoped they would.

Therefore, I never assume that a history of prostatitis is accurate. In fact, I often assume it is not, until I find evidence of a tender prostate or true acute prostatitis as described above.

CHANGING NAMES

The National Institutes of Health (NIH) has tried to classify the above complex categories into three categories. The first two are true infections—*acute prostatitis* (category one) and *chronic bacterial prostatitis* (category two).

Prior to the NIH classifications, the traditional terms for noninfectious symptoms—*chronic (nonbacterial) prostatitis* and *prostadynia*—described inflammation and pain, respectively. However, as discussed above, they often describe symptoms that may be completely unrelated to the prostate. The NIH now groups these into the classification of *chronic prostatitis/chronic pelvic pain syndrome*. Its acronym, *CP/CPPS, category 3*, is not as user friendly but is more accurate in its depiction of a situation lacking clarity. You may see it used more as physicians move away from randomly treating men for a prostate infection.

STRESS

Most disease conditions associated with vague symptoms and episodes of relapses that may or may not respond to treatment are in some way stress related. Chronic prostatitis and pelvic pain are no different.

Sometimes stress is the result and sometimes it is the cause. In the former, stress might make you contract the pelvic floor muscles in a manner similar to clenching your teeth. The former results in pelvic pain, while the latter results in headaches. In addition, stress reduces the pain threshold.

Pelvic pain might also *cause* stress due to concerns that more serious conditions are being overlooked, or if pain is severe enough to produce stress on its own. This is an example of a vicious cycle that should be nipped in the bud. A vicious cycle occurs when one problem causes another, and the second problem in turn causes the first one to get worse.

GRADING PROSTATITIS SYMPTOMS

The NIH-CPSI (National Institutes of Health Chronic Prostatitis Symptom Index, which is shown below) is a validated scoring system that is used to quantify such symptoms. Although there are no agreed-upon levels that define severe versus mild CPPS, the symptom score is useful to quantify symptoms and to assess a response to intervention.

Pain or Discomfort

1. In the last week, have you experienced any pain or discomfort in the:

	Yes	No
a. area between rectum and testicles (perineum)?	1	2
b. testicles?	1	2
c. tip of the penis (not related to urination)?	1	2
d. below your waist, in your pubic or bladder area?	1	2

2. In the past week, have you experienced:

	Yes	No
a. pain or burning during urination?	1	2
b. pain or discomfort during or after sexual climax (ejaculation)?	1	2

3. How often have you had pain or discomfort in any of these areas over the last week?

0	Never
1	Rarely
2	Sometimes
3	Often
4	Usually
5	Always

4. Which number best describes your AVERAGE pain or discomfort on the days that you had it, over the last week?

0	1	2	3	4	5	6	7	8	9	10
No Pain										In Pain as Bad as You Can Imagine

Urination

5. How often have you had a sensation of not emptying your bladder completely after you finished urinating, over the last week?

        0   Not at all
        1   Less than 1 time in 5
        2   Less than half the time
        3   About half the time
        4   More than half the time
        5   Almost always

6. How often have you had to urinate again less than two hours after you finished urinating, over the last week?

        0   Not at all
        1   Less than 1 time in 5
        2   Less than half the time
        3   About half the time
        4   More than half the time
        5   Almost always

Impact of Symptoms

7. How much have your symptoms kept you from doing the kinds of things you would usually do, over the last week?

        0   None
        1   Only a little
        2   Some
        3   A lot

Quality of Life

9. If you were to spend the rest of your life with your symptoms just the way they have been during the last week, how would you feel about that?

        0   Delighted
        1   Pleased
        2   Mostly satisfied
        3   Mixed (about equally satisfied and dissatisfied)
        4   Mostly dissatisfied
        5   Unhappy
        6   Terrible

Scoring the NIH-Chronic Prostatitis Symptom Index Domains

Pain: Total of items 1a, 1b, 1c, 1d, 2a, 2b, 3, and 4 =   _____
Urinary Symptoms: Total of items 5 and 6 =   _____
Quality of Life Impact: Total of items 7, 8, and 9 =   _____

(Reprinted with permission of the American Urological Association and the *Journal of Urology*.)

TREATING CHRONIC PROSTATITIS

You now know that most of the time the diagnosis of prostatitis is one of exclusion—when some doctors don't find anything else wrong they use their "kitchen sink" explanation for the problem and call many such symptoms "prostatitis." A majority of men receive antibiotics or prostate medications because their doctors feel the pressure to "do something." I don't believe in the existence of this form of "prostatitis."

I recommend treatment with antibiotics primarily for men who have tenderness *in the prostate*. A minimum of ten days is appropriate, and four to six weeks if your doctor is convinced there is a serious infection. If he suspects you could have an atypical or resistant infection, he may try a different antibiotic such as doxycycline.

Failure to respond to antibiotics suggests the possibility of other problems and might warrant testing (see chapters 4 and 7). These might be used to determine whether urinary obstruction or other bladder problems are the source. X-rays or other tests might be needed. If the symptoms bother you enough you should see a specialist.

However, after seeing a urologist you might choose to accept the fact you have already been checked and nothing serious has been found. It might be time to move on and not chase the symptoms with antibiotics and other medications directed at things that are not the problem. Consideration of stress, normal changes of aging, or simply the aches and pains of life might be in order. But of course you should not assume anything until you have been properly examined by a physician.

TREATING PROSTADYNIA

One of my most insightful patients with such conditions was a physical therapist named Edward. Approaching fifty, he mentioned severe problems that he was having with "prostatitis" to a physician whom he was treating for a rotator cuff tear. The physician, a friend of mine, wasn't a urologist but recognized that five courses of antibiotics in the past few months didn't sound right. Relief with each course had been fleeting at best, followed by resumption of pelvic pain. The symptoms had crescendoed in the past week to the point that he had gone on leave because his pain prevented him from doing his job. By that time he was developing nausea and diarrhea. "I'm taking leave of absence until I find out what's wrong," he declared. "I think it might be cancer."

I agreed with Edward's assessment for the most part, although a normal PSA led me to believe cancer was unlikely. Another course of antibiotics made no sense.

Rectal examination made the diagnosis obvious. Pressing on the rectal wall overlying Edward's prostate caused him significant discomfort, but confirmed the prostate to be normal. However, the true site of tenderness was in his perineal body, *the central tendon of the pelvic floor. Pinching it between the forefinger and thumb of my gloved hand made clear that a strain of this tendon was the problem.*

I explained the situation and reassured Edward cancer was not the source of his symptoms. Indeed, the prostate was not even the source. "You'll be fine, but the reason it hasn't cleared up is that you have strained a tendon and its muscles in a place that is difficult to overcome."

"That's what I thought!" he almost blurted as he recognized the logic of my conclusion. "But the doctor kept giving me antibiotics." He noted that he had been examined only on the initial visit. Tenderness on DRE had been the determining factor and a failure to improve had been followed by multiple ill-fated attempts involving antibiotics.

We discussed ways to manage his problem. I stopped the antibiotics, which I was sure were the source of his nausea and diarrhea. "Your occupation deals with similar situations all the time," I explained. "When people strain a muscle or tendon they come to you for help just as you are here now for me to help. The difference is that the most significant things you do for your clients are administration of heat, exercise, and massage to the muscle. That's not so easy for the pelvic floor muscles," I explained.

His eyes lit with full understanding. "You're right," he said. "I didn't want to tell you—I thought you'd think I was nuts—but I already began treating it myself." I expected him to say he was taking over-the-counter anti-inflammatory medications. He instead described a logical regimen for this muscular problem. He recognized the area of tenderness was just behind his scrotum, so had begun massaging the site. He said he had considered internal massage, but couldn't bring himself to do that. He had begun using hot baths to improve circulation to the area, and found significant relief by performing a couple of hot water enemas. He had not wanted to describe the self-treatment, believing I would disapprove. It was probably the best thing he could have done.

***

When infection has been ruled out and it becomes clear the problem is in the pelvic musculature, you are essentially dealing with a muscle strain and must be treated as such. If a muscle strain is in a hamstring, you try to rest it, use heat and anti-inflammatory medications, and massage. The pelvic floor muscle is no different. This muscle bundle called the *levator ani* is a hammock of muscle and tendon that supports the entire abdominal contents—the Atlas of pelvic anatomy. Therefore, it is easily strained by daily activities that cause it to contract, such as lifting and straining.

However, unlike the hamstring, the levator ani forms the floor of the abdominal enclosure, so it is affected by a couple of unusual activities. First is a big sneeze. Yes, when you sneeze the abdominal wall contracts quickly and almost violently. As the most fragile portion of the abdominal wall (really the abdominal floor if you will), the pelvic floor muscles tighten and easily tear small muscle bundles or their central tendon, the perineal body. The same thing can happen during a difficult bowel movement, when straining can cause injury. Finally, any movements that contract this muscle can lead to problems as easily gotten as straining a neck muscle.

Following any pulled muscle (or tendon), you feel pain. Unlike other muscles there is no way to rest the levator ani. The pelvic floor must work the entire time you stand, or even sit. Another sneeze or cough will cause reinjury. A bowel movement will stretch it.

In contrast to relieving the hamstring or external muscles, there is no easy way to massage the levator ani and perineal body. You may place a finger rectally combined with external massage of the perineum and perineal body, but this is neither easy nor popular. Applying heat can be a problem. Like Edward, some men report relief with hot water enemas.

Although Edward as a physical therapist found the seeds of success through home treatment, most men will not be as attuned to principles of massage and heat for muscular problem. They will probably be better served by consideration of specialized physical therapy if such symptoms persist unacceptably long. Unfortunately, very few physical therapists have learned such specialized techniques. In many communities there may not be one, which presents an access problem. Still, if you and your urologist determine pelvic floor dysfunction is the underlying issue, you might discuss it with a physical therapist prior to seeing if there is a problem.

***

I offered Edward some simple suggestions regarding timing and how to perform his own heat and massage treatments. I also offered to refer him for physical therapy if he failed to respond. Reassured his methodology was reasonable (and that he didn't have cancer) he told me he would let me know if he felt that he needed the additional help. I still await the call.

PROSTATE MASSAGE AND OTHER FALLACIES

A time-honored method to treat men with chronic pelvic pain is prostatic massage as described above. For years men have visited doctors' offices for treatment. For unclear reasons (since there is no scientific basis for it, so it is probably a placebo effect) some of these men felt better after their massage and left to return another day. This practice diminished.

To be fair, I have occasionally met men who swore such massage helped them and actually requested it. This usually happened after they relocated into the area or their previous urologist retired. I even respected their request on a *very* rare basis. However, once I explained that they probably felt better because of a placebo effect and I saw no medical reason to perform this procedure, they either decided they agreed or decided to find another urologist. My suspicion is that most who improve have pelvic floor strain as discussed above, and that it was actually the levator ani that felt better, not the prostate. As such, they may have received the right treatment for the wrong diagnosis.

The other practice that doesn't work is the revolving drug trick. Most of the men who practice this have received countless prescriptions for antibiotics in addition to prostate drugs. If the problem is neither infection nor prostatic abnormalities, these agents will clearly work no better than an appendectomy will correct a hernia.

Too many men (and their doctors) believe the medications are worth it and might help. Without scientific evidence to suggest these agents work, they appear to make some men feel better because of the *placebo effect*, which is a powerful tool. A placebo is something (often a sugar pill or other inactive ingredient) that is given to a patient that has no known medical effect on the condition being treated. Interestingly, about one-quarter of people will experience improvement in a medical condition purely because they've been given something. In their mind, they *are* being treated, and the mind is a powerful broker. If convinced they should be getting better from a treatment, around one-quarter will say they are, even if the treatment consists of a placebo. This effect can be especially pronounced for conditions such as chronic pelvic pain, which has such a vague nature.

The placebo effect is responsible for the fact that so many unproven treatments have testimonials to their effectiveness. Therefore, in proper medical studies, some patients are given the treatment while a *control group* is given a placebo. Neither group gets to know if it is taking the drug or the placebo. If the symptoms of one-quarter of the patients in each group improve, a placebo effect is clearly the reason. However, if one-quarter of the patients in the placebo group are improved, but one-half of the patients receiving the tested substance are improved, the tested substance is clearly helpful for the symptoms in some patients with that condition. The placebo effect causes about one-quarter of patients to report improvement during most drug studies, even if they are in the placebo group.

A good example is found in the studies on Viagra. The trials used to obtain FDA approval for Viagra found that 25 percent of patients taking the placebo reported improvement in erections, while about 80 percent of those taking Viagra reported improvement. Therefore, the FDA agreed that the studies showed a clear benefit to Viagra in treating erectile dysfunction, so it was approved for use in the United States. Of course, the manufacturer also has to determine that it was safe for most men.

CHARLATANS AND QUACKS

> *The functional form of impotence fills the coffers of the quacks.*
> —Rutherford Morison, 1965

Because of the vagueness of its symptoms, prostatitis has led to an embarrassing amount of charlatanism over the years. A few clinics were founded purely for treatment of these men, knowing they were a captive audience almost certain to become frequent flyers. Electrical stimulation, magnetic therapy, and most other snake-oil-type interventions became the highlight of a fascinating but embarrassing chapter in urological history.

A clinic in the Midwest in the twentieth century did essentially nothing except direct injection of antibiotics into the prostate. The underlying theory was that the prostate was hidden so deep and was so protected in the pelvis that medications could reach it only if injected directly through large needles. Despite the obviously painful experience, men traveled from far and wide to seek these treatments. Many of these men continued to have pelvic pain not only because of their initial problems, but also because of multiple injections. Many have nodular prostates due to scarring—this mimics cancer and can cause unnecessary alarm. I have performed prostate biopsy in some of these men simply to confirm that their firmness was due to scarring and not from cancer.

To my knowledge, these clinics were not manned by urologists.

HOPE: MOVING ON BEYOND THE PROSTATE

Men with the diagnosis of chronic prostatitis are often the most frustrated patients I see. They have often visited several physicians and have never received a satisfactory answer. Only when someone tells them the truth— their prostate is not the problem—do they see the first signs of hope.

Hope for these men arises when they are able to move on beyond the prostate. Those with true infections do find hope through antibiotics. The vast majority without infection find hope when they begin to address the actual problem for the first time.

If the problem is pelvic floor muscle spasm or perineal body strain, treatments aimed at a musculoskeletal problem are in order. Just like a severe ankle sprain, these injuries take a while to resolve. If steps are taken to allow recovery and avoid further injury, both conditions usually do so fully.

If stress or other nonurological sources are the cause of such symptoms, hope is revealed when the source is addressed. Directing attention away from a healthy prostate and toward an unhealthy mental state takes more work than popping a pill. However, addressing the true problem allows permanent resolution and paves the way to a better future.

KEY POINTS:

- Prostatitis actually describes two different conditions. The first (acute prostatitis) is a serious bacterial infection that arises suddenly and resolves completely through antibiotics. The second (chronic prostatitis) is an inflammatory condition in the prostate that is usually unrelated to infection.

- Most men diagnosed with "prostatitis" actually have chronic pelvic pain, urinary difficulties, or other noninfectious symptoms.

- Men with chronic pelvic pain usually fail to respond to antibiotics because infection is not the source of their problems. Addressing muscular strains, stress, or other causes of vague pelvic symptoms is more likely to yield successful relief.

WHY NOT JUST GIVE EVERYONE ANTIBIOTICS?

It is tempting to simply prescribe antibiotics to every man with possible prostatitis symptoms. On the other hand, there are some strong reasons not to do so in the absence of infection. First, antibiotics cost money. Second, they can cause side effects, which occasionally become severe.

This danger is demonstrated by the experience of one of my favorite patients. I had the pleasure of caring for a legendary and delightful entertainer who left a good urologist because of problems with a common antibiotic. The gentleman had no infection, but was given a "safe" antibiotic for a presumed but inaccurate diagnosis of prostatitis. After the first few doses this celebrity broke out in the most horrendous rash I'd ever seen. He had developed *Stevens Johnson Syndrome,* an allergic reaction where his skin essentially sloughed.

After several painful weeks he returned to normal and requested a second opinion for his presumed diagnosis of prostatitis. I respectfully disagreed with the diagnosis and confirmed my suspicion with a prostate biopsy. We avoided the responsible antibiotic and started successful prostate cancer treatment.

Another concern with such antibiotic use is the risk of developing drug resistance. Bacteria adapt quickly and develop resistance to antibiotics. Every time a new antibiotic is introduced, it is capable of killing almost any bacteria known to man. However, after just a few years we begin to find bacteria resistant to its effects. You also don't want to have antibiotics become useless in defending you against infection in the future.

Flouroquinolones such as Cipro and Levaquin are good examples. Early in my career I knew I could prescribe one of them for almost any infection. However, it is common now to find resistance to these antibiotics. Overexposure to bacteria for noninfectious reasons such as "chronic prostatitis" is responsible.

7.

BENIGN PROSTATIC HYPERPLASIA (BPH): THE ANNOYING PROSTATE

Male urination really is a kind of accomplishment, an arc of transcendence.
—Camille Paglia, 1990

Extra trips to the restroom during the night were the first sign. Ellen didn't complain, but teased Ron regularly about the awakenings. Her self-conscious husband knew Ellen was a light sleeper. He wanted to avoid disturbing her so badly that he regularly tried to hold off the inevitable. Each time he felt nature's call, he would try to lie still and fall back asleep. It became a miserable cycle as he predictably reawakened within minutes.

First he dropped his evening cup of Irish tea, believing that the caffeine simply made him sleep lightly enough to sense the bladder. Then he dropped the glass of wine they shared before bed each night. He finally stopped drinking any fluids after dinner. Nothing helped.

***

Although cancer is the most common prostate-related fear, far greater numbers of men experience the urinary effects of benign prostate changes. When men suffer urinary troubles, the prostate is the first and most likely suspect. Almost one-third of all men over fifty experience moderate to severe voiding symptoms caused by prostate problems.[1] This chapter explores these changes, while the next discusses management of them.

105

THE PROBLEM

The most clear-cut symptom of a prostate problem is a slow stream. This is usually due to the prostate compressing the **urethra** it encircles, thereby causing obstruction. The problem may be due to either a muscular contraction or physical compression from excessive growth. A combination of both is usually involved. The man experiences a weak stream, like when someone steps on a garden hose. He may tie up the restroom, taking more time to empty his bladder. (At baseball games, knowledge of this problem helps urologists get through the restroom more quickly than the uninformed. We know to avoid the lines with old men and to stick to the lines with young men whose prostates haven't yet started to cause problems.)

After slowly developing over a few years, these symptoms may change. The bladder can initially compensate for mild blockage simply by pushing harder. This overcomes the acute problem, but may lead to secondary symptoms. The bladder is like any other muscle—when it works harder it gets bigger and stronger. Individual bands of muscles enlarge, causing a condition known as trabeculation. Contraction of such muscles becomes the source of **irritation**, leading to urinary **urgency** and **frequency**. These symptoms may be confused with feelings of incomplete emptying. At night, multiple awakenings known as **nocturia** are especially annoying results of these muscle contractions since they disturb the man's sleep and likely that of his wife. As in Ron and Ellen's case, this annoyance is often the symptom that leads to the first complaint or doctor's visit.

In the later stages, feelings of incomplete emptying may not simply be sensations. The bladder really may not be completely empty. When this occurs, some portion of the bladder contents remains after voiding—an elevated **residual volume**. At that point the bladder has lost its ability to simply squeeze harder and starts to decompensate.

WHAT'S IN A NAME?

Like many things in medicine, prostate problems are often described in inconsistent ways. Layman's terms and medical terminology often align poorly. Physicians have long used the term **BPH**, or benign prostatic hyperplasia, to describe this condition. This is because this overgrowth, or *hyperplasia*, is usually the source of the symptoms. Laymen are more likely to use terms such as "enlarged prostate" or "prostate trouble" to describe the same thing.

The problem with these terms is twofold. First, we're talking about the same condition almost as if using two different languages. Second, none of these phrases is accurate. BPH is a poor term because it really describes a microscopic change in the prostate. However, such symptoms may be the result of a number of factors, including growth, constriction, or (rarely) late-stage cancer. Thus, BPH is a vague, catchall phrase. Similarly, "enlarged prostate" and "prostate trouble" may have nothing to do with the symptoms.

Since BPH isn't very accurate, many urologists have used (and still use) terms such as prostatism, obstructive uropathy, and urinary difficulties. Another descriptive phrase, bladder outlet obstruction (BOO), may be scary but is uncommonly used. None of these terms is universally accepted, but your doctor might use these or other terms for lack of anything better.

In order to more accurately discuss this condition, leaders in urology have tried to develop more descriptive terms. Unfortunately, the best one they have come up with—*lower urinary tract symptoms (LUTS)*—may be even worse! This catchall phrase that we're supposed to use could mean any symptoms, from bleeding to burning to leakage. The intent is good, but the outcome didn't get us any closer to terms that doctors and patients can use to talk the same language.

For the time being the abbreviation **BPH** continues to be the most common term applied—until a larger group of doctors gets together again and tries once more to come up with a better one.

SIZE MATTERS—BUT NOT AS MUCH AS YOU THINK

"Do you really have to do that?" Ron asked Dr. Merritt as the doctor put on the examination glove. "I hate it."

The doctor insisted. "We need to check for cancer . . . or enlargement." After a quick DRE he reassured Ron, "Your prostate is pretty small. It must be something else." A long discussion ensued, but as long as he was sure the prostate was normal, Ron didn't want to pursue the issue further. He declined the offer of a urology consult and left for a lunch date with Ellen.

"Dr. Merritt says I have the prostate of a twenty-year-old," the fifty-three-year-old bragged to his wife, taking great liberties with the doctor's assessment. "Nothing needs to be done."

***

The other issue with prostate size is that perception is usually based purely on DRE. This invokes the experience of the group of blindfolded observers describing an elephant by touch. The one in front would describe his subject—the trunk—as long, thick, and wet on the end. The one on top would articulate his feeling as a leathery mound, while those touching the legs would have the impression of something like tree trunks. The final observer would describe the tail as long, ropelike, and stinky.

Like those describing one aspect of the elephant, a physician performing DRE feels only one side of the prostate. We perceive only one facet—the posterior aspect adjacent to the rectum—but have no idea how thick the gland is. We cannot tell if it has an *intravesical median lobe* growing into the bladder, or two *lateral lobes* compressing the urethra. We can tell if it is absolutely huge, but this is uncommon.

In order to demonstrate this principle to medical students or physicians in training, I often recommend they estimate the prostate volume based on DRE prior to performing a prostate ultrasound (as described in chapter 12). Ultrasound can calculate size relatively accurately based on measurements taken during the procedure. It usually takes only one or two cases for them to recognize their perception of size based on a single aspect of the prostate is mostly guesswork. Thus, size is not the critical factor most men believe, so I try to steer their focus onto obstruction.

When men have symptoms related to their prostate, most assume the problems have to do with its being enlarged. Size is the first thing most men ask about when I perform a DRE. They blow right by concerns of cancer to find out—"Is it enlarged?" This male societal obsession makes me wonder if there is a reward offered somewhere out there for men with large prostates.

My answer is almost always a variation on one theme: size really doesn't matter (at least not that much). As we get older the prostate grows. As long as this growth is controlled and causes no symptoms, it is no big deal.

The only reason growth would matter is if it pushed on something else. Recall that the prostate sits right in the middle of a neighborhood of *soft tissue*. If it grows outward, it might push something away, but this rarely has consequences. If it grows upward into the bladder, it simply sits inside taking up space that would otherwise fill with urine. This might diminish bladder capacity, but not much. It might also push the bladder up, but approximately twenty feet of flexible, mobile intestine sits above the bladder. The intestines simply move to the side if anything pushes upward. They do this several times a day when the bladder fills, only to slide right back into position after the bladder empties. The prostate pushing everything up would be unnoticeable. The same concept holds for the back. The rectum is a hollow tube with plenty of extra room.

Growth to the front will simply push the prostate away from the pubic bone toward the rectum. If growth expands to each side, there is a lot of fat and muscle to serve as padding. The gland must really grow to epic proportions before it becomes large enough to reach side to side in the pelvis. Because of all this room for expansion, the prostate (unless cancerous) can sometimes grow like a wildflower without causing problems. It is only when this growth pushes inward that problems occur. Such inward growth can obstruct the urethra and cause **obstructive** symptoms.

SO WHY ALL THE NOISE ABOUT "ENLARGEMENT"?

As noted above, enlargement is not really the issue except when growth turns inward. Then the prostate compresses the urethra running through its middle, like a foot stepping on a garden hose. If all growth turns inward toward the urethra, obstruction occurs rapidly. Conversely, growth primarily occurring away from the urethra may progress a long time before it finally compresses the urethra.

I tell several men each workday that their prostate is normal for their age. They are routinely taken aback because someone somewhere told them that their prostate was enlarged.

"I've had an enlarged prostate for years," is the common response. They think I'm missing something.

The only honest explanation I can give (and do routinely) is that I rarely meet a man of their age who has not been told his prostate is enlarged. Either (almost) every man on Earth has an enlarged prostate, or a lot of men have been alarmed about its size unnecessarily. You can obviously guess my theory on that.

***

Things only got worse for Ron in the coming months. He hadn't recognized the severity of his problem, since it took years to become almost unmanageable. He finally became concerned when coworkers teased him during the annual meeting. They noted he tied up the urinal longer than anyone else. Male colleagues avoided lining up behind him in the restroom. After dismissing their teasing initially, he began to observe his colleagues and noted that they were right. He stood for several minutes before he could generate a stream. It cut off intermittently before he finally dribbled out the last few drops. Unless he waited each time, the final drops ended up in his shorts.

"Have you noticed anything different when I go to the bathroom?" he sheepishly asked Ellen that night. She tried to not be anywhere nearby when he voided, but couldn't help noticing some things while waiting to use the restroom herself.

"It takes time for you to start . . . and it sometimes seems like you're never going to finish. For that matter," she thought out loud, "it sounds like you're barely getting anything out while you're going." She concluded with her displeasure at the misdirected drops she had to clean up.

With his suspicions confirmed and his concern finally out in the open, Ron made the urology appointment.

WHY OBSTRUCTION MATTERS

Most people (including many physicians) confuse the term *obstruction* with total blockage. The difference between *obstruction* and *total blockage* can be illustrated by the example of a river dam. The dam rarely stops flow completely. Instead, water pressure builds up as the level rises. When enough builds, flow simply continues at a slower rate. Thereafter, a wide reservoir forms and water stagnates. Progress of boats, fish, or other passersby slows but continues despite this obstruction. Although water and other objects eventually make it through, there is a price to pay. Egress takes longer. Stagnation causes silt to form, leading to less efficient cleansing of the watershed. Some objects such as debris may never pass.

A similar situation occurs when partial obstruction dams the urinary stream. Water (urine) eventually makes it through, but a wide reservoir may accumulate above the dam. It takes longer for water to pass, so voiding takes longer and wastes time.

Stagnation leads to inefficient cleansing of the urinary tract watershed. This may allow infection to arise if bacteria, that normally would be readily expelled, are allowed to hang around and reproduce.

Silt eventually settles into solid mud at the river bottom, whereas bladder stones form when "silt" accumulates due to urinary stagnation. Finally just as debris may never pass the river dam, a bladder stone may never pass through the dammed prostatic urethra.

Disaster can occur eventually in either scenario. The Mississippi River floods of the nineties were examples in nature. When the reservoirs became too full, the water had to go somewhere so it spilled over the banks. Such backup in the urinary tract can lead to dilation of the **ureters**. This is called *hydronephrosis* (meaning "water on the kidney") and shows up as a widening on imaging tests such as a CT scan.

When urinary obstruction reaches this severity, it places undue pressure back against the kidneys—in essence spilling over the banks upstream. Kidneys cannot function effectively in that scenario, and they lose their ability to cleanse the bloodstream. Unless reversed in time, this can lead to permanent kidney damage or kidney failure. Dialysis or kidney transplant are the only means of survival thereafter. Such partial obstruction can occur anywhere in the urinary tract. The prostate is the most common location.

WHAT ACTUALLY HAPPENS?

Ron wrote "bladder problem" on the medical history form at the urology clinic. After reading half an article on prostate cancer in the reception area, he went to give a urine sample and was then shown to an exam room.

"Tell me what you mean by 'bladder problem,'" I inquired after introductions.

"My wife and my coworkers have all noticed how bad my bladder is," he answered. "I get up three or four times at night. I get back to sleep okay but my getting up is really affecting my wife. Sometimes she ends up in the guest room. At work I spend most breaks during meetings in the bathroom instead of networking. It's really affecting my job and I need to have something done about my bladder."

After a few more questions, he balked when I reached for the gloves. "You don't need to do that," he asserted. "My prostate isn't enlarged. Dr. Merritt already checked."

***

Two circumstances can lead to obstruction. The first and most common is indeed related to prostate growth. This explains why "enlargement" gets such a bad rap. Individual prostate cells multiply, creating islands or nodules of

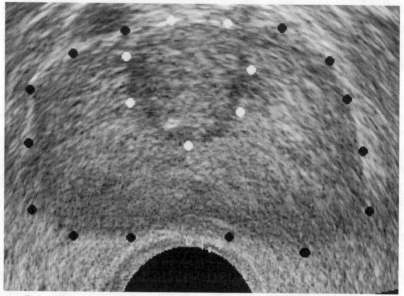

Figure 7-1. Ultrasound image demonstrates the inner central or transition zone (outlined with white dots) and the surrounding peripheral zone (outlined with black dots).

tissue that compress the urethra. These nodules are typically in the *transition* or *central zone*, which encircles the urethra. This location makes the urinary stream particularly vulnerable to their growth (see figure 7-1).

A second cause of partial urinary obstruction is the result of muscular contraction around the urethra. So-called smooth muscles are particularly common in and around the prostate, especially at the urethra and bladder neck. These involuntary muscles may pay no heed to their owner, maintaining low-amplitude contractions even during voiding.

Such contractions often explain why a man whose prostate size is completely normal or even small may experience LUTS. This can lead to unnecessary suffering if unrecognized. I often meet men such as Ron seeking a second opinion for classic obstructive symptoms who have been told that the problem cannot be with their prostate since it is small. These men often believe they may be hypochondriacs until tests clearly demonstrate obstruction. Medications or surgical intervention provide a seemingly miraculous solution for the long suffering. A combination of growth and muscular contraction is usually involved, which thus presents two targets for therapy.

***

"Let's start from scratch," I suggested after Ron gave it his best shot at avoiding the DRE. "No assumptions." This wasn't really true, because I had my own preconceptions. I simply wanted to overcome his. Since he was a fifty-three-year-old man with significant **obstructive** *and* **irritative** *urinary symptoms, I knew what his diagnosis would most likely be.*

It wasn't rocket science—most men his age and above with such symptoms have obstruction from BPH. "Let's just check," I recommended. Indeed, his prostate was normal size, perhaps even small. More important, through the combination of my normal DRE and the normal PSA I subsequently ordered, I was comfortable that prostate cancer was not part of the situation. "Let's talk about your options."

I asked my nurse to check a postvoid residual volume using the portable ultrasound as described below. Even after he voided, almost a pint of urine remained in his bladder. No wonder he voided often and had to get up several times at night. The minute he left the restroom, his bladder was already almost full. Everything suggested obstruction.

LESSONS FROM DOUGHNUTS

My friend and partner, Dr. Jim Ulchaker, offers my favorite explanation for the above concepts. He is recognized nationally and internationally for subspecialty work in the innovative treatment of men with BPH. He uses the metaphor of the prostate as a doughnut. A big one might have a big hole or a little hole. The same can be said for a little doughnut. Regardless of total doughnut size, if the hole is big, it is easy to pass something through the middle. If the hole is small, it is not.

"I don't care how big your doughnut is," he repeats several times a day to patients with prostatic obstruction. "I care how big your doughnut hole is." If their doughnut hole is too small—whether because of enlargement, muscular contraction, or both—he addresses the problem. If the hole is adequate, he confirms that their doughnut (or prostate) presents no problem. Everyone can understand that metaphor.

WHY ARE SYMPTOMS DIFFERENT FOR DIFFERENT PEOPLE?

Recall that urinary obstructive symptoms belong to two separate categories—**obstructive** and **irritative**. Irritative symptoms such as **urgency**,

frequency, and **nocturia** (frequent or excessive voiding at night) are signs that the bladder is overactive in response to partial obstruction. This is similar to the situation in nature where incoming upstream water eventually builds enough height and pressure to keep water flowing over or through the river dam. Similarly, the bladder simply creates more pressure by contracting forcefully in order to overcome partial obstruction. This increase in contractility is sensed as an urge to void. If contractions occur with minimal filling, urinary frequency results. Such contractions during sleep lead to nocturia.

Irritative symptoms are often the earliest signs of partial obstruction. Such bladder contractions may eventually become so severe that they push beyond the prostate at inappropriate times. This is called **urge incontinence** because the man usually senses the urge to void but doesn't make it to the restroom before it is too late. By the time this symptom arises, obstruction is usually advanced.

In contrast, obstructive symptoms are similar to the situation in a corroded pipe. The slow stream is often noted first. Water (urine) molecules must compete for limited space to exit. They become similar to Archie Bunker and his son-in-law trying to get through the kitchen door at the same time. A decreased force of stream is the most obvious sign of obstruction. Instead of crashing against porcelain, the urinary stream begins backing off and may soon pose more threat to your shoes. **Hesitancy** often comes next as a man stands several seconds before urine begins to pass. This indicates that the prostate is constricting the urethra significantly and opens enough to pass urine only after several seconds of bladder contraction. *Dribbling* occurs following voiding as the prostate begins to back up while the bladder attempts to push the last bit of urine past. Care must be taken to avoid a spurt of urine *after* the penis returns to the underwear.

Intermittency is a late obstructive symptom that occurs when the prostate slams open and shut. Bladder contractions can push hard enough that if the man is patient and persistent he may eventually get most of the urine out. This is a late obstructive symptom suggesting that the disease is advanced. In a way it is actually an example of intermittent **urinary retention**, the final stage when urine is trapped completely. Only at the stage of urinary retention does *complete* obstruction occur. Misery strikes at that point and the patient begs for relief.

Occasionally patients reach this point with minimal symptoms. Although stoicism may be the reason for many to ignore symptoms, others simply do not have normal sensation to perceive a problem. Diabetics are classic examples of the latter because diabetic nerve damage inhibits sensation. They may develop massively distended bladders without realizing it. Another group that commonly develops such symptoms includes men who hold urine so long that its pressure causes sensory nerve damage, rendering them unable to perceive sensations. Truckers are candidates for this because they are on the road and cannot easily stop to void. In addition, time is money, so pulling over cuts into the paycheck. Teachers and nurses are as likely to have such problems in my experience, since they tend to be committed professionals who keep working with those who need them instead of running out for a break.

The worst combination is a diabetic truck driver who is motivated to hold urine for as long as he can and is capable of doing so because of impaired sensation. I have had several such patients tell me they could drive most of the way across the country without stopping to void. With that story I usually know the diagnosis even before checking.

URINARY RETENTION: FOILED BY PHYSICS

The final straw is urinary retention. It may occur spontaneously, but often occurs after a man who is barely getting by experiences something to throw him over the edge. This may occur following anything that weakens the rest of the body, such as surgery, injury, or a heart attack. When retention is imminent, any of these may allow the bladder to decompensate.

Not only is the bladder (as part of the complete body) weakened, but other factors come into play. The most significant is related to a physics lesson many of us forgot after high school—the *Law of Laplace*. In class we learned that $P = 2T/r$. To the physics teacher (and to Dr. Laplace) the formula meant that the pressure (P) inside a sphere (i.e., the bladder) is equal to twice the wall tension (T) divided by the radius (R). Most of us don't care about that. To a kid, the Law of Laplace means that it's hard to start blowing up a balloon. The first puffs will hardly make a difference, but once it is started (the radius increases), it is easy to keep putting more air in until it pops.

To the urologist (or the man with urinary retention) the Law of Laplace means that the more distended the bladder becomes (the radius becomes greater), the less pressure it takes to keep the wall overstretched. This limits its ability to contract and empty. Not only that, but the bladder wall muscle will become thinner. Therefore, it is weakest at the moment it needs to squeeze the most to overcome not only obstruction, but also the Law of Laplace. Therefore, allowing the bladder to overfill is a recipe for disaster.

SETUPS FOR URINARY RETENTION

A few circumstances can predispose one to sudden urinary retention. The first involves the use of medications that constrict the urinary tract. Such meds are useful for the respiratory tract, where constriction actually opens channels. Typically marketed as cold and allergy medications, these agents also tighten the prostate and bladder neck/internal sphincter. That is why they carry the warning, "Ask your doctor if you have prostate problems." When taken by a woman or a by a man with no prostate problems, the effect on the urinary tract is barely noticeable. However, it will close off the stream in a man with near obstruction, leading to urinary retention.

Another scenario involves a man with BPH who drinks too much alcohol. Not only is he weakened by the substance, but his bladder becomes over distended because of the fluid volume. The implications are obvious.

A prostatic *infarct* can also cause sudden urinary retention. Complete loss of blood flow to an area is called an infarct. In the *myocardial* muscle of the heart, it is known as myocardial infarct. Doctors usually abbreviate it "MI," while patients call it a heart attack. Heart tissue swells and dies, leading to the serious consequences we all know. When the same thing occurs in the prostate it is called a prostatic infarct (although no one calls it a "PI"). Prostate tissue swells and dies, leading to urinary retention if the swelling overwhelms a urinary stream barely adequate at baseline.

The final and *least common* reason that a man develops retention is prostate cancer. Twenty or more years ago, when prostate cancer often went undetected until advanced, cancer would sometimes obstruct the prostatic urethra and would eventually lead to *rapid* progression of urinary symptoms and retention. With current screening techniques this rarely occurs—most men with cancer are detected well before they reach that stage. Therefore, most urinary obstructive symptoms are from BPH and *not* cancer.

"MY HEMORRHOIDS SAVED MY LIFE"

Urinary retention occasionally signals more serious problems. Allan is a forty-year-old African American man who was sent to my office urgently a few hours after hemorrhoid surgery. The operation went fine and he went home soon after it was completed, but he could not void when he got home. Fortunately, his operation was the first case of the day so he recognized the problem before lunch. When he called the surgeon's office, the staff told him to come directly to my office downstairs.

This scenario is common because of a combination of things. Anesthesia and surgery weaken the entire body, including the urinary tract. The bladder may become distended during surgery because IV fluids are going in but the patient is not awake to empty on command. Finally, an operation on that part of the body is painful so it is difficult to relax enough to empty.

When Allan arrived, the nurse gave him one more chance to void before he saw me. Abdominal examination revealed a distended bladder. But I wouldn't even consider a DRE immediately after hemorrhoidectomy. I reassured him that this problem was common following surgery and that most men who experience urinary retention immediately after surgery will resume voiding unless they were having substantial problems before surgery. He assured me he had not and was relieved to learn that the prognosis was good. I started him on an alpha blocker (as discussed in the next chapter), and my nurse taught him how to do self-catheterization.

A combination of things allowed him to resume spontaneous voiding within twenty-four hours. Medications relaxed his prostate and bladder neck. Time away from the operating room allowed his body to remove the anesthetic agents. The pain began to subside. Catherization allowed his bladder to return to a normal filling size or radius. Two days later he was voiding better than pre-op and was back to normal.

During our initial discussion I made it clear that follow-up was absolutely necessary. Although I acknowledged that it was an issue, I was only minimally concerned that prostate cancer could be playing a role. This was heightened a little bit by the fact that men with prostate cancer can develop sudden onset of urinary retention as discussed above. However, knowing it was rare, especially in a man of forty, my concern was more that he was an African American man in the age range at which many urologists recommend screening for prostate cancer. I am one of those urologists who do.

I scheduled an appointment for a few weeks later in order to be assured that he had resumed normal voiding and to check his PSA. A DRE at that time was finally tolerable and it was normal, but the PSA was not. It was 2.5 ng/dl, slightly high by most standards and certainly high for his age. I hoped that perhaps the catheterizations had caused a misleading elevation, so I simply recommended it be repeated in another month. If it was going down I would try to hold off on a biopsy. The opposite occurred. The repeat PSA was 3.7. This was suspicious for cancer. Even more so, the percent of his PSA that was free (or unbound to protein) was 11 percent. As discussed later, this left no doubt that a biopsy was in order.

Allen tolerated the biopsy very well since I used an anesthetic block. The *diagnosis was more challenging—cancer. Fortunately, Allen is a rock. He wasn't happy to hear the news, but he cut to the chase. "I have an eleven year old son. I want to watch him grow up," he said. "Tell me what it will take to get there." After a long discussion regarding all the options, Allen chose to proceed to surgery.*

After recovering from the operation, Allen had the opportunity to brag that his hemorrhoids—or at least the problems he had experienced after surgery for them—had possibly saved his life.

MAKING THE DIAGNOSIS

Most medical diagnoses are based on analyzing symptoms. This is especially true for BPH. In order to quantify complaints, the American Urological Association has developed a questionnaire that is similar to several others used by specialists around the world.

Although not specific to BPH, the **AUA Symptom Score**, as shown below, uses seven questions to define severity. In general, a score of 0 to 7 is considered mild. Moderate symptoms fit a total score of 8 to 19, while a score of 20 to 35 is thought to represent severe symptoms. Many urologists, including me, actually fudge a little on those formal recommendations and consider anything below 10 as mild.

There is no score that automatically warrants treatment. If tests show that the kidneys function normally and the bladder empties adequately, some people with significant symptoms will be comfortable with remaining untreated. Others will request therapy though having symptoms generally regarded as mild.

The International Prostate Symptoms Score (IPSS) is a similar index that uses the same seven questions, plus a *quality of life* question or "bother score." It asks simply: *If you were to spend the rest of your life with your urinary condition just the way it is now, how would you feel about it?* Possible responses range from delighted to terrible on a zero-to-six-point scale. The question is about the closest urologists get to being "touchy-feely," and its severity helps the urologist decide whether to recommend therapy.

The American Urological Association (AUA) Symptom Index for BPH

AUA BPH Symptom Score						
	Not at all	**Less than 1 time in 5**	**Less than half the time**	**About half the time**	**More than half the time**	**Almost always**
1. Over the past month, how often have you had a sensation of not emptying your bladder completely after you finished urinating	0	1	2	3	4	5
2. Over the past month, how often have you had to urinate again less than two hours after you finished urinating?	0	1	2	3	4	5
3. Over the past month, how often have you found you stopped and started again several times when you urinated?	0	1	2	3	4	5
4. Over the past month, how often have you found it difficult to postpone urination?	0	1	2	3	4	5
5. Over the past month, how often have you had a weak urinary stream?	0	1	2	3	4	5
6. Over the past month, how often have you had to push or strain to begin urination?	0	1	2	3	4	5

	None	**1 time**	**2 times**	**3 times**	**4 times**	**5 or more times**
7. Over the past month, how many times did you most typically get up to urinate from the time you went to bed at night until the time you got up in the morning?	0	1	2	3	4	5
					Total Symptom Score	**=**

Printed with permission of the American Urological Association and the Journal of Urology.

TESTING FOR BPH: UROFLOWMETRY

Recall that men and their physicians are tempted to blame any symptoms below the collarbone on the prostate. If they avoid the temptation to blame problems on prostatitis, they will often attribute pain or urinary difficulty to an "enlarged prostate" or BPH. They will often be right, because of the frequency of prostatic obstruction, but not always. However, since a diagnosis isn't always straightforward, testing is sometimes needed.

Effective emptying is different from *efficient*. The former indicates the bladder empties completely, whereas the latter indicates how well it does so. A bladder that empties slowly but completely is effective but not efficient. A bladder that shoots urine out quickly but still contains half its volume when voiding stops is efficient but not effective.

Urine flow rate (efficiency) can be easily measured by voiding into a funnel-shaped flowmeter (**uroflowmetry**) that quantifies the volume released per second. This allows the urologist to tell if the bladder empties efficiently.

The uroflowmeter should normally show a peak as the stream hits its maximum flow during the first few seconds. Flow should remain almost as strong and steady until the bladder is almost empty, when the flow should decrease to a trickle. Some patients can force out a little squirt at the end as indicated.

A low flow indicates inefficient voiding. This is most often due to **obstruction** or blockage. A sawtooth pattern as shown in the tracing suggests obstruction is the culprit, caused by the patient's straining to push out spurts of urine. However, a weak bladder muscle that is incapable of pushing hard enough to generate adequate pressure can also give the same slow flow.

Telling whether poor flow is due to obstruction or a weak bladder muscle can be difficult through uroflowmetry, so the patient may require **urodynamics** (as discussed below). The advantage of uroflowmetry is that it is noninvasive and a simple test to perform, so it serves as an excellent screen. If the test is normal the patient usually has minimal difficulty from either obstruction or bladder weakness (*atony*). If it is abnormal and doubt of the cause remains, urodynamics may be the next step.

RESIDUAL VOLUME MEASUREMENT: THE BLADDER SCAN

Ineffective or incomplete bladder emptying leads to a number of problems. The first may be **frequency** because the bladder is already half full when the

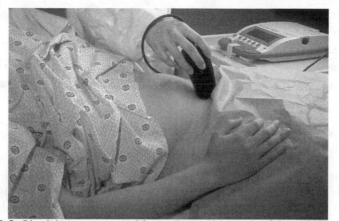

Figure 7-2. Bladder scan machine allows the urologist to determine how much urine remains in the bladder after voiding without placing a catheter. (Courtesy of Bladder Scan™)

patient leaves the restroom. A quick return trip is likely if you start out that way. Infection can result if the bladder doesn't receive a fresh flushing to remove occasional bacteria that enter; if bacteria are given enough time to grow they may replicate and eventually lead to a clinical infection. Bladder stones can form from stasis. This is similar to salt or sugar building up inside a container that isn't stirred adequately.

For these reasons it is helpful to measure the amount of urine remaining in the bladder after voiding. This is called the **postvoid residual volume**, and is often measured by a noninvasive ultrasound probe placed onto the lower abdominal wall. Therefore, it is also often referred to as the **ultrasound residual volume** (USRV).

A simple method to measure USRV is called a **bladder scan**. A small machine that reads the amount of residual urine automatically is placed over the bladder (as shown in figure 7-2). This machine will kick out a tracing in seconds, which allows the urologist to determine if the amount of residual volume is acceptable. It can be followed over time to determine the success of therapy or progression of the disease.

***

Recall that Ron had an USRV (the amount remaining in his bladder after voiding) of almost 500 cc. In medicine we use cc from the metric system, but most Americans think in terms of ounces, quarts, etc. Think of a two liter soda or a one

liter water bottle. Ron's USRV was almost half the latter, or about a pint. That is
pretty full, considering it was the volume remaining after he emptied.
    He wasn't convinced. "Are you sure?"
    I reassured him of my suspicion and recommended uroflowmetry to lend
supporting evidence. His voiding pattern revealed a classic case of obstruction.

URODYNAMICS

Urodynamic testing is the gold standard assessment of urinary function. It
may give the final answer if the diagnosis remains in doubt following the less
invasive testing discussed above. Although it requires catheterization, it is
generally well tolerated and very useful if indicated. Most men with prostate
problems will not need such testing, since the diagnosis can usually be rea-
sonably established through assessment of the symptoms.

    Most urodynamic testing is performed in specialized urodynamic cen-
ters, which may be in a urology office or the hospital. Trained urodynamic
nurses usually perform the procedure.

    Upon arriving at the office or urodynamic center, the nurse will ask you
to change into a gown, and ask you to provide a urine sample to rule out
infection. She may give you an antibiotic to prevent infection. You will initially empty your bladder so the **residual volume** can be measured. A
catheter will then be placed through the urethra into the bladder, and another
will be placed into the rectum. Pressure in the bladder can be differentiated
from the pressure applied in squeezing the abdomen by subtracting bladder
from rectal measurements. This difference is called the *detrusor pressure*,
and indicates the bladder's contraction.

    Next the bladder is filled. When the volume and pressure give you the
first sensation of filling, the amounts are noted. As capacity is approached,
measurements are taken to indicate either a contraction or an abnormality in
its ability to stretch, called *compliance*. The total volume is measured when
you say you are so full you can stand no more.

    At that point you will be asked to void. The pressure generated inside the
bladder will then be measured, along with flow and completeness of emptying. A low flow despite high pressure indicates that obstruction is the
problem; whereas a low flow with a low pressure indicates the bladder is too
weak to push hard enough. A combination of the two is possible, especially
in the late stages of obstruction, when long-standing overworking has weakened the bladder muscle.

Some urodynamic studies are performed using x-ray *fluoroscopic* monitoring. This is often unnecessary but is helpful if there is a concern of an open bladder neck or some other abnormalities. If x-rays are used, a lead shielded room is required.

Patients understandably want to avoid discomfort, so some will request that the studies be performed under anesthesia. This is inappropriate, as the study is meant to replicate the symptoms. Therefore, you must be awake throughout the study. The good news is that the test performed by professionals usually entails minimal discomfort.

TIME TO TREAT

Ron had asked if I was sure. I couldn't be absolutely but was very close to it. With no history of diabetes or other neurological conditions that would cause his bladder to malfunction, there were few other possibilities. The only other condition even remotely likely would be a urethral stricture—scar tissue constricting urinary flow. Cystoscopy would confirm its absence, but with no history of catheterization or other instrumentation of the urethra, he simply had no reason to have one.

I was sure enough to convince him that the only other information we could obtain would involve invasive testing that I didn't feel was necessary. It was time to consider treatment.

KEY POINTS

- Symptoms due to an obstructing prostate may be irritative (nocturia, urgency, frequency) or obstructive (hesitancy, slow stream, intermittency). The presence of either suggests the possibility of BPH and warrants consideration of the diagnosis.
- Whether any given man experiences irritative or obstructive symptoms is variable and unpredictable. Obstructive symptoms are suggestive of obstruction (obviously), but irritative symptoms in men often result from obstruction as well. The latter are less classic and might warrant testing prior to treatment if the diagnosis is substantially in doubt.
- There are several terms to describe prostatic obstructive symptoms including BPH, LUTS, prostatism, and bladder outlet obstruction (BOO). They usually mean the same thing.

- Size matters when considering prostatic symptoms, but it isn't every-thing. I agree with Dr. Ulchaker. We don't care how big your doughnut is—we care how big your doughnut hole is. If the hole is too small for adequate passage, you will experience problems.
- The harmful aspect of such conditions is obstruction. Partial obstruc-tion can lead to bladder damage and stones, infections, hydronephrosis, and kidney damage.
- Response to medications can essentially confirm the diagnosis. If in doubt, then uroflowmetry, residual volume measurement, cystoscopy, or urodynamics can clarify the diagnosis. These tests are also some-times used prior to therapy.

8.

TREATING BPH

Since I came to the White House I got two hearing aids, a colon operation, skin cancer, a prostate operation and I was shot. The damn thing is, I've never felt better in my life
— President Ronald Reagan, 1987

Two questions arise when a man experiences prostate symptoms. The first is whether the symptoms are serious and require treatment. Since most are not, the second question is whether they bother him enough to justify treatment. If the answer to either question is yes, this chapter describes the options involved when choosing management.

WATCHFUL WAITING: THE SIMPLEST APPROACH

Unless obstruction is so severe that urinary retention develops or kidney failure is likely, most men can choose whether to treat or not. If the bladder empties adequately and kidney function is normal, nothing has to be done. Therefore, the simplest option is **watchful waiting**. In other words, it is acceptable simply to wait to see whether symptoms bother you enough to be worth treating. Once reassured their symptoms are not serious, many men will be willing to put up with the nuisance. This avoids the cost, effort, and possible side effects of medications or surgery.

When I find a man's symptoms are bothersome but not harmful, I explain that medications will probably relieve their condition but are not absolutely necessary. Those willing to wait may rest assured of the benign nature of the condition, and that they may return to reassess the situation either if things worsen or on a yearly basis. They can change their minds at any point if their symptoms make them feel like it is worth undergoing treatments as described below.

BEHAVIORAL CHANGES

Men with prostate symptoms can achieve some improvement through some simple measures. Limiting fluids lessens urinary frequency in most men. However, such limitation may become so drastic that urine becomes concentrated enough to irritate the bladder. Therefore, simply drinking a normal amount of fluid is appropriate.

Unfortunately, there is no such thing as a *normal* fluid intake. The guidelines you hear about eight glasses of water a day are fictitious. Someone somewhere came up with that amount arbitrarily, and like lemmings, many doctors and patients have followed the recommendations ever since. This amount might be normal for you, but it also might not. It could be too much if you are eighty pounds and have kidney problems, or too little if you work in the hot outdoors and sweat profusely all day.

Since there is no universal definition of normal fluid intake, a better guideline would be to listen to your body. Drink when you are thirsty. Drink more if you are physically active to prevent dehydration. Drink more if your urine becomes visibly concentrated and dark yellow (although be aware that vitamins or other substances such as beets can artificially color the urine, misleading you to believe that the urine is concentrated).

What you drink (and eat) makes a difference, but perhaps not as much as believed. Every urology office has a list of substances you should avoid if you have prostate or bladder problems. Most contain acidic foods such as citrus and tomatoes. Most contain spicy foods and alcohol. All are mostly made up!

As it turns out, the only substance that we know is unequivocally related to bladder irritation is caffeine. It releases calcium into muscle cells, causing their contraction. Since a bladder contraction is the source of most **irritative** bladder symptoms, caffeine can be a culprit. Sitting at the coffee shop all day won't likely kill you, but may keep you running to the restroom.

Despite this, occasionally people find that one or more of the other items commonly listed as "bladder irritants" actually seems to be just that for them.

My advice is to listen to your body. If something you eat or drink seems to bother you, it is reasonable to avoid it. However, unless you are the rare person who can tell a definite difference in urinary symptoms with intake of substance other than caffeine, you can disregard lists of "bladder irritants."

TREATING BPH: ALPHA BLOCKERS

If symptoms bother you enough to treat, the most effective option for obstruction involves a class of drugs called **alpha blockers.** Their effectiveness comes from the fact there are chemical *alpha receptors* in the prostate and bladder neck that cause contraction or narrowing. Blocking them with the drugs listed below allows the bladder neck and prostate to relax, creating an easier egress for urinary flow.

Patients often try to bargain when we discuss caffeine intake. "How much can I drink?" is the usual line. I tell them that caffeine is not bad, nor is there a specific dose that causes problems. It is just that caffeine will stimulate bladder contraction. If you drink it and it doesn't bother you, there is no urological limit. If it bothers you, the more you drink, the more you will be bothered.

I also tell them that I probably drink more caffeine than they do (a cup of hot Irish breakfast tea is currently at my side). The difference is that they are in my office complaining of their prostate and bladder—I'm not in their office complaining of mine. Therefore, sometimes it is a matter of choice. You may choose to run to the restroom more often in order to enjoy your caffeine.

The effect of alpha blockers was first recognized in the eighties. Men who took such drugs—designed to relax muscular walls of blood vessels to lower blood pressure—found their prostatic symptoms were also relieved. Investigation found this was due to relaxation of similar muscles in the bladder neck and prostate. We know that 80 to 90 percent of men—who previously would have had surgery as their only option—responded and tolerated the medications well.[1]

Side effects are relatively uncommon with alpha blockers. Because the nonselective ones (*prazosin,* **terazosin,** and doxazosin) also lower blood pressure, they can occasionally cause dizziness or lightheadedness. This is very uncommon, and usually occurs only during the first few days of taking it as the body becomes accustomed. Thereafter, most men will feel normal. Essentially all medications known to man have been reported to cause tiredness, headache, upset stomach, or similar nonspecific side effects on occasion, but these are fairly uncommon with these medications and usually resolve.[2]

One occasionally annoying side effect is called *retrograde ejaculation*. This occurs when semen gets lost on the way out and turns into the bladder instead of coming out the urethra. Some alpha blockers cause this by relaxing the bladder neck. Since fluid will follow the route of least resistance, it simply runs into the bladder and is expelled on the next void. Unless the patient wishes to father children, this should not this be cause for concern. If he does, he will need reproductive assistance from an infertility specialist. As a result of a **transurethral resection of the prostate (TURP)** operation (as discussed later in this chapter), the opening from the prostate into the bladder is enlarged. This also results in retrograde ejaculation. Regardless of the cause, these men can still enjoy a normal orgasm (the pleasurable feeling), they just don't have emission of semen, or ejaculation. Fortunately, most are beyond the age when childbearing is desired. Retrograde ejaculation is uncommon with nonselective alpha blockers, including *afulzosin*. It is most common with *tamsulosin* because it exerts essentially all its effects on the bladder neck and prostate. Such strong relaxation will inevitably cause about 5 percent of men to experience such symptoms. Unless trying to father children, most men note it as a simple curiosity. However, in men attempting paternity or in some men who simply don't like the absence of semen for personal reasons, a switch in the doctor's prescription to *afulzosin* will often correct the situation.

OPTIONS FOR ALPHA BLOCKADE

Early versions of these medications were actually developed to treat high blood pressure. Their effects on either blood *press*ure or the *card*iovascular system are evident in a couple of their brand names—Mini*press* (e.g., "pressure") and *Card*ura (e.g., cardiovascular). These drugs block alpha receptors throughout the body, so are called *nonselective*. (Receptors are sites on cells that are stimulated by chemicals to create an action, such as constrict a blood vessel or the urinary tract.) All have some effect on the cardiovascular system, although the newest options (afulzosin and tamsulosin) are more specific to the urinary tract because they exert most of their effect on the specific receptors located there. They are marketed with brand names designed to indicate this *uro*selectivity—*Uro*xatrol and *Flo*max.

Typical Doses of Alpha Blockers Used to Treat LUTS	
Name	**Common Dose**
Prazosin (Minipress)	2 mg twice daily (used uncommonly)
Terazosin (Hytrin)	5 or 10 mg daily
Doxazosin (Cardura)	4 or 8 mg daily
Afulzosin (Uroxatrol)	10 mg daily
Tamsulosin (Flomax)	0.4 mg daily

HOW TO TAKE ALPHA BLOCKERS

Because alpha blockers lower blood pressure, they have the possible side effect of lightheadedness, so doctors generally recommend taking them at bedtime. The logic is that the time when blood pressure is lowest will be the time you are flat in bed.

This theory originated in a most unscientific way. A research nurse apparently noticed that some of her patients during the early studies became dizzy. She suggested they take the pills before bedtime, when they indeed stopped experiencing lightheadedness. The tricky part is that this also occurred with subsequent doses; lightheadedness usually occurs only following the first or second dose. Therefore, most of these men would have had no further side effects with subsequent doses anyway. However, this piece of *uromythology* still drives our prescribing habits and may never go away.

More logical is to address the so-called first-dose effect by starting nonselective prazosin, terazosin, and doxazosin with smaller doses. If a doctor gives only 1 to 2 mg of each for a few days, most patients will adapt without lightheadedness.

During the nineties the companies that make terazosin and doxazosin supplied doctors with sample "starter packs" that had smaller doses for the first few days, building up to effective doses. This helped the doctor avoid writing prescriptions for several different doses and allowed patients to reach effective levels before they paid for a prescription. These became unavailable when patent protection expired and generic competition arrived. As a result, one of the primary obstacles to using these nonselective drugs is the complexity of the first few doses.

Note from the table above that all of the medications except terazosin and doxazocin come in a single strength. Although most men need the 10 mg strength of terazosin, the 4 mg strength of doxazosin is adequate for most

One memorable patient disregarded my instructions to start his doxazosin cautiously. I told him that as an elderly man, he should hang out around the house for the first couple days in case he became dizzy.

He skipped the starting doses and took 8 mg the first night. This presented no problem until the following afternoon, when his wife heard him yell for help. A quick look around the house left her clueless of his location. She ran outside to find him clinging to the center of the roof with both hands. After climbing the ladder to do some repairs, he had become so dizzy he could not return.

The fire department rescued him like the proverbial cat, unharmed, using their truck with a swinging basket. When his wife called, I asked to speak to him to determine what had led to this fiasco.

"You told me to hang out around the house," he explained.

people. Many physicians prescribe the 8 mg tablet of doxazocin and suggest that their patients cut the pills in half in order to keep down the costs. If half a tablet is not strong enough, the patient can simply take the entire pill.

Similar milligram doses don't mean the same thing for different medications. Therefore, don't feel that a 4 mg dose of one medication will necessarily be less strong than 10 mg of another. They are different chemicals, so the numbers don't correlate when comparing drugs. *Always* be certain to discuss medications with your physician prior to taking them. Also keep him aware of your progress or problems related to the drugs.

TWO BIRDS WITH ONE STONE

Jonathan had taken high blood pressure medications for almost twenty years before I saw him for BPH. The diagnosis was straightforward—he had a slow stream, hesitancy, and dribbling that had been getting worse throughout his sixth decade. He rarely got a full night of sleep. A USRV revealed that his bladder emptied only about halfway. Over 200 cc remained after he urinated. Watchful waiting seemed inadequate.

When I checked his medication list for potential drug interactions I noticed the blood pressure medication. He took a drug called a beta blocker, which lowered blood pressure by blocking the other (nonalpha) receptors in blood vessels. It had done a decent job of controlling his hypertension, although the dose had recently been adjusted upward and his pressure was still on the borderline of being high. In addition, he recognized it made him tired and seemed to inhibit erections so had begun using Viagra.

Although I usually use a selective alpha blocker to treat LUTS, I suggested switching from his beta blocker to a nonselective alpha blocker in order to kill two birds with one stone. I felt doxazosin or terazosin would treat both problems with one pill, avoiding the cost, side effects, and nuisance of being on two separate medications.

"I don't want to take anything stronger for my blood pressure," Jonathan protested. "This one makes me feel poorly enough." He didn't mention erections, although I knew from earlier conversations what was on his mind.

*** *** ***

Since alpha blockers were initially developed for treatment of high blood pressure, they offer a particularly appealing combination for men with both hypertension and BPH. We know that they cause only insignificant changes in blood pressure in men without hypertension, but can normalize blood pressure in those with hypertension.[3] In other words, they simply bring blood pressure to normal in most men, rarely causing it to go below normal.

If the combination effect is desired, your physician would likely opt for a nonselective alpha blocker such as prazosin, terazosin, or doxazocin. The others work specifically on the lower urinary tract, so they will not adequately treat blood pressure.

Afulzosin is an anomaly because it is technically not specific to the urinary tract. However, it appears to have minimal effect on blood pressure so it cannot treat hypertension. This also minimizes side effects.

In addition to the ability to treat both hypertension and LUTS, there is some suggestion that the uroselective options afulzosin and tamsulosin may actually have a positive impact on erections. It is unclear whether this is simply because men feel better once their LUTS are improved, or whether there is a direct effect on erections. Regardless, I have had a few patients who have reported anecdotal improvement in their sex lives when taking these medications.

*** *** ***

I talked Jonathan into trying doxazocin because it does a good job at managing blood pressure. He broke an 8 mg tablet in half, and then divided each half similarly, in order to get his first four days' dosage. Instead of dizziness, he actually felt better by the third day. His strength was better and he found that erections were a little better once the beta blocker was out of his system.

By the second week he was on 4 mg of doxazosin and his urinary symptoms were essentially gone. However, when I checked his blood pressure the following week, it was still borderline. I discussed it with his internist, who agreed that 8 mg was a good idea. The last time I saw Jonathan his blood pressure was perfect, his urinary symptoms were a memory, and he had not needed Viagra in the past year!

SHRINKING THE PROSTATE: 5-ALPHA REDUCTASE INHIBITORS

Alpha blockers are the mainstay of therapy for BPH, but they only treat symptoms. As a result, a class of drugs called **5-alpha reductase inhibitors** has been developed that actually reverses prostate enlargement.

Eunuchs and men who are born without testosterone (because of any number of birth abnormalities) do not develop BPH. This observation led to successful treatment of BPH using surgical or chemical castration. After six months, the prostate will shrink by about one-third, relieving urinary obstruction in many men. The only problem is that few men would be willing to accept castration for BPH.

A second observation was that men who have a genetic defect making them unable to convert testosterone to its active form, dihydrotestosterone (DHT), are also immune to the development of BPH. This led to efforts to block this conversion, resulting in the development of **finasteride**. Within six months the same effect on prostate volume could be expected.

Unfortunately, the effect on urinary symptoms has been less reliable. With further experience we now know that many men who fail to respond to finasteride actually have normal-size prostates to begin with. In retrospect, they would not be expected to have improvement in urinary symptoms when their problem is actually not an enlarged prostate. The men with smaller prostates usually simply have too much contraction based on their alpha receptors, so it is not surprising that they respond better to alpha blockers.[4]

In addition, finasteride lowers PSA by about 50 percent, so this should be adjusted in your mind if taking the drug. In other words, if you take finasteride or **dutasteride** (see below) you should double your measured PSA to determine what its "real" value is. A PSA of 2.2 ng/dl in a man on these medications is really a PSA of 4.4 ng/dl, so beware and make sure your doctor recognizes this.[5]

OTHER BENEFITS

Finasteride reduces the chance that a man with BPH will eventually require surgery from 10 to 5 percent. Whether this is worth taking a pill for years is controversial. In addition, 5-alpha reductase inhibitors can shrink enlarged prostate tissue that is causing hematuria (blood in the urine). Several months' administration can stop this frightening symptom. The *Prostate Cancer Prevention Trial* also showed that men who take finasteride have a lower chance of being diagnosed with prostate cancer. Finally, one side effect of finasteride is actually good for most men. It causes hair growth, and is actually prescribed in the smaller (1 mg) dose for treatment of baldness. This form of the exact same drug is marketed as *Propecia*.

DUTASTERIDE: BLOCKING TWO RECEPTORS

The newest 5-alpha reductase inhibitor is *dutasteride* (*Avodart*). Its selling point is that it blocks both *type one* and *type two* 5-alpha reductase receptors. The logic is that blocking both receptors should be more effective, though it remains theoretical at this point until studies elucidate if there is a difference in dutasteride and finasteride. Several in progress will determine their relative roles and the impact of dutasteride on prostate cancer prevention.

WHICH IS BETTER: ALPHA BLOCKERS OR 5-ALPHA REDUCTASE INHIBITORS?

Determining "better" is often complex, but we can establish some differences. Alpha blockers work almost immediately and are successful in a vast majority of patients. These benefits make them the first line of therapy most of the time.

Men with large prostates, typically greater than forty grams, benefit more from 5-alpha reductase inhibitors. Certainly of the size requires a transrectal ultrasound measurement or other imaging study, although DRE can detect an obviously huge gland that is a good candidate for their use. Some physicians will use them as first-line therapy in such patients. In addition, the risk of side effects with 5-alpha reductase inhibitors is very low. The most significant are retrograde ejaculation, impotence, or a decreased libido, all of which happen in less than 5 percent of patients.[6]

To summarize, alpha blockers will be the mainstay of therapy for most men. Those with very large prostates who cannot take alpha blockers are candidates for 5-alpha reductase inhibitors. In addition, men who wish to reduce their risk of disease progression and surgical intervention may choose to take them as well after conferring with their physicians. Finally men with hematuria caused by BPH may find relief using the latter.[7]

WHAT ABOUT TAKING BOTH?

It is appealing to use the combination of alpha blockers and 5-alpha reductase inhibitors to both *relax* and *shrink* the prostate in an effort to avoid surgery for men with severe LUTS. However, some studies have suggested that combination therapy may only add cost, not benefit. This has changed recently with publication of an analysis called Medical Therapy of Prostate Symptoms (MTOPS).[8] This large study contradicted earlier reports and showed that two drugs (one alpha blocker and one 5-alpha reductase inhibitor) might be better than one. Men who added a 5-alpha reductase inhibitor had a lower risk of urinary retention and were half as likely to eventually require surgery.

It can be difficult to decide whether the cost and possible side effects of the second pill are enough to justify taking it for years, knowing that there is a 90 percent chance you will not need surgery anyway. For many men, the decision may be influenced by how well you tolerate them as well as your insurance coverage.

COMPLEMENTARY MEDICINE

A billion-dollar industry offers promise to men with LUTS—a promise to take your billion dollars. After decades of men taking stinging nettle, pygeum, zinc, and other supplements, we still have no proof they are worth it. Despite these concerns, more than one-third of urology patients may be using complementary medicine supplements for prostate cancer and BPH.[9]

Some studies have shown effectiveness for a number of natural products. However, just as many studies have failed to do so. Most that have shown benefit are poorly designed, so their positive results are questionable. Other studies show that the actual dosage of the purported ingredients is unpredictable, so men usually have no idea if they are even taking what they believe they are. Therefore, many who sense improvement may primarily experience a *placebo* effect. Moreover, the quality of these agents may vary from batch to batch since there is no regulatory quality control.

Please do not interpret the above to mean that there is no effect of these agents. The point is that without proof of their effectiveness despite a long history of observation, the effect must be questioned. Without rigorous double-blind testing (in which neither the tester nor the subject know if the agent is real or a placebo), we cannot judge their efficacy. Compared to the proven benefit of prescription medications, it is difficult to advise people to spend money on supplements when we know of neither their effect nor potential risks.

The Complementary and Alternative Medicine for Urological Symptoms (CAMUS) study is a three-thousand-patient trial taking place that compares placebo to the most commonly used alternative options—saw palmetto and *Pygeum africanum*. Its results will be eagerly anticipated.

MINIMALLY INVASIVE TREATMENT OF LUTS

The lack of a lavatory in the cockpit never bothered Brian during his two decades as a navy pilot. Even on long flights, he knew that a trip to the restroom before takeoff was enough to get him through the flight. However, in his final years of military service he noticed that he began avoiding coffee to make the end of each trip more comfortable.

After retiring from the military he accepted a job with a major airline flying out of Cleveland. After five years, his seniority enabled him to fly the long-distance routes he most coveted.

Over the North Atlantic one evening he noticed urgency, *but turbulence necessitated he remain at the helm for longer than he wished. He trusted the copilot implicitly, but his sense of responsibility was stronger than his sense of urgency. He remained in his seat until they cleared the area. An adrenaline rush had blocked the urge, but when that abated, he had to make a mad dash to the restroom. The movie had just ended, so a passenger was already occupying each of the first-class lavatories. He thought he was about to pop.*

When he finally found an open lavatory, he unzipped his pants and prepared for relief. Nothing happened. He stood for several minutes but simply could not void. He turned on the water in the sink to stimulate his bladder, but the faucet turned off automatically after a few unsuccessful seconds. Nothing helped.

It became clear that his bladder was not going to empty. Panic set in. Fortunately, an intercom request for a doctor identified an internist in seat 16C. The doctor searched the airplane's emergency kit and found a catheter and lubrication. An airborne clinic was set up in the galley (thank goodness for those curtains), and the floor became a medical table. Relief was at hand as the catheter slipped in easily. The copilot handled the landing duties into Heathrow, and Brian was off to a hospital.

A review of events revealed that Brian had taken an over-the-counter allergy medication prior to flying the night before. The urologist educated him that the fine-print warning for men with prostate troubles was intended to prevent this occurrence. As soon as it was out of his system he would probably return to normal.

*When Brian returned home he came to my office to have his catheter removed. My assistant filled his bladder with sterile water and took the catheter out. He voided into a **uroflowmetry** machine, emptying the entire amount that she had placed. He said it was consistent with his normal voiding pattern. The flow pattern was slow and suggested that normal for him was actually not normal. It was clear that obstruction had been present for years—allergy medication had simply been the final blow.*

As a forty-eight-year-old man, Brian almost certainly would live long enough to experience urinary retention again, so my goal was not only to improve symptoms, but also to prevent a similar incident in the future. We discussed options and I recommended doxazocin because his blood pressure was borderline high. I warned him about lightheadedness and suggested he begin therapy during an upcoming week when he was not scheduled to fly.

Two hours after Brian took his first dose—a low starting dose—he stood up quickly and fell back into his chair. This happened several times, until he learned to arise slowly. He was convinced that the "first-dose effect" would recede. He noted a significant improvement in urinary symptoms but three days later remained dizzy. Flights were scheduled in a few days and this would not do.

Brian called on the fourth day to see if I had any suggestions. I did—stop taking doxazocin. It was a great drug and relieved his symptoms and his hypertension completely, but as a pilot, he could not take the chance of being dizzy on the job. I switched him to tamsulosin because of its very low risk of dizziness. He would have to deal with the blood pressure separately, but this drug would most likely relieve urinary symptoms with minimal risk.

Two days later Brian called again, frustrated. Urinary symptoms remained in check, but he had two other side effects. Whereas new onset headaches would be simply a nuisance for most people, for Brian they meant an inability to fly and earn a living. Moreover, retrograde ejaculation became an issue until I reassured him this was not a problem unless he wanted to become a father, which he did not. However, the headaches were not acceptable so I offered a final attempt to treat with alpha blockade using afulzosin, but he was done.

"Is there another option?" he asked. We discussed 5-alpha reductase inhibitors, but he was tired of playing musical prescriptions.

"Let's talk about surgery."

***

With a majority of men eventually developing BPH it is predictable that physicians and the industry have developed a number of interventions aimed at relieving obstruction with minimal side effects. The process began in the early twentieth century, when the only option was to open the patient through an abdominal incision and cut out the obstructing tissue found in the middle of the prostate—the central zone. This larger channel allowed urine to pass freely but was a major operation associated with bleeding and prolonged recovery. Doctors began using scopes placed through the urethra that would scrape out "chips" of prostatic tissue until the opening was adequate. This became known as a **TransUrethral Resection of Prostate,** or **TURP**. It avoided an abdominal operation and quickly became the first "minimally invasive" option for treatment of urological diseases.

TURP remained the gold standard for treatment of LUTS until the late twentieth century when an explosion of challengers arose. Medications allowed most patients to avoid surgery. Even if medications didn't work, a number of less invasive options were developed.

TUNA

Radiofrequency energy can be placed into prostate tissue using fine wires in an office-based procedure called *TransUretral Needle Ablation* or *TUNA*. Its appeal is based on the ability to apply this energy in the office setting.

A special cystoscope is placed into the urethra, which allows the urologist to put small needles into the prostatic tissue under direct vision. A special electrical generator is turned on. Over a few minutes, an area of approximately one centimeter is burned into the prostate. This may be repeated several times for larger prostates in order to remove enough tissue to void better. A sedative or local anesthetic helps make it tolerable in the office.

Symptom improvement of more than 50 percent is expected.[10] However, temporary urinary retention and/or **irritative** voiding symptoms occur in 10 to 40 percent of cases. Between 12 and 14 percent of patients require further surgery or repeat treatment within two years. To date, there are no adequate long-term studies to indicate if the effect lasts beyond that. As a result of potentially lower success rates and the development of other technologies, a minority of urologists routinely employs TUNA.

MICROWAVE THERAPY

A catheter similar to the one used for bladder drainage can be equipped with a microwave tip that heats the prostate to 42–44° C (108–111° F). This heat treatment is called **TransUrethral Microwave Therapy (TUMT)**. A balloon holds the heat generator in place at the bladder neck and directional microwaves heat the prostate for thirty to sixty minutes. Most men will experience enough swelling that a catheter is required for a week or longer.

TUMT relieves LUTS in some men, although the exact percentage that responds to it has been a cause of controversy. Some studies suggest success occurs in a majority of patients, while others find equal success from sham (fake) surgery, even if the machine is not even turned on. Others show that placement of a nonmicrowave catheter for an hour gives improvement in symptom scores equal to that of TUMT after three months. This suggests the placebo effect is strong for urinary symptoms.[11]

Although the mechanism of action is not completely understood, it may be that this temperature is enough to damage the nerves causing prostatic contraction, but not hot enough to actually shrink or damage the prostate. As a result, many urologists believe TUMT is simply a minimally invasive way to block alpha nerves in the prostate and bladder neck in a manner similar to giving alpha blocker medications. This has led some to advocate TUMT as a temporary alpha blockade that allows men to avoid medications instead of a replacement for surgical therapy. The long-term effectiveness and significant cost of TUMT should be considered regarding this approach.

My personal observation with TUMT is that most men are better for awhile, but most will not experience prolonged symptom relief and are likely to undergo other forms of therapy within two to three years. This experience has led many urologists to abandon microwave therapy. However, to be fair,

I have urologist friends who have had great success with the procedure and continue to advocate it for their patients. Therefore, the jury remains out on the role of TUMT.

LASERS

"Can't you use a laser?" Brian asked one of the most common questions I hear when I proposed surgical correction of BPH.

***

Patients love lasers. They sound cool, new, space-agey, and cutting edge. For certain applications they are all these things, while for BPH they have had mixed results. I was chairman of a hospital institutional laser committee in the nineties as multiple laser machines were released for treatment of BPH. We reviewed too many to count. The original ones used laser energy that simply penetrated deep into tissue and caused its death, leading to a larger channel through the prostate after a period of sloughing. Subsequent versions used laser energy applied directly into or onto the prostate in order to create a more immediate opening. Acronyms such as TULIP (TransUrethral Laser Incision Prostate), VLAP (Visual Laser Ablation Prostate), ILC (Interstitial Laser COagulation), and HoLAP (HOlmium Laser Ablation Prostate) dominated the scene. The first one is already gone, and many others have largely disappeared because of a combination of side effects, improvements in competition, and sometimes unreliable results. Three versions currently compete for first place in the race to be the preferred minimally invasive option for LUTS.[12]

The first is ILC, a laser fiber placed directly into the prostate through a cystoscope in a manner similar to TUNA. Its energy can cause cell death of small areas in the prostate, leading to enlargement of the channel and improved voiding within weeks. Swelling necessitates a catheter to drain the bladder for a few days similar to the protocol following TUMT and TUNA. A major appeal of these three options is that they may be performed in the office instead of the operating room. The disadvantage is that their results do not appear to be as marked or as prolonged as can be obtained when tissue is actually removed.[13]

These limitations led to development of laser applications that actually remove tissue instead of simply damaging it. HoLAP uses a laser to remove large areas of prostate tissue through a combination of vaporization (literally) and enucleation (removing a portion of the obstructing prostate). Enucleation is similar to cutting pieces of pie and removing it instead of forking out individual bites. Whichever method is used, a large defect in the prostate allows urine to flow through easier.

The latest generation of such lasers is called Photo Vaporization Prostate (PVP). Because of the color of its laser light, many physicians and patients call it the "green light laser." This laser indeed has a Buck Rogers allure to it since it specifically vaporizes the target (BPH tissue) but stops at the "surgical capsule," the part of the prostate that the surgeon would like to leave in place. This method is based on the absorption of its specific light wavelength in soft tissues such as the prostate. The tissue of the surgical capsule absorbs this wavelength light poorly because of blood flow characteristics, so the laser usually removes only the tissue that it should.

As a result of the above physics, the green light laser creates the desired open channel through the middle of the prostate with minimal risk of bleeding, incontinence, impotence, or other risks of TURP. Although these risks are very low, in medicine there is essentially no such thing as zero. Still, these risks appear low.

DISADVANTAGES OF LASER THERAPY

There are four main disadvantages to lasers. Most are slower than TURP as discussed below. This is least significant with ILC. All can create (usually) temporary **irritative** voiding symptoms as side effects, and may be more likely with ILC or VLAP (rarely used anymore). All have the risk that the laser energy penetrates deeper than it appears to the naked eye, potentially damaging deeper tissues (least with HoLAP or PVP). Finally, all are expensive.[14]

Expense has been an issue with all forms of minimally invasive therapy. Because TUMT, TUNA, and all lasers except HoLAP and PVP leave significant amounts of tissue in place, their long-term results appear limited. Therefore, these expensive technologies often require repeat treatments, sometimes on a serial basis. This is especially true in men with large prostates. This downside makes many urologists believe that a procedure that actually removes the problem and creates an adequate channel is more appropriate for most men, especially those with prolonged life expectancies.

TURP: THE GOLD STANDARD

We now return full circle to the original minimally invasive option for LUTS—**TransUrethral Resection of the Prostate** (**TURP**). It used to be the most common operation performed by urologists. Since surgery was the only successful treatment option, urologists used this method to help almost all men with such problems.

This all changed in the nineties. First we recognized the ability to treat most men with medications. About 90 percent of my patients can be adequately managed with a simple prescription. Thus, half of men who previously would have seen a urologist to consider surgery are treated by their primary care physicians.[15]

Next, the above-mentioned options arrived. Because this combination of new drugs and minimally invasive treatments, the frequency of TURP has dropped dramatically. In 1987 250,000 TURP procedures were performed in the United States. By 2000 that dropped to 88,000, and the trend appears to be continuing.[16] An ongoing discussion among urological educators shows concern that future urologists may not obtain adequate experience to learn this age-old operation.

Urologists nonetheless almost universally agree (a bold statement for us!) that the most effective treatment for the relief of BPH is the TURP. Using a special scope called a *resectoscope* (see figure 8-1), the urologist can create a wide-open channel through the area where BPH had previously caused obstruction (see figures 8-2 and 8-3). He usually leaves a catheter overnight to allow irrigation to clear minor bleeding, and most men will be able to void normally as soon as the catheter is removed. After a few weeks' recovery, the area usually heals completely and long-term relief is at hand.

WHY NOT A TURP FOR EVERYONE WITH BPH?

The primary disadvantage of TURP is that it requires spinal or general anesthesia, plus hospitalization, although usually only overnight. In addition, since it uses electrical energy it may be more likely to cause scarring, and may *rarely* cause permanent impotence or incontinence. Finally, it is possible to absorb enough irrigating fluid to cause dilution of the chemicals in the bloodstream. This is called *TUR syndrome* and is usually reversible, although occasionally it can be more serious. This can apparently be avoided by using newer resectoscopes (as described below in the section on TURIS).

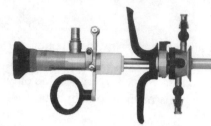

Figure 8-1. A resectoscope is an instrument that allows the urologist to remove the inner (central) portion of the prostate without an incision during a TURP. (Courtesy Olympus, USA)

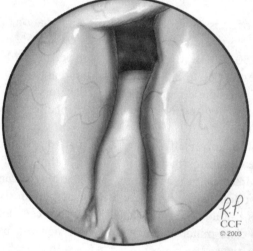

Figure 8-2. Prostatic urethra prior to TURP. Lateral lobes are encroaching on the channel, obstructing urine flow.

Figure 8-3. Prostatic urethra following TURP. Removal of inner central zone of the prostate opens an adequate channel for voiding.

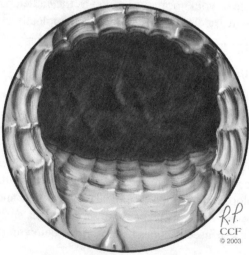

Studies disagree on the frequency with which BPH will recur following TURP, but my experience is that approximately 10 percent of men will eventually require repeat surgery if they live long enough. This is usually due to regrowth of BPH. Occasionally a patient will develop a **bladder neck contracture**, scar tissue that narrows the bladder neck. Reopening it with a simple incision usually does the trick.

A final concern with TURP is that some earlier reports suggested the risk of dying in the months following the procedure was higher in men who had TURP. This has been shown more recently to simply be related to other age-related diseases in these men, so we believe the operation poses no such risk.[17]

Despite the above relatively minor concerns, one fact is clear. TURP remains the *gold standard* treatment for BPH. Success rates range from 70 to 96 percent, with an average reported success rate of 88 percent, better than that for any of the less invasive options.[18] This may be challenged soon, however, as Photo Vaporization of Prostate (PVP) and newer lasers arrive.

TRANSURETHRAL RESECTION IN SALINE: TURIS

Recall that absorption of fluid used to irrigate during TURP can cause the *TUR syndrome*. In response, endoscopes have been developed that allow the urologist to resect in saline—a fluid with electrolyte content close to that of the body's natural fluids. Absorption of this fluid will therefore cause no serious problems. Even if massive amounts get into the bloodstream, the kidneys will normally flush the excess. This safety margin allows the urologist to resect larger glands that previously would have taken too long and risked too much fluid absorption.

I regard the TURIS as simply a modification or improvement of the TURP. The operation appears to be identical with the exception of decreased risk of TUR syndrome. Without this risk urologists can take their time and complete a good job even in very large glands.

The main disadvantage is that the scopes are more expensive. Hospitals that already have good scopes in place will be slow to replace them as long as they continue to do a good job. In addition, TURIS seems to take a little bit longer (usually a matter of minutes more) to perform.

TRANSURETHRAL *INCISION* OF PROSTATE: TUIP

An even less invasive version of TURP for men with small glands (probably less than forty grams as measured on transrectal ultrasound) involves simply making two incisions into the prostate through a scope. Cuts at the five and seven o'clock positions all the way through the prostate and its capsule allow the prostate and bladder neck to pop open (see figure 8-4). This can be performed in minutes. Moreover, appropriate candidates will respond almost as well as if they had undergone a full TURP resection.

The downside of TUIP is that it is appropriate mainly for men with small prostates or a rare condition known as **primary bladder neck obstruction**. In addition, data regarding long-term success are lacking. However, with success rates within 10 percent of those from the more aggressive TURP, TUIP will maintain a role in BPH care.[19]

OPEN PROSTATECTOMY

All the options discussed to this point have been minimally invasive, avoiding an open operation (using an incision). However, men with huge prostates (150–200 grams or larger) still sometimes require the oldest operation—open prostatectomy. This operation involves a lower abdominal incision similar to that used during radical retropubic prostatectomy. The prostatic capsule is

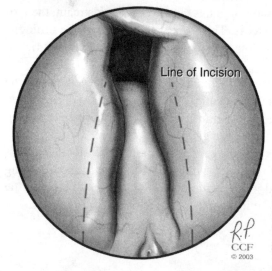

Line of Incision

Figure 8-4. TUIP involves incisions on each side of the prostate as shown, instead of resecting the entire central zone.

opened and the obstructing tissue physically removed. This provides the largest opening in the prostatic channel, but also the produces the most morbidity.

Few urologists continue to perform open prostatectomy because it is rarely needed. Many will perform a staged TURP instead, resecting as much tissue as they safely can from one side then returning a few days later to resect the remainder. The advent of TURIS may obviate the need for staging since the risk of TUR syndrome will be eliminated.

DEALING WITH COMPLICATIONS OF BPH TREATMENT

Incontinence and impotence are fortunately uncommon following BPH treatment. Management of these problems is discussed in chapter 20.

URINARY RETENTION

Urinary retention is a medical emergency. Kidney failure may be present or impending. This leaves no choice but to begin treatment immediately. The most common way to empty the completely obstructed bladder is by placement of a urinary catheter, often called a **Foley catheter**. This is a soft rubber tube, as shown in figure 8-5. It contains a large channel that drains urine into a bag. A smaller channel runs through the wall of the large one and allows injection of fluid through a syringe in order to fill a balloon at the other end. This setup assures the catheter remains securely in place until no longer needed—when a syringe can empty the balloon so it can be easily removed.

A permanent route for a Foley catheter can be surgically placed through the skin of the lower abdomen into the bladder if there is a problem with the urethra that limits its use for a catheter. Because of its location in the lower abdomen, it is then called a *suprapubic catheter*. This tube is reserved for rare permanent situations, and can be replaced by a nurse every month as long as needed.

The final and best method to drain the bladder actually involves **clean intermittent catheterization** (CIC). Instead of leaving a catheter in the urethra to constantly drain the bladder, the patient puts one in just long enough to empty the bladder and then removes it. He washes it off with soap and water and puts it back in his pocket (preferably in a zipped plastic bag). Each time his bladder is full he repeats the process.

CIC has been used only since 1971, when Dr. Jack Lapides of the University of Michigan reported its use in patients with uncorrectable bladder problems. Prior to that, urologists believed that each time a catheter was placed through the urethra it would push bacteria inside and risk infection. Dr. Lapides went in the face of urological conventional wisdom and came up with some surprising findings. Instead of an increase in urinary tract infections, his patients had *fewer* infections![20]

As it turns out, a Foley catheter remaining through the urethra serves as a nice conduit for bacteria. Cleansing, antibiotic ointments, silver coating, and many other maneuvers have been tried to stop this, but nothing keeps bacteria from entering along the catheter. Therefore, placing the catheter just long enough to empty the bladder may pull a few bacteria in, but not as many as would travel this bacterial autobahn if a catheter remained in place.

Perhaps even more surprising is the fact that the catheter is reusable and does not need to be sterile. Nonprofessionals can place the catheter with bare hands (after washing with soap and water) and do not need to use sterilizing solutions. This not only limits the cost, but also does not increase the risk of infection. This technique has led to markedly lower risk of infection and is now the *standard of care* for long-term bladder drainage.

Another advantage of CIC is that the patient has the discomfort of a catheter for only a few minutes a day, instead of twenty-four hours a day. The lifestyle advantage should be obvious, and becomes even more so at night when you can sleep without a catheter in place.

The main disadvantage is the preconception that you cannot do it. Men think self-catheterization will hurt or be too complex for them to do. Those convinced of this will probably be right. However, those willing to consider the possibility will usually be much better off than they would be if they had a catheter in them full time.

Another advantage exists for the man with temporary urinary retention, such as that following surgery. This situation will often resolve, but if a catheter is in place there is no way to know when it has resolved. You may end up having it in longer than needed. If performing CIC, then you simply stop doing it when you regain the ability to void spontaneously.

MEDICAL MANAGEMENT OF URINARY RETENTION

Although it sounds appealing simply to start medications when men develop urinary retention, it is often not successful. Most men will require surgery even if medications are prescribed.[21] Success is higher if something reversible

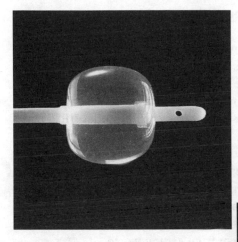

Figure 8-5. A catheter is a soft rubber tube with an inflatable balloon that drains the bladder. The balloon prevents its accidental dislodgement. (Courtesy of Cook Urological.)

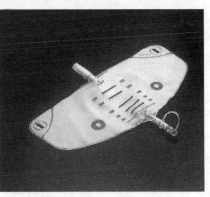

Figure 8-6. A leg bag attaches to the leg to collect urine from a catheter. (Courtesy of Cook Urological.)

caused urinary retention, such as cold medications, surgery, or temporary weakness from injury.

WHY DON'T SYMPTOMS ALWAYS GO AWAY WITH TREATMENT?

Recall from the discussion above that even in the best-case scenario, some men fail to respond to interventions including medications, minimally invasive procedures, or surgery. This may be because obstruction persists despite the simpler options. However, even if obstruction is conclusively removed during surgery, some men continue to experience symptoms.

This is not surprising since treatment is aimed at prostatic obstruction, which may not be the only source of symptoms. The bladder also plays a role. It may be weak and unable to push strongly enough to generate a good stream no matter how wide open the channel is. If the problem is severe enough despite surgery, you may not be able to void at all, requiring inter-mittent catheterization.

In addition, the bladder may be overactive leading to persistent **irritative** symptoms. Uninhibited contractions can cause **urgency, frequency, nocturia,** and even **incontinence**. These symptoms persist because any damage to the bladder is already done. Removing obstruction cannot change that.

Such bladder damage is the reason that you should not let BPH symptoms go too long, especially if you are developing severe irritative symptoms, or if the bladder doesn't empty completely. Doing so only risks further bladder damage. Think of the bladder as a piece of clothing. If overstretched for too long, it never returns to normal.

I tell men that irritative symptoms are not the reason to perform surgery. Arresting their progression is the reason. They may not get better, but at least we should usually be able to keep them from getting worse.

Irritative symptoms can be managed postoperatively by a group of medications called anticholinergics, such as Detrol LA or Ditropan XL. Newer medications recently released are Enablex, Vesicare, and Sanctura.

NEUROMODULATION

The final treatment for men with LUTS involves neuromodulation—electrical stimulation designed to affect urinary function. An electrical wire surgically placed into bladder nerves at the point where they exit the spine can bring their activity back to normal if it is either underactive or overactive. This paradoxical concept is poorly understood, but can restart some bladders that fail to empty even after prostate surgery. In addition, overactive bladders that contract too readily and fail to respond to anticholinergic medications can be regulated using this technology as well. Although it requires minor surgery to implant what is basically a pacemaker for the bladder, it is a major advance for complex cases.

LESS FAVORED OPTIONS

For purposes of completeness I will mention some alternatives that you may hear about. The International Consultation on BPH, held in July 2000, evaluated all alternatives and felt several were unacceptable for most patients. Balloon dilatation, hyperthermia, and high-intensity focused ultrasound were not judged of adequate value to be used as routine therapy. Injection of alcohol or botox were both too new to garner a stamp of approval, although both may be promising.

Prostatic stents, devices designed to pop open and hold obstructing lobes apart, were judged acceptable with restrictions. However, problems with these devices have prevented their widespread use either temporarily or long term. Work continues, so stents might become important at some point, but they are useful only rarely at present—typically only in men who are too ill to undergo a TURP.[22]

THE PILOT CHOOSES LASER SURGERY

Earlier, Brian found medications were not an acceptable option. Dizziness at thirty-seven thousand feet simply wouldn't fly. After discussing several options, he chose a PVP green light laser procedure. After tests to confirm he was a good candidate, I referred him to Dr. Ulchaker, who is internationally known for his work with BPH surgery. The procedure was performed as an outpatient in our ambulatory surgery center. After the procedure, he voided well in the recovery room and was discharged without a catheter.

After a week at home, he had a normal voiding pattern and was bored to tears. When the call came for an extra flight to the West Coast, he jumped at the chance. Just before landing at LAX he realized this was the farthest he had flown in years without a trip to the lavatory. He looked forward to an in-flight cup of coffee on his flight home.

KEY POINTS

- Men with mild or moderate BPH may choose behavioral changes and watchful waiting.
- Most men with BPH will respond to alpha blocker medications. Side effects are uncommon.
- Men with very large prostates are candidates to treat symptoms by shrinking the gland through 5-alpha reductase inhibitors.
- The combination of alpha-blockers and 5-alpha reductase inhibitors maximizes the chance of long-term success and minimizes the chance of complications and eventual need for surgery. Whether this is worth the additional cost and possible side effects is controversial, but it is gaining in popularity because of recent studies.

- Minimally invasive treatments such as TUNA, microwave therapy (TUMT), and laser surgery can treat many men with LUTS. Long-term effectiveness remains the concern with these technologies.
- TURP, or its modern version, TURIS, is the gold standard treatment for prostatic obstruction. Both require more aggressive therapy than medications or minimally invasive options, but their success is unequalled.

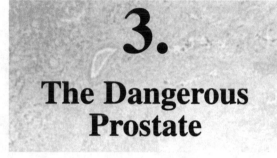

3.
The Dangerous Prostate

9.

PROSTATE CANCER OVERVIEW

A conquered nation is like a man with cancer: he can think of nothing else.

—George Bernard Shaw

Greg looked ill. Even if I weren't a physician, this would be obvious. He was shaking as I entered the room to give him a second opinion. Sweat beaded on his forehead. He was pale, blurry eyed, and almost hyperventilating. "What's wrong?" I asked. "Are you sick?"

"I've got cancer!"

***

Cancer is one of the scariest words in the English language. Fear of developing—or suffering from—"the big C" exceeds that of practically every other human ailment. Most people are more afraid of cancer than of heart disease. To put it in perspective, a man's chance of dying from heart disease is ten to fifteen times greater than his chance of dying from prostate cancer.

PROSTATE CANCER BY THE NUMBERS

The lifetime chance for men of being diagnosed with prostate cancer is about 17 percent, but the chance of dying from the disease is only 3.4 percent.[1] Therefore, most men who develop the disease die *with*, and not *from*, prostate cancer. In other words, when they die their bodies may harbor prostate cancer, but most of the time something unrelated to the cancer leads to their demise.

These numbers are evolving for a number of reasons. Prostate cancer mortality increased at an annual rate of 3.1 percent between the late eighties and early nineties, but then decreased by 1.9 percent annually through most of the nineties, according to the most recent data available.[2] Paradoxically, this decrease occurred as even greater numbers of men reached the ages at which prostate cancer occurs. As a result, the American Cancer Society predicts that the number of prostate cancer deaths will decrease 25 percent or more as this trend continues. This drop in mortality is real, but the cause is subject to debate and is covered in more detail in the coming pages.

Encouragingly, if you have recently been diagnosed with cancer, your chances of survival and doing well are better than the chances for any group of patients in history. We know that irrespective of all factors covered in the following chapters, a later year of diagnosis is a favorable prognostic sign. In other words, *everything* else being equal, your prognosis is better now than it would have been even a few short years ago.[3]

This trend has not yet been seen in Europe (where screening is less widespread), suggesting early diagnosis efforts in the United States are at least part of the reason. In addition, we continue to develop improved treatments. Whatever the reason, you can see that, in perspective, most men *will not die* of prostate cancer.

***

If only Greg could believe that. . . .

PROSTATE CANCER: TWO DISEASES

There are really two forms of prostate cancer. The first is the one urologists know about and treat. It releases PSA into the bloodstream or becomes a palpable nodule that can be detected by **Digital Rectal Examination (DRE)**. This is the type that can become dangerous—or deadly. Therefore, we call this form **clinically significant prostate cancer**. This form is the one we are concerned with, and it is the major focus of this book.

The other form is the one no man hopes to know about. This so-called *latent* or *occult prostate cancer* eventually develops in most men if they live long enough. It is sometimes called autopsy prostate cancer due to the fact that many men who die of unrelated causes will be found to have insignificant small deposits of low-grade cancer if they undergo autopsy. They lived their entire lives without knowing they had cancer, even though it may have been there for years. The very fact that it was never suspected until autopsy is a clear sign of its nonthreatening nature. Its indolence allows us to call this **clinically insignificant prostate cancer**.

Since the second form never becomes a problem, and is rarely detected, it might even be a little misleading even to call it cancer. If it can't hurt you, it seems unfair to characterize it with that word. However, it indeed fits some *histological* (microscopic) criteria to qualify as cancer, so we're stuck with the label. Still, it is better if any of us never even knows it is there in order to avoid not only the anxiety it might cause, but also to avoid unneeded treatment.

Interestingly, latent prostate cancer occurs in similar prevalence worldwide and effectively shows no preference for any ethnicity, race, religion, or region. In contrast, clinically significant prostate cancer shows great variations in these parameters. We will try to make sense of that in the following pages.

Unfortunately, *it is currently impossible to determine with certainty whether a given case of prostate cancer is clinically significant or clinically insignificant.* Neither a pathologist looking at the tissue on a microscopic slide nor the urologist can be absolutely sure. Nevertheless, you will learn in the coming pages the factors that lead physicians to suspect a case is one or the other. This will help you and your physician to make treatment decisions.

***

As it turns out, Greg had a cancer that was unlikely to lead to his demise. As a seventy-five-year-old diabetic smoker recovering from a recent heart attack, his life expectancy was limited. Even the worst prostate cancer was unlikely to grow rapidly enough to cause problems during his expected lifetime. In addition, his cancer was a small, low-grade tumor detected coincidentally during a TURP—theoretically clinically insignificant. In that setting, it was likely that he had already been cured regardless of his life expectancy. Indeed, he had cancer but was going to live—if he didn't die as a result of stress first.

PROSTATE CANCER: TWO DIFFERENT SITUATIONS

As noted above, prostate cancer can be considered to be two different diseases—one serious and one not. A different way prostate cancer can be separated into two categories is by location. The first and most common today is **organ-confined** or **localized prostate cancer**, meaning that the only known cancer cells are confined to the prostate or its immediate vicinity. This is very different from advanced or **metastatic** prostate cancer, which is defined as cancer that has spread to other areas. The implications are fairly obvious, insofar as cancer that is confined to the prostate can be cured, while advanced cancer usually cannot. Moreover, treatments directed at the prostate such as surgery, radiation, or cryotherapy are usually not appropriate or helpful for men whose cancers are outside the treatment area.

When I was in medical school in the early eighties, we were taught that half of all cases of prostate cancer were of the second type—detected after the cancer had spread. This half of the men had an incurable disease. Prostate cancer care at that time was often not satisfying.

That statistic has changed dramatically in the past two decades, theoretically because of improved screening techniques. Currently, a vast majority of cases are of the first type (organ confined), since those cases are detected while the cancer is localized. This means that most cases are curable. Most of our attention here will focus on the group of men who have organ-confined cancer.

UNEQUAL OPPORTUNITY

Prostate cancer is the most common cancer in men. According to the World Health Organization (WHO), 542,990 cases of prostate cancer arise each year, and 204,313 men die each year worldwide.[4] Of those diagnosed, 230,110 are Americans.[5] Almost 30,000 of them will die.

How could almost half of all cases of prostate cancer occur in the United States, which has less than 5 percent of the world's population? There are several reasons. The least significant is that Americans tend to live longer than citizens of some countries, thereby surviving things that might shorten their lives until they grow old enough to develop cancer.

The far greater reason is that Americans are more likely to see a doctor. There's a medical adage that "if you don't want to find a fever, don't take the temperature." This adage applies to other medical conditions as well, including prostate cancer. As noted above, we know that many men harbor prostate cancer for years without developing symptoms. Therefore, unless they undergo DRE, PSA testing, and prostate biopsy, we may never know they had prostate cancer—and that's often okay. In fact, one concern with our aggressive screening approaches today is that we may detect cancer in some men who have only the second type, latent prostate cancer. Had we not looked so closely, these men would have never known they had a problem; or, more correctly, they didn't really have a problem in the first place. Finding their cancer may have simply created one.

AGING AND PROSTATE CANCER

As alluded to above, cancer may be inevitable if men live long enough. Before panicking, slow down to consider that the previous statement may not be all bad. Think about it—cancer was rare when the average life expectancy was thirty to forty years. Long before cancer had time to develop, a saber-toothed tiger would eat most people, or at least they would die from disease or famine. Today in Western societies, we usually outlast those as well as other *competing mortalities*, allowing us to reach the age when most cancers occur.

Most of our bodies wear out or develop other causes of death first, but none of our tissues is meant to last forever. If nothing else gets us first, eventually cancer will develop somewhere in the body; the prostate is one of the most likely spots. The average age of prostate cancer diagnosis is seventy-one years—with the average age of death from the disease being seventy-eight (according to the U.S. Preventive Service Task Force).[6]

Most urologists have a bias that prostate cancer is more serious in young men than is it is in older men. This is probably because the potential loss of life expectancy is greater in a man with more potential years to lose. However, this bias may be incorrect, and there is some evidence that cancer may actually be more aggressive in older men.[7]

To summarize, we will all die someday. Prostate cancer is rarely rapidly fatal. In many men, some competing mortality will take over before prostate cancer does.

WHEN DOES PROSTATE CANCER BEGIN?

One of the most common questions men ask following diagnosis of prostate cancer is, "When did it start?" The answer may be, "A long time ago."

This answer is based on some interesting data from a large autopsy study. Men who died of traumatic and other unrelated causes underwent autopsy. Previously unsuspected prostate cancer was present in 8 percent of men in their twenties, and in 31 percent of men in their thirties. This is consistent with the known slow progression of prostate cancer, where few men younger than forty develop clinical disease, but some percentage of these men will do so and potentially die of prostate cancer.[8]

Dr. Paul Lange, chairman of urology at the University of Washington, has a useful illustration of how some cancers behave very differently than others. He says there are three types of prostate cancer—turtles, rabbits, and birds. All three are inside the imaginary fence of the prostate. Turtles grow more slowly, and must get very big before they can escape. They will be able to do so rarely. Birds grow quickly, and escape as soon as they are big enough to fly. They are often out by the time you realize they are present. Rabbits are in between, so can usually be contained if detected early and managed appropriately.

If these animals were prostate cancer, they would demonstrate its variability. The birds cannot be stopped and will excape not matter what, but are fortunately rare. Rabbits can be contained if you catch them in time. Tortoises are at no risk of escape, and may simply be observed.

HOW DOES PROSTATE CANCER OCCUR?

How prostate cancer occurs is a difficult question. Since most men will develop prostate cancer if they live long enough, one issue we must consider is what triggers it to occur in the first place. This may be preprogrammed, since the risk seems fairly even among all men of all cultures and regions. Given that a majority of men will develop **clinically insignificant** cancer, it's perhaps a matter of drawing one of *many* short straws. In any case, the odds don't seem to change with anything other than advancing years.

The short straw is usually caused by **oxidative DNA damage**. In other words, harmful *oxygen free radicals* (toxic by-products of various normal cellular processes or from environmental exposure) circulate through the body. They disrupt DNA, leading to a change in the cell's genetic makeup.

This is similar to what occurs when a computer's DNA—its software—has minor disruptions or glitches. In either case, minor damage is usually easily repaired and leads to no permanent harm. The person involved probably never even knew that the ongoing repair process occurred. However, sometimes the damage is more than can be repaired routinely. In the computer's case, if the damage is severe enough, the hard drive locks up or crashes. In the body's case, the tissue might become malignant.

The second issue to consider is the question, Why do most of these men never develop **clinically significant** prostate cancer (as defined above), while a few do? Why do very few develop it in some cultures, whereas a larger few develop it in others? This suggests that the first step is triggering the development of cancer in the first place, whereas the second step is triggering significant growth. The first step is called **initiation**. The second is **progression**.

Initiation refers to the conversion of normal cells to abnormal, potentially cancerous cells. This process probably occurs regularly in the body, but our immune system usually corrects the glitch before it can become dangerous. The immune system thus keeps these changes in balance. In regard to prostate cancer, initiation may lead to a tumor, or collection of such cells. Any growth is called a *tumor*, but that doesn't mean a tumor is a cancer. A tumor may be benign (or noncancerous). An example might be a bump on the skin or a thickening of a bone due to a previous fracture. Conversely, a tumor may be *malignant*, meaning cancerous.

Progression occurs when the balance is lost and cancer overcomes the body's immune system. It can then grow, possibly spread, and potentially lead to death. This occurs in a minority of prostate cancers, which explains why many men will have incidental prostate cancer if they undergo autopsy, but few will die of the disease. The $64,000 question is why some cancers progress and most don't. This is explored in more detail in the following chapter.

GENETIC VERSUS SPORADIC PROSTATE CANCER

Most cancers occur spontaneously or sporadically. In other words, they are not based on genetics and simply occur with a given frequency in any population. However, about 10 percent of cancers are hereditary, based on any of a number of genetic defects that have been identified. (This is discussed in the next chapter.)

KEY POINTS

- Prostate cancer is the most common cancer in American men, diagnosed during the lifetime of at least one in six or seven men.
- Prostate cancer is the second most common cause of cancer death in American men.
- Prostate cancer can be considered two diseases. The first (**clinically significant**) is the focus of this book. The second (**clinically insignificant**) is inconsequential. If we are lucky, we never even know it existed. Unfortunately, it is impossible to be definite about which type a man has.
- Prostate cancer occurs in two different situations. The first is when cancer is **organ confined**. The second occurs after advanced cancer spreads to other areas, or is **metastatic**.
- Most men who develop prostate cancer will die of something else.
- **Initiation** of prostate cancer occurs in large numbers of men, but doesn't necessarily mean that the cancer will ever become clinically significant. **Progression** is much less common.

10.

CAUSES OF PROSTATE CANCER: A ROAD TO PREVENTION?

> *Prevention is so much better than cure, since it saves the burden of being sick.*
>
> —Thomas Adams, 1618

"I don't understand how I could get prostate cancer," Dan blurted after I told him that that his biopsy was positive. "I eat right, exercise, and don't smoke. How could this happen?"

I quickly reassured the fifty-eight-year-old that it's usually just a matter of chance—bad luck. He drew the wrong card. "Most cases 'just happen.'" The explanation didn't help much; despite having followed a healthy lifestyle, he now defined himself as a cancer patient and couldn't fathom how this was fair.

Sometimes life isn't. I recalled that Dan's father was diagnosed with prostate cancer at the age of fifty-two. Unfortunately, this was before widespread screening was available, so he sought attention only after he developed back pain from a tumor that had spread to his spine. As in the case of half of all men diagnosed in that era, his cancer was detected at an incurable stage. His father fought for almost two years before leaving Dan an orphan at the age of thirteen. This was clearly the only thing Dan could focus on as we talked.

"Hold on," I broke in as his wife began weeping. "Remember what I told you the day we scheduled the biopsy—you're in an entirely different situation than your father." Neither looked reassured. "I told you that if the diagnosis turns out to be cancer, we've caught it early; I would expect it to be curable."

Since he knew how things had turned out with his father, Dan had followed aggressive early detection recommendations. He began having a serum PSA drawn yearly from the age of forty. The first time it became abnormal, he actually came in asking me to perform a biopsy. As a result, we found the cancer while it was confined to the prostate. I could honestly reassure him that most men diagnosed in this situation will eventually die of old age. "Don't start getting your affairs in order."

"Then how did this happen?"

***

Dan's prostate cancer clearly didn't "just happen." Apparently the genes that cause a propensity to develop prostate cancer ran in the family's chromosomes. For most men it's not as simple as that. Moreover, even men with a family history of prostate cancer may have their risks increased or decreased by a number of factors. Therefore, it can be said that the cause of prostate cancer is *multifactorial*; in other words, it is usually due to several different causes in each patient. We must understand all the factors if we hope to try to control the ones that are responsible in any given person.

LOOKING FOR CAUSES—IT'S COMPLEX

Many cancers are related to the causative risks we take. Smoking is the worst cause of several types of cancer (*not* including prostatic). Others are poor diet, lack of exercise, exposure to environmental toxins, and so forth. Even if any of these things isn't *solely* responsible for the development of cancer, it places individuals at increased risk.

On the contrary, prostate cancer appears to be influenced more by factors that we cannot control. Therefore, most cases appear to arise spontaneously. However, although most of the process is inalterable, there are some things that that can be influenced by our behaviors.

THE BIG THREE RISKS

Age

Being a male is actually the greatest risk factor for prostate cancer (women don't have a prostate so they cannot develop the disease), but age is a strong second and the first one that we actually consider. Some sobering statistics reveal that prostate cancer changes begin in some men while in their twenties. Recall the autopsy study that found that prostate cancer was present in 8 percent of men in their twenties. Latent cancer was present in 31 percent of those in their thirties.[1]

One urological truism spread by word of mouth is that the likelihood of a man having prostate cancer roughly parallels his age. In other words, at age fifty, up to half of men may harbor small areas of cancer. Most of these are **clinically insignificant** as discussed earlier. By the time a man is a century old, the chance he has microscopic cancer somewhere in his prostate approaches 100 percent.

Obviously, far fewer men die of the disease, so don't let such statements cause you undue stress. Likewise, don't assume that such high rates of clinically insignificant cancer mean that your cancer is insignificant if diagnosed at an age when you are young enough to be at risk for **progression**.

It's (Sometimes) in the Genes

There are two primary paths in which prostate cancer arises. Most commonly it arises spontaneously. This occurs when a combination of factors allows normal cells to lose their normality. They then turn on their *host*—the body of their owner. They begin to grow rapidly and uncontrollably. They lose their natural tendency to stop growing when they run into another structure, so they dig into normal tissues or spread and cause all kinds of problems.

Less commonly, the man's genes seem to be programmed to allow this to occur. In families with such genes, several men may develop prostate cancer. Around 10 percent of cases of prostate cancer are inherited.[2] This typically happens at an earlier age than it would occur in most men.

The risk is higher when multiple men in the family have prostate cancer. Men with one close relative (a brother or father, known as a *first-degree relative*) who has prostate cancer have double the risk of developing it as men with no family history. The risk implied by a brother may be a little greater than that from having a father with prostate cancer. Moreover, men with two or three first-degree relatives have a five- to elevenfold risk.[3] Those statistics are impressive, demonstrating why most urologists will aggressively evaluate men with such a family history for early detection.

Men diagnosed at a particularly young age (typically below the age of fifty-five, but that is changing, as noted in the sidebar) present an even more concerning family history. Their families will sometimes have a pattern of inheritance that suggests a single gene is responsible. This is called *auto-*

Our understanding of "young" or "early-onset" diagnosis is changing. The high numbers mentioned above were from times when we often didn't catch prostate cancer at its earliest stages. As noted, the disease takes several years to become manifest without an aggressive early diagnosis program. Therefore, many men had cancer at these ages but didn't know about it until they were in more typical ages of diagnosis, usually after age sixty. Now that we find many of these cases several years earlier in their development, these men may be diagnosed at an age that previously would have been atypically low. These men aren't the same as those found two or three decades ago whose cancer had already advanced while in their forties or fifties. Thus, carrying a diagnosis of prostate cancer at these ages may now simply reflect improved detection rather than a worsening genetic makeup of the family.

Therefore, if you have a relative with prostate cancer in his forties or fifties, don't assume you have the genes. Rather, count it as a blessing that they were well served by physicians who found it while it was still curable, and schedule your own checkup similarly early.

somal *dominant* inheritance of a gene; though rare, it apparently causes cancer in up to 88 percent of its carriers. Up to 9 percent of all prostate cancer cases may be due to this gene, but almost half of early-onset cases may be. Several genetic mutations have been identified, but these are still largely being investigated at this point.

It is controversial whether hereditary prostate cancer has a worse prognosis than spontaneous cases. Studies disagree. A study of patients at the Cleveland Clinic who have familial prostate cancer appeared to have a worse prognosis,[4] but other studies have not found this to be the case.[5]

Another issue regarding genes is to understand the difference in a tumor-causing gene (*oncogene*) versus a gene that protects us from cancer (*tumor suppressor gene*). An oncogene actually stimulates either the **initiation** or **progression** of prostate cancer, whereas a tumor suppressor gene inhibits this stimulation from occurring. Therefore, possessing an oncogene might cause cancer, but losing a tumor suppressor gene because of **oxidative DNA damage** might do the same thing. This loss can be the mechanism that enables oxidative DNA damage to create malignancy. Such damage underlies several of the risk factors discussed throughout this chapter, and has been postulated as a reason *chronic inflammation* might be related to prostate cancer risk.

Finally, you should understand the difference in **hereditary prostate cancer** and *genetic prostate cancer*. Hereditary cancer is the result of genes that run in the family. These genes are present at birth, and exhibit their behavior later in life. Since these genes are present in all cells, they may be passed on to offspring. On the other hand, genetic prostate cancer really describes all cancer cases, since DNA (genetic) damage underlies malignant transformation in individual cancer cells. However, these abnormal genes are acquired later in life because of oxidative DNA damage, and are present only in malignant cells, so they can't be passed on to offspring.

Uncles, Cousins, Etc.

Men commonly ask about increased risk of prostate cancer when someone other than a first-degree relative is involved. Uncles, grandfathers, cousins, and other second- or third-degree relatives with prostate cancer don't impart the same concern. Although their cases may be a sign of genes in the family, if there are significant prostate cancer genes they will usually manifest in closer relatives. Therefore, cancer cases in these men should make you alert, but certainly not alarmed.

RACIAL DIFFERENCES IN PROSTATE CANCER

No one fully understands why, but African American men are about twice as likely as Caucasian men to develop prostate cancer.[6] They are about twice as likely to die of the disease as well.[7] This contrasts with the low risk in native Asian men; African American men are *sixty times* more likely to develop prostate cancer than native Chinese men.

The reason black men are at risk is complex. Poverty can limit access to medical care, and is more common in the United States among African Americans than among Caucasians. Some behaviors inversely related to socioeconomic status such as smoking and fatty diet are also general health-risk factors.

Independent of the above risk factors, it seems black men in America and other countries may be at risk purely based on race. It is possible that this is related to vitamin D levels based on sun absorption, although this is purely a hypothesis.[8] Studies continue to explore the risk to African American men.

STILL NO EASY ANSWERS

As noted previously, this and chapter 5 ("Maintaining Prostate Health") were the hardest to write, because the information available on causes and dietary or other factors that might affect the risk of prostate cancer is inconclusive. As you read these two chapters, you must keep in mind that some studies support the role of issues that other studies contradict. I have tried to clarify when a majority of urologists have concluded that a preponderance of evidence supports an approach. Although a majority may share certain views, it is rare in such topics that there is universal agreement.

Recall the warning for concrete thinkers. The role of the topics covered in these two chapters will remain controversial and under investigation for years to come. You should consider the information with this understanding, and decide with your doctor whether you believe any approach herein is in your best interest. Thereafter, you must keep up with developments in research that may affect interpretation of these factors, and adjust accordingly.

LESS CLEAR FACTORS

Diet

All mothers provide admonition to their children—you are what you eat. However, it's tricky to tie dietary intake to disease processes. It is true that people in parts of the world with differing diets have vastly different rates of many cancers, including prostate cancer. If only the diets were different, we could draw some easy conclusions. However, these people also have different air quality, sun exposure, habits, and genes. Therefore, their risks may simply reflect who or where they are instead of what they've eaten.

Prostate cancer incidence and mortality have increased in concert with Westernization of Asian nations, although they still have lower rates than Americans.[9] This implies that there is more to it than simply diet, but that dietary changes have an impact. Many researchers, including my colleague from Singapore, Dr. Christopher Cheng, are considering why prostate cancer rates are appearing to rise rapidly in Asian countries.

The effect of making dietary changes is complicated. We know that many men have *occult* or latent prostate cancer. The risk of having these **clinically insignificant** tumors is about the same in all societies. However, the risk of having a cancer that causes problems that lead to a troubling diagnosis is vastly different among societies. Interestingly, men who migrate from low-risk areas such as Asia to high-risk areas such as the United States develop **clinically significant** cancers at increasing rates over time. This suggests that diet may not actually cause prostate cancer (since initiation rates of clinically insignificant cancer are similar throughout the world), but rather may influence its progression into the significant form. In the following sections, we look at various dietary issues that may be important.

Fat

Prostate cancer rates correlate with dietary fat consumption around the world. This may be related to several issues. First, fat can increase testosterone and *sex hormone binding globulin levels*,[10] which can serve as growth factors for prostate cancer. Second, fat is a source of *oxygen free radicals*, which are known carcinogens. Third, fatty acids may induce *inflammation*, which may lead to prostate cancer.

The role of fat is complex. Physicians in the Health Professionals Follow-up Study who consumed a high-fat diet were at increased risk of prostate cancer.[11] The worst problem identified in this study was red meat. However, a review of all the major studies found that the relationship to a high-fat, meaty diet was circumstantial and not absolutely convincing.[12] Dairy products in that review were not associated with cancer risk.

Studies of Seventh-Day Adventists and Hawaiians found lower prostate cancer rates in both groups of men among those who avoided meat. However, they also found increased risk with the use of dairy products. Thus, the risk with both fat and dairy products remains unclear.

Recall that it is never easy to determine the role of diet in heath issues. Perhaps it's not really the fat, or even the meat, that is related to increased cancer risk. Diets high in meat and fat are necessarily low in vegetables and fruits, so maybe it's a loss of their protective effects. Zinc and calcium from meat might be the culprits, as they may be related to cancer development.

In summary, most urologists interpret the above information to conclude that dietary fat is a risk factor, but that dairy products are probably not. This will remain controversial until definitive studies clarify these risks.

Vitamin D

Vitamin D is a steroid hormone that inhibits the growth of prostate cancer. Men with lower levels of vitamin D appear to be at higher risk of prostate cancer.[13] We receive vitamin D both from diet and from a chemical reaction to ultraviolet light exposure. This leads to the theory that vitamin D deficiency could be related to the interesting finding that men in far northern countries have higher risks of prostate cancer than comparable men in southerly, sunnier climes.

Vitamin D and calcium balance each other. Increased cancer risk is associated with large amounts of dietary calcium intake. The mechanism could be related to other substances found in association with calcium (e.g. milk), but may also be related to calcium-causing decreased vitamin D production. Studies have failed to prove the ability to alter cancer risk with either vitamin D or calcium. Some believe that vitamin D levels may play a role in the increased risk of African American men, but this has not been proven.

Testosterone

Although testosterone encourages the growth of prostate cancer, it is not clear whether the male hormone causes the disease. Some studies have indicated it does, but others do the opposite. Moreover, it is difficult to be certain of the results because measurement of testosterone is difficult. Sure, it's easy to do a blood test. However, interpretation of its results can be misleading.

Testosterone levels fluctuate throughout the day and over time. If I draw blood from a man every hour for a week, three things will be obvious. First, that he will be annoyed and bruised from all the blood drawn. Second, the levels will generally be higher in the morning than in the evening. Third, the levels even on different days at similar hours will fluctuate. Moreover, no one knows how much all this matters.

In addition, it is nearly impossible to measure testosterone levels inside the prostate, so varying blood levels may not be meaningful if they don't affect the actual amount of hormone reaching the prostate. Also,

POLITICS, MILK, AND CANCER

Politics hit below the belt in the discussion of milk's possible role in prostate cancer risk. After former New York City mayor Rudy Giuliani announced he had prostate cancer during his campaign for the United States Senate in 2000, the animal rights group PETA (People for the Ethical Treatment of Animals)—opposed apparently to any use of animal products—put up billboards showing the mayor with a milk mustache. They played on the milk industry's catchy ad campaign ("Got Milk?") by attaching the words, "Got Cancer?" Giuliani smiled, drank a glass of milk at a press conference, and proceeded to undergo apparently successful cancer treatment.

we don't know whether it is exposure to the prostate throughout a man's life-time or just at crucial points (such as adolescence or late in life) that makes a difference.

Finally, there is some counteracting evidence that a low testosterone level may actually be a cause of prostate cancer.[14] Whether this is true, or is related to changing testosterone levels or balancing levels with estrogens associated with aging is unclear, so research will continue.

Obesity

Irrespective of dietary intake of the various agents suspected of having either a causative or preventative role, obesity (in contrast to dietary fat alone, which continues to have a confusing role in the risk of prostate cancer) appears to be a risk factor and is related to prostate cancer incidence and mortality.[15] Researchers have found that obese men have a worse prognosis.[16]

The impact of obesity may be related to the chronic state of *oxidative stress* and the *inflammation* it causes. These factors increase the chance of cancer and many other diseases. Obese men also have hormonal abnormalities that may affect their risk. Such obesity related hormone changes may also play a role in the increased risk in African American men.

ISSUES THAT DO NOT CAUSE PROSTATE CANCER

Uromythology is rife with things that someone claims causes prostate cancer. In the preceding pages, we discussed those factors that appear to play a role. Now let's dismiss some that there is no reason to believe do play a role.

Relationship of Vasectomy to Prostate Cancer

Two reports in the early nineties found increased rates of prostate cancer in men who had previously undergone vasectomy. This caused understandable alarm among those of us who perform vasectomies, as well as those who had it done to them. Several studies began in earnest. Fortunately, no link was found in any of the studies that were conducted in several countries.[17]

Each September urologists and other health professionals nationwide mark *Prostate Cancer Awareness Week (PCAW)*. During that time, free screenings take place to offer DRE and PSA testing en masse. A few weeks later the patient receives a letter saying either that everything was normal, or that something of concern was found on either the DRE or PSA. Urological consultation should follow if either is the case. Following the first studies that indicated a possible causal relationship with vasectomy, all men undergoing screening during PCAW were asked about a history of vasectomy. After more than a decade of investigation, hundreds of thousands of men have been tested. If a true relationship between vasectomy and prostate cancer existed, a group that large should have validated it.

Fortunately, there has been no linkage established in this or multiple other studies performed worldwide. Although proving that two things are *not* related is almost impossible, this is as close as we can come to doing so conclusively. Therefore, any risk would have to be so small that it would pale in comparison to the known factors discussed above.

Thus, it appears that vasectomy is only a risk for prostate cancer in its predictive capacity. Men who have vasectomies typically are intelligent and healthy. They have jobs and seek medical care (by definition). They usually aren't the types to be dying young of risk-seeking behaviors. Therefore, they are at risk of prostate cancer because they are at risk of living long enough to reach the age when men develop it.

Alcohol, Sexual Activity, Vices, and Other Rumors

There is nothing moral or immoral about prostate cancer. However, several habits and behaviors have mistakenly been considered factors, as if God might punish men with prostate cancer for their indiscretions. Apparently not.

Overdoing alcohol consumption increases estrogen, which can decrease testosterone by its feedback to the pituitary gland; if estrogen is present, the brain senses adequate levels of *sex hormones,* so it turns off production of testosterone. This would theoretically decrease the likelihood of developing prostate cancer. At any rate, no direct link has been found to alcohol use, although its overuse leads to a number of other serious consequences. As discussed in chapter 5, smoking has a huge negative impact on overall health, and makes radiation therapy less effective against prostate cancer, but does not play a clear causative role.

Some doctors have suggested a link with sexual activity early in life, which might be a surrogate measure of a man's likelihood to either be more sexually active in his lifetime or his likelihood to have multiple partners. However, recent findings suggest the opposite is true, as discussed below.

Similarly, sexually transmitted diseases have been investigated. The human papilloma virus (HPV) causes most cases of cervical cancer in women. Therefore, it is logical that the same virus might cause male cancers as well. It does appear to increase slightly the risk for penile cancer, which is mercifully rare. Infection with the *Chlamydia* bacteria has also been suspected but never proven.

Some studies have shown that taller men have a greater risk of prostate cancer and a worse prognosis, but the links are weak and probably disproven.[18]

Dr. Robert Atkins introduced us to the concept of insulin resistance in relation to his widely successful books advocating carbohydrate limits. Soon after his death another risk was identified when a multi-institutional study showed an increased prostate cancer rate in people with insulin resistance.[19] Further study will be needed to corroborate these findings.

THE GOOD NEWS?

One prostate cancer risk factor that is beginning to gain supporting evidence is *lack* of sex. According to a recent study in the *Journal of the American Medical Association*, men who ejaculate less often have higher rates of prostate cancer than do men who ejaculate more often.[20] This is supported by the finding that priests have an increased risk.[21] The risk is decreased most by sexual activity later in life, clearly indicating that sexual activity should not slow down later in life if a man is to minimize his risk.

A recent study from Wales (ancestral home of the Jones clan) looked at the role of sexuality on overall health. Men were half as likely to die in a given time period if they had over one hundred orgasms a year.[22] Therefore, even if you don't feel like it, try your best to have intercourse twice a week. If you have to miss a few television reruns to achieve that goal, so be it. Your prostate health and longevity are worth it.

POTENTIAL UNFORESEEN BENEFITS TO PREVENTION

The Prostate Cancer Prevention Trial created an interesting dilemma. There was a 25 percent reduction in total cancer cases when finasteride was administered, but critics point out that the reduction was only in lower-grade cancers that might not be life threatening anyway. Therefore, one interpretation might be that there may not be an eventual impact on prostate cancer mortality.

Another viewpoint was pointed out to me by Dr. Eric Klein, head of the Section of Urological Oncology at the Cleveland Clinic Foundation. His interpretation is that there is a clear benefit to preventing a diagnosis of prostate cancer regardless of impact on longevity. Doing so avoids the *burden of cure*. In other words, 25 percent of men at risk may never have to undergo the stress, cost, and potential side effects of treatment. If these men are not at risk of prostate cancer death, they would therefore logically be better off not having to deal with all that. This alone may be the most powerful argument for prevention strategies.

SUMMARY

Now the hard part—do I recommend prevention strategies? The answer is an unequivocal "I don't know." The potential benefits are obvious, but the risks of long-term finasteride or the other prevention strategies listed in this book are unknown. There is a long list of concepts and drugs littering the historical road to prevention. Drugs that were once believed safe have been withdrawn from the market when long-term side effects were revealed only after years or decades of use. Natural products sometimes appear safe, only to be deemed harmful at some point. (Remember that tobacco was believed harmless by most people, including physicians, for longer than we have castigated it.)

Thus, you should discuss prevention strategies with your urologist, especially if you have a family history of prostate cancer. Then, you should keep up with emerging information and adjust accordingly.

KEY POINTS

- Most cases of prostate cancer arise spontaneously.
- Hereditary prostate cancer is responsible for about 10 percent of cases.
- The concept of early diagnosis is evolving. Before accurate screening techniques were adopted, it was rare to identify prostate cancer in men younger than sixty. However, we now detect cancer in many men in their forties and fifties. It is unlikely that the cancers are occurring earlier; rather, we now detect them much earlier in their growth cycle and usually while curable.
- The goal of cancer prevention is usually thought of as prevention of death. However, because most people with prostate cancer will not die

of the disease, prevention can also prevent the *burden of cure* for many.

- Vices and vasectomy appear to play no role in prostate cancer risk.
- Prostate cancer cause and prevention are complex, and there will probably be no consensus anytime soon. Despite this, many of my colleagues believe a reasonable strategy might involve a low-fat diet high in cooked tomatoes and soy. Adding vitamin E and selenium in accordance with your doctor's recommendations may also decrease cancer risk.

11.

SUSPECTING PROSTATE CANCER: PSA AND SCREENING

Patients don't get cancer—families do.
—Anonymous

A PSA reading of 3.8 caught the attention of Tom's internist. Although technically within official "normal" limits, the internist was concerned because he knew Tom's father had died from prostate cancer. "It is probably all right," he reassured. "But, just to be sure, let's send you for a urology consult."

Tom was nervous when I introduced myself. His father had not painted a pretty picture. A biopsy ten years prior had been no fun, and he had adequately described the humility of the event to Tom. He had undergone the procedure in a hospital radiology department with minimal confidentiality. He felt that the doctor had been rough in placing an ultrasound probe into the rectum. Each of six passes of the needle into the prostate had been more painful than the one before. An annoying loud click accompanied each one. "Do I have to go through that?"

"You never have *to do anything," I replied, "but let's discuss whether biopsy is in order." Most importantly, I reassured him that if a biopsy were in his future, his experience would not be that of his father's. "We've come a long way."*

***

The urologist will be able to predict the likelihood of prostate cancer based on an elevated **PSA** or abnormal **DRE**. Still, this will still only be a prediction of that likelihood. But we now have additional measures to help clarify

175

the likelihood of having cancer, including *percent* **free PSA**, **complexed PSA**, *pro-PSA*, and possibly some newer markers under investigation. Despite all these tools, when suspicion exists, a **biopsy** is the *only* way to definitively clarify the picture.

PSA: THE BEST TUMOR MARKER KNOWN TO MODERN MEDICINE

First, let's consider exactly what PSA is. PSA is an abbreviation for **prostate specific antigen**. This protein is produced by the prostate to turn semen into its more liquefied form several minutes after ejaculation. Liquefaction releases sperm for their journey toward the egg.

After completing procreation, PSA really doesn't do anything. Scientists didn't even discover the molecule until the seventies. For the first few years after discovery, it was a simple curiosity. Then we found that certain disease states of the prostate released PSA into the blood stream in higher amounts. Cancer is the one of the most obvious interest.

Our understanding of PSA is still in the works, but we know that it is the best screening tool available at this time to detect prostate cancer. In addition, it is useful for evaluation and surveillance of men diagnosed with prostate cancer (as discussed in the following chapters).

PROSTATE SPECIFIC—NOT CANCER SPECIFIC

The greatest criticism of PSA is that it is not specific enough. It may be elevated from prostate cancer, but may also be so because of prostatitis, BPH, infarcts, or several other factors. In addition, the PSA may be elevated on one reading but then return to normal. How often this occurs is controversial, but some reports indicate it may occur as often as one-third of the time.[1] In my own experience, this occurs much less often—fewer than one time in ten. Perhaps that is because I see a group of preselected patients whose primary care physician has repeated it, so if it returns to normal I may never even hear about the patient. Nevertheless, when I see men who have had only one previous PSA, I usually recommend confirming it prior to further investigation.

One study even suggests that variable PSA levels might be under genetic control in some men and not indicative of cancer.[2] If this is true, some men may simply have an elevated PSA that is normal for them.

Finally, a couple of behaviors can trigger an increase in PSA. Occasionally patients will cause trauma to the prostate during bicycle riding which increases PSA. This is probably uncommon. Moreover, an ejaculation will also cause a *slight* increase, but not enough to make a normal PSA convert to abnormal.[3]

The bottom line is that PSA is a chemical in the bloodstream—nothing more and nothing less. It just happens to be released in response to any disorder of the prostate, including cancer. As such, no one ever died of PSA.

***

Based on the above concepts, the first recommendation I made to Tom (after confirming that his DRE was normal) was to repeat the PSA. It had been 1.3 the year before, so it was feasible that the higher level was a laboratory error. I also ordered a free PSA (as discussed below) to be obtained at the same time.

I explained that laboratory values do fluctuate a little bit. He might also expect that our laboratory might repeat the test using a different method, so the number was unlikely to be exactly the same. As long as the variation was small, however, the results were apparently accurate.

WHAT PSA LEVEL IS NORMAL?

This question is more complex than it appears. When PSA testing was approved in the eighties, the original studies found that men with cancer usually had a PSA above 4 ng/dl. As unscientific as this was, it still influences our perceptions of "normal."

Multiple subsequent studies have tried to define the normal level of PSA, leading to a plethora of factors to consider in deciding whether your PSA is normal. In the early nineties, researchers at Washington University demonstrated findings that became part of the lexicon. They reported that men with a PSA between 4 and 10 have an approximately one in four chance of having cancer, while those with a PSA of 10 or higher have a two-thirds chance of having cancer.[4]

We now know that these numbers underestimate the chance of cancer for reasons discussed in this chapter. Nevertheless, the race was on to find ways to decide who was likely to have cancer and who was not, based on laboratory studies.

One such study looked at serum samples frozen in 1980 from men who were subsequently found to have prostate cancer. This was a unique opportunity, since their serum was frozen before urololgists even knew to look for PSA. They found that men with "abnormal" PSA levels (greater than 4 ng/dl) were twenty-seven times more likely to have prostate cancer in the future than men with a PSA level less than 1 ng/dl. However, an unexpected finding also came out in the same study. Men with a PSA between 1.3 and 2.5 ng/dl were three and a half times more likely to develop prostate cancer in the coming years.[5] This suggests that these men may have already undergone **initiation** of prostate cancer, and subsequently underwent **progression**, leading to the diagnosis of cancer. These are sobering numbers to those of us who rely on PSA to rule out prostate cancer.

Such increased risk has been confirmed in other studies, which have shown that men with PSA between 1 and 1.5 have a four times greater relative risk of developing prostate cancer than those with PSA below 1. Those with PSA of 1.5 to 2 are nine times more likely, and those with PSA of 2 to 3 are fifteen times more likely to develop prostate cancer in the coming decade.[6] In other words, a "normal" PSA is all relative, and deserves careful interpretation. Confusion created by the difficulty in defining a normal level of PSA has led to consideration of aging changes in regard to PSA, as well as PSA density and velocity.[7]

RISING PSA WITH RISING AGE

PSA does appear to rise with aging. The prostate grows, producing more PSA and releasing more into the bloodstream. The only problem is that it remains unclear what the natural progression is. In addition, the tables used to classify normal values of PSA are based on broad categories by decade. The most common age-specific ranges suggest that normal is below 2.5 ng/dl for men in their forties, 3.5 ng/dl for those in their fifties, 4.5 ng/dl for those in their sixties, and 6.5 ng/dl for those seventy or older.[8]

Since it is unlikely that the normal PSA jumps the day a man turns fifty, sixty, or seventy, the tables probably give readings inaccurately low at the later years of a decade of life, while potentially high at the early years of each decade. In addition, we know that using these cutoffs we miss many cases of cancer, so they should not be considered absolute values.

Instead of the above age-specific ranges, I regard a PSA greater than 2.5 to be abnormal in any man under the age of sixty. This is based on many studies and my own experience that makes it clear that many men with a PSA greater than 2.5 will continue to develop increasing PSA over the next few years and will eventually hit the arbitrary cutoff level that calls for a biopsy. Therefore, waiting for the PSA to go from 2.6 to 4 only delays a biopsy likely to find cancer at an earlier stage, when cure is most likely.

Even in men over sixty, it is clear that the numbers above are not absolute, so most urologists have abandoned the use of age-specific values until their accuracy is validated. Most remain aware that a mild elevation of PSA above 2.5 ng/dl is possibly related to aging, but not reliably so.

BE WARY OF PERCENTAGES: THEY ARE ONLY PREDICTORS

No matter how much information is used to calculate the possibility that any given man has prostate cancer, the bottom line is that it is still just a prediction of likelihood—not a diagnosis. No matter what the likelihood is, we still must find out whether cancer is really the cause. A biopsy (see below) is the only way to know.

For example, the urologist might tell you that there is an approximately 50 percent chance that you have prostate cancer based on the above factors. That is kind of like the weatherman telling you that there is a 50 percent chance of rain. No matter what the chance of it happening, in the end, either it rains or it doesn't.

If it rains, you still get wet whether the chance was 10 percent or 90 percent. When the prediction is the likelihood of cancer, either you have it or you don't.

Similarly, if the chance of cancer is 90 percent based on your clinical scenario, it doesn't matter how likely it was if you don't end up having cancer. It matters only that you don't have cancer. Therefore, try to avoid focusing on the probabilities and simply know that you will need a biopsy if the numbers are suspicious and if you want to find out whether you have cancer. Biopsy is the only way to know.

WHAT ARE THE PERCENTAGES?

As discussed above, the probability of cancer is just that—a probability. Nevertheless, everyone wants to know what that probability is. If you have a nodule detectable on DRE and a completely normal PSA, the chance that a biopsy will show cancer is about 10 percent. That is markedly different than the probability before PSA became available. Without knowing the PSA level, we knew that half of all nodules turned out to be cancerous.

In the early years of PSA use we found cancer in about one-fourth of men with a PSA of 4 and 10 ng/dl. This was misleading, as we now know that almost as many men had cancer but it was not identified during traditional **sextant biopsy**. (This is discussed in detail in the next chapter.)

Currently we believe that almost half of men with a PSA level between 4 and 10 have prostate cancer. One of the best reports was by Dr. Joseph C. Presti Jr. at Stanford University. He studied biopsies of 2,229 men and found that appropriate biopsies (as described later) detected cancer at the rates shown in table 1.

Table 1.
Likelihood of Cancer at Various PSA Levels[9]

PSA	Percent of patients found to have cancer
2–4	34
4.1–7	44
7.1–10	50
10.1–20	49
> 20	68

FREE YOUR PSA

In an effort to enhance our ability to predict the likelihood of cancer, some newer versions of PSA have been developed. The most common is **free PSA**. Unfortunately, free doesn't mean you aren't charged for it. The term is based on the fact that a majority of PSA in the bloodstream is bound to *alpha-1 antichymotrypsin* and other serum proteins. This portion is called *bound (or protein-bound) PSA*. The remaining portion floats *free* in the bloodstream, so it is called free PSA.

We know that PSA released by prostate cancer is more likely to be attached to proteins. Therefore, a high percentage of bound PSA (which is the same thing as saying a low percentage of free PSA) suggests a higher likelihood of cancer.

Although it is easy to measure the total amount of PSA in the bloodstream, it has traditionally been difficult to measure bound PSA. Therefore, we usually simply use free PSA as a percentage of the total PSA. An example might occur when a man has a PSA of 10 ng/dl. If one-fourth (2.5 ng/dl) of this PSA is free, his free PSA *as a percentage* is 25 percent.

The fact that the ratio is a calculation can lead to confusion. Notice that the free PSA reflects a percentage of the total. As a result, if the man above has the same *amount* (2.5 ng/dl) of free PSA, but has a *total* PSA of 20, his free PSA is 12.5 percent. Similarly, he might have the same *amount* of free PSA with a total PSA of 5 ng/dl. In this scenario, his free PSA would be 50 percent.

As is common in medicine, it is unclear what percentage should be considered abnormal, but most accounts put it at somewhere between 11 and 25 percent of the total. Studies have primarily looked at the use of free PSA when the total PSA is in the moderately elevated category—between 4 and 10. In this range, a free PSA below normal as defined in the previous sentence, suggests a likelihood of prostate cancer. Recent evidence suggests a low free PSA also indicates tumor aggressiveness. Further studies will be needed to confirm this.

***

The repeat PSA on Tom was 3, with 10 percent of that being free PSA. For a fifty-two-year-old businessman, it was technically abnormal on the original reading of 3.8, but potentially normal on repeat testing. The free PSA was abnormal by any parameter, although its accuracy when the total PSA is less than 4 ng/dl has not been established.

PSA DENSITY, VELOCITY, AND OTHER CONFUSIONS

A number of other PSA-related issues are pertinent to determine the probability of prostate cancer. **PSA density (PSAD)** is a concept based on the ratio of PSA to the size of the prostate. The logic is that a large prostate produces more PSA, so a man with a prostate five times normal size may make enough PSA to raise the blood level to five times normal without indicating cancer. There is some truth to this, but the overlap is too great to direct many decisions.

PSAD is calculated by dividing the PSA by the prostate gland size as measured on transrectal ultrasound. For example, if a man has a PSA of 8 and a prostate gland volume of eighty grams, his calculation would be $8 \div 80 = 0.10$. A PSAD of 0.15 or greater is considered abnormal, although some people regard 0.10 as the level. Whichever number is used, we know this is not accurate enough to justify avoiding biopsy.[10]

PSAD of the transition zone (PSA-TZ) is higher in men with prostate cancer,[11] but has also not been reliable enough to make the decision on whether to biopsy. The same calculation can determine PSA-TZ by using the volume of the **transition zone** instead of the volume of the entire prostate. Although perhaps more accurate, it is still not enough to dictate decisions.

PSA velocity, or rate of rise (also called *PSA slope*), has also failed to gain widespread acceptance for the same reason, although that may be changing. It is based on seeing a trend over several readings. The rate of rise generally considered abnormal is 0.75 ng/dl per year and its significance is emphasized by the fact that the National Cancer Care Network recommends biopsy be considered for any man who has a PSA velocity of that rate regardless of their total PSA. It may be more important prognostically than diagnostically, as men with a rise of 2 ng/dl in the year prior to diagnosis appear to have more aggressive cancers than men whose PSA rises more slowly in that duration. Therefore, PSA density, velocity, and PSA-TZ do add information. However, since they aren't specific enough to base decisions on, their use is limited.

***

PSA velocity can easily be misleading, especially at lower levels. For example, a man might have a PSA that rises from 0.2 to 0.4 in the year between checks. It would be easy to interpret this change as doubling, but both are still well within normal limits. On the other hand, a PSA that rises from 4 to 8 is much more significant. If this trend is confirmed to be real by repeated testing, it is very possible that cancer is the explanation.

PSA velocity requires at least three separate readings to establish a clear trend. Since Tom's PSA bounced from 1.3 to 3.8 to 3, there was no clear trend. As is common, PSA velocity was of no help.

MAKING IT EVEN MORE COMPLEX

In the nineties, the Bayer Company (Leverkusen, Germany) finally found a way to reliably measure PSA complexed (bound) to protein. The assay, which is called **complexed PSA**, now offers a commercially available alternative to directly measure the part of PSA that is related to cancer risk (bound) instead of measuring the part that is not (free). Even better, instead of measuring a percentage based on the total, this assay measures bound PSA directly, so it gives an absolute level instead of a percentage.

As with other tests, the level defined as abnormal is inexact, but is probably somewhere between 2.3 and 3.7 ng/dl of bound or complexed PSA. The lower of those two numbers is the value I use, but others would recommend using higher numbers, with 3.6 ng/dl used as the official "normal" cutoff.

A limitation of the complexed PSA assay is that it has not been proven significantly better than what can be obtained by simply calculating the same information from measurement of free and total PSA. If a man has a total PSA of 20 ng/dl and 25 percent of it is free, we know that 5 ng/dl is free (25 percent of 20 is 5). If 5 of the 20 ng/dl are free, then 15 of the 20 are bound or complexed (20−5=15.) The Bayer assay will measure this directly, but its value compared to simply determining it as a calculation as shown remains under investigation.

***

With 10 percent of Tom's PSA being free, we could calculate that 90 percent was bound or complexed. Therefore, we could calculate his complexed PSA by taking 90 percent of 3. (This would be 0.9 × 3 = 2.7). Therefore, his calculated complex PSA was greater than 2.3, so it was abnormal.

LIKE A PRO

A promising version of PSA recently introduced is *Pro-PSA*—a precursor that is quickly converted into PSA. It accumulates in prostate tissue so is a promising marker that is not in wide use at this writing. There are indications it may be more sensitive for detection of aggressive tumors. Another form is *BPSA*, the B standing for **BPH**. This and other forms under investigation may play a role in cancer diagnosis in the future.

WHO NEEDS A BIOPSY?

This is one of the most difficult questions we must answer. In short, men with an abnormal PSA or DRE who are healthy enough to benefit from treatment should consider having a biopsy. The long version is much more complicated.

First, no one can agree on a universal definition of abnormal PSA. The traditional cutoff of 4 ng/dl is clearly not as set in stone as some might wish. A more likely automatic cutoff is probably 2.5.

The patient's age also comes into play since we know PSA rises during a man's lifetime. In addition, we sometimes will take into account PSA density, velocity, free PSA, complex PSA, or other factors when trying to decide whether to recommend biopsy.

One clear indication for biopsy is when a nodule is present on DRE in a man healthy enough to benefit from therapy. Even with a normal PSA, this indicates a chance of prostate cancer of at least 10 percent.

Some men may not want to know they have prostate cancer. They know that most prostate cancers are not dangerous, so they simply choose to take their chances. Conversely, some men with a life expectancy of less than ten years will be unwilling to leave the diagnosis unknown. I address the issue by asking the man bluntly whether he wants or needs to know if he has prostate cancer. I explain that even if I knew he had cancer I would probably recommend **watchful waiting**. Therefore, if he is willing to make that same decision without knowing the diagnosis, it is acceptable to simply follow his wishes. We will do so unless symptoms develop or the PSA shoots so high it implies cancer is advancing rapidly (for example, over 50 ng/dl).

Many such men will understand the issues but will be unable to make such a decision until they know the diagnosis. Biopsy can help them move forward in such circumstances. Moreover, knowing the extent and grade of cancer may also shape their decision. A biopsy showing a small volume of low-grade cancer will allow the man to know the diagnosis, but also know the good prognosis. In the rare event that high-grade cancer is identified, the biopsy will allow him to consider aggressive therapy. Therefore, the long answer is that the decision must be individualized, and should involve an open and detailed discussion with your urologist on the issues involved.

WHAT LEVEL PSA ASSURES THERE IS NO CANCER?

None. Nada. The only level that assures there is no cancer is total absence of PSA. Otherwise, it is always possible to have prostate cancer, although the chance is low when the PSA is at very low levels.

The best evidence is from the Prostate Cancer Prevention Trial. Men in that study were biopsied at the end of the investigation regardless of PSA or DRE findings. Some interesting numbers came from that in men with normal PSA levels. Men with levels of 3 to 4 ng/dl—defined as "normal" until recently—had cancer 27 percent of the time. A rising PSA within the normal limits or a family history of prostate cancer made a positive biopsy even more likely. Even men with a PSA of 0.5 ng/dl had prostate cancer 6.6 percent of the time! Therefore, a low PSA doesn't rule out cancer—it just rules out a high PSA.[12]

How is this possible? To understand it, you must go back to the basics of what PSA is. It is simply a protein made in the prostate and released into the bloodstream in disease states of the prostate. Therefore, a cancer might arise that doesn't disrupt the prostatic membranes, so it doesn't release PSA. In that circumstance the PSA may remain normal.

SCREENING: THE DILEMMA

The greatest controversy in urological oncology surrounds prostate cancer screening. Some people find inadequate proof of its value. First, there is concern regarding cost. There is the chance that potentially unnecessary testing may result from a positive screening PSA in a man who ultimately turns out to have no cancer. In addition, there are risks to such testing as discussed in the next chapter.

There is also concern that screening may lead to overdiagnosis. Recall that most men with prostate cancer have **clinically insignificant** cancer. If screening identifies these cancers, men who are not at risk of dying from cancer will have the stress of learning they have a disease which sounds frightening but doesn't need to. It would actually be better if they never even knew it existed.

As noted earlier, diagnosing men whose cancers are not threatening creates a *burden of cure*. In other words, some men who don't need a cure (because their disease will not require it) may undergo surgery, radiation, or other treatments that may cause more harm than good. Thus, there is no consensus that screening accomplishes its ultimate goal—saving lives. If it does not, then screening adds cost, stress, and possible risk without payoff.

Although most urologists believe screening is of great value, you need to understand the controversy in order to decide for yourself whether prostate cancer screening is for you. The remainder of this chapter will attempt to present a fair and balanced view of the controversy.

SCREENING VERSUS EARLY DETECTION

It is important to understand the difference between **screening** and **early detection**. The terms are often used interchangeably. This is misleading, in that most such testing is actually more accurately described as early detection. *Early diagnosis* is another term appropriately applied.

Screening is randomly looking for disease. An example might involve performing a chest x-ray on everyone in your community. With little reason to suspect anyone in town has lung cancer, this screening program would probably not be successful. It would be costly and time consuming, and might not find anyone with lung cancer. Everyone in town would experience the stress of waiting for results that almost surely would be normal.

Some citizens *without* lung cancer might have an abnormal chest x-ray. This could be due to scarring from previous infections, or might simply be a spot that is inexplicable but not malignant. This is called a *false positive* test—it is read as positive but there is actually no cancer. These people would require further costly testing, including biopsies or other x-rays to prove they don't have cancer. With any medical test there is risk, so some of them might suffer consequences despite being perfectly healthy in the first place.

No medical test is perfect, so the screening program might miss some people who actually do have early lung cancer. Their chest x-ray might be normal even though they have cancer (*false negative*).

The only people who would benefit in that scenario are those with early lung cancer who wouldn't have known about it otherwise. Nonetheless, lung cancer is an especially virulent disease that is often incurable, so screening might have not even helped those with the disease.

In contrast, *early detection* involves identifying disease in people who are either symptomatic or at high risk. In the above example, replacing the screening program with an early detection program would change a lot. First, everyone under the age of fifty might be excluded. Nonsmokers at low risk might be left out as well. An early detection program might focus further on those with a chronic cough and/or weight loss. This would save the cost and unnecessary testing on most members of the community, concentrating resources on those who were most likely to benefit. If successful, some smokers with a cough might be found to have early lung cancer. With luck, some of them would be caught in time for cure.

Applying the above criteria to prostate cancer, **screening** would involve checking a PSA and DRE on everyone. In contrast, an *early detection* program would automatically eliminate all women (obviously), and those too young to be likely to have prostate cancer. It would emphasize at-risk groups, such as men with a family history of prostate cancer and African American men. Men presenting to the doctor with urologic symptoms or concerns of prostate cancer might be tested as well. Finally, men of an age known to be associated with prostate cancer would be included.

Unlike a virulent disease such as lung cancer, an early detection program for prostate cancer would also take into account the fact that it is typically a slowly progressive disease. Therefore, a man's life expectancy should be in the equation. Men whose health or age are such that they could not live long enough for the cancer to become life threatening would be excluded because they would not gain from knowing of a disease they didn't need to treat. This might leave out all those over a certain age.

Such are current recommendations for prostate cancer early detection, usually referred to as screening. The American Urological Association (AUA) recommends that all men over age fifty be tested. Men at increased risk—those with a family history of prostate cancer and African American men—should be evaluated beginning at the age of forty. The American Cancer Society has similar recommendations, although forty-five is the age suggested for men at increased risk.

The above organizations simply recommend screening as shown. The National Cancer Care Network takes it a step further, recommending a PSA test be performed on all men at age forty. If their PSA is 0.5 ng/dl or less, a repeat at ages forty-five and fifty is recommended. However, if the PSA is 0.6 ng/dl or greater annual screening is indicated, based on the knowledge that even minimal rises in PSA could be an early sign of prostate cancer. In addition, it is recommended biopsy be performed for any man with PSA of 2.6 ng/dl or greater.

Some other organizations take a less dogmatic view. The American Academy of Family Practice has deemed that there is no standard to recommend. The American College of Physicians recommends the doctor describe the "potential benefits and known harms of screening, diagnosis and treatment; listen to the patient's concerns, then individualize the decision to screen." The American Medical Association suggests providing information regarding the risks and potential benefits. Because the term "screening" is so prevalent, we will use it interchangeably with "early detection."

REASONS TO SCREEN

We have already noted that there are several problems regarding screening. However, there are also strong reasons to do so. The best evidence that screening saves lives comes from the National Cancer Institute's (NCI) SEER database. This large nationwide representative survey that looks at cancer incidence and death derives its name from the acronym for surveillance, epidemiology, and end results. The database shows a decreasing mortality curve occurring around the midnineties. The timing corresponds to the time frame one might expect if cancer screening were to have an impact—a few years after PSA screening became widespread.

As noted in figure 11-1, SEER identified an increase in cancer cases as well as cancer deaths around the time screening began in the late eighties.[13] Fortunately, there was a reversal soon thereafter, with prostate cancer diagnosis and deaths falling significantly, as shown in figure 11-2. Some critics point out that the decrease in mortality may be too soon to be the result of screening. They suggest that better treatments or undefined factors may be responsible for the drop in death rate. Thus, this remains controversial.

Nevertheless, we know that prostate cancer mortality has dropped between 22 percent and 69 percent in Austria,[14] Quebec,[15] and Olmstead County, Minnesota[16] in the presence of aggressive screening programs. To be fair, sporadic areas have reported decreased prostate cancer death rates without screening programs in place, but the purposeful nature of these programs combined with these impressive results leads to a compelling argument for the potential of screening.

Prostate cancer is the most age-dependent malignancy. As we age, the incidence goes up—period. Therefore, as the population ages overall, more men develop cancer. This makes the decreasing death rate even more significant as a smaller number of those developing the disease eventually succumb to it.

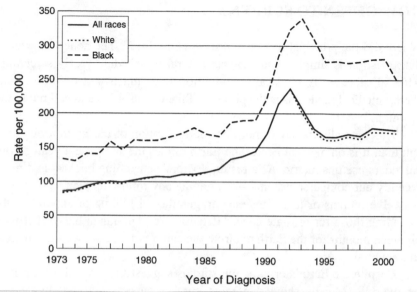

Data from the National Cancer Institute's SEER database shows that the incidence of prostate cancer rose significantly following the identification of PSA as a screening tool (figure 11-1, above). Prostate cancer mortality was rising around the same time. However, note that the incidence began to decrease significantly within a few years. More importantly, mortality began to decrease and is now lower than it has been in years (figure 11-2, below).

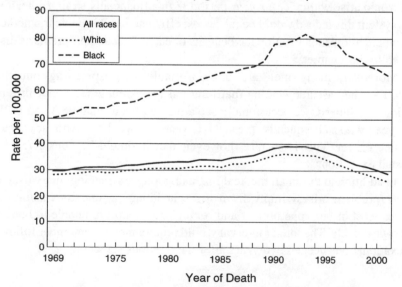

HOW OFTEN TO SCREEN?

Where did the principal of yearly testing come from? The honest answer to that question is simple. It just *seems* natural to schedule yearly screening. After all, the yearly physical examination is as much part of the Marcus Welby medical model, as is the phrase, "Take two aspirins and call me in the morning."

This mentality is based more on the revolution of the Earth around the sun than it is on medical need. The Earth circles the sun once a year, so our calendars use this metric. As a result, doctors' scheduling books—and more recently our computer systems—can handle any follow-up plan as long as it is twelve months or less. This encourages the scheduling of appointments, including those for prostate cancer detection, on an annual basis. If it took eighteen months for the Earth to circle the sun, I am sure we would screen at that interval.

Despite the Earth's orbit, some studies suggest that annual testing may be overkill. Models show that *most* curable cancers detected by annual screening will also be curable under a screening program performed every two years.[17] Other studies suggest that screening might yield higher cure rates and decrease unnecessary testing if started at even younger ages. In that model, lower-risk men based on low PSA values would be tested less frequently, focusing resources and attention on those men likely to benefit.[18]

One study found that a single PSA measurement identified most cancers that would arise within a *four-year* period.[19] In a financially strapped healthcare system this indeed would be more cost efficient, but it is unclear whether this would allow men to enjoy the benefits of early detection programs as discussed in this chapter.

Moreover, many men are uncomfortable with spreading out the schedule. They assume waiting that long risks something bad happening in the interim. Indeed, we occasionally see a man with a normal PSA and DRE one year who subsequently presents a year or two later with advanced prostate cancer. This is so rare, however, that it should be considered an unusual exception.

In addition to the small medical risk using longer screening intervals, the bigger problem arises simply from the scheduling complexity mentioned above. Most of our appointment and reminder systems are unable to handle a two-year cycle. The longer interval would require men to remember follow-up examinations needed two years after the previous screening.

WHAT ABOUT THE WARNINGS ABOUT SCREENING?

Although you now know my advocacy for early detection, it is only fair to discuss the alternative standpoint. Opposition has softened as more data accumulate on the value of early detection. The United States Preventive Services Task Force originally opposed screening in the nineties because of insufficient proof of its merit, but has softened its stance to neutral as evidence mounts. Instead of opposition, the task force now feels that the data do not yet prove whether we should screen or not.

Critics want the patient to know that screening is controversial. They want him to know that PSA is imperfect—it may be elevated in the absence of cancer, or may be normal in its presence. They want him to understand that further testing may be required to determine whether the elevated PSA is caused by cancer or something else. Finally, they want him to understand that **clinically insignificant** cancer may be exposed, leading to over treatment and all its implications. Unfortunately, once detected, it can be difficult to determine whether your cancer is truly significant unless it is very low grade.

Some primary care groups advocate the position that the patient should be informed of the risks and benefits prior to screening, and some even advocate having the patient sign a consent form acknowledging he understands all the risks, benefits, and alternatives to screening.

This book demonstrates my agreement with these concerns—each man should make an informed decision in collaboration with his doctor on all issues regarding the prostate. That includes the decision on early detection. Several pages are devoted herein to the information required to make the decision.

However, some of these groups' recommendations sound fine on a position paper but don't work in the real world. Primary care physicians are overextended; their focus is (appropriately) divided among concerns for every organ system. During the time available for a routine checkup, there is no way they can adequately meet the demands required by such recommendations. The facts are complex, ranging from cost to risk to the controversial value to the risk of overdiagnosis. Meanwhile, their visit must also encompass management of the entire patient. Cardiovascular, lung, kidney, gastrointestinal, and any number of other issues must be considered. The recommendations are laudable and idealistic, but not always realistic.

As a result, an early detection program must be simple and complete if there is any hope of success. Therefore, annual testing remains our best alternative at present.

WHEN TO STOP SCREENING?

This issue is a sensitive one. Recall that most recommendations are based on the expectation that a man will live long and well enough to benefit from early detection. The logical extension is that screening should be discontinued when that is no longer the case. A common cutoff applied is somewhere between seventy and eighty years old.

Not surprisingly, most men who reach that empirical cutoff age don't consider themselves unfit for screening. "Are you saying I'm too old?" is a common objection. More biting is "age discrimination."

Neither is the case. It is simply a matter of honestly facing the fact that prostate cancer in a man with a life expectancy of less than ten years is unlikely to cause enough problems to justify investigation. Men screened in that circumstance may undergo the risk, cost, and stress of testing that has little or no chance of improving their quality or quantity of life. Therefore, finding out they have clinically insignificant prostate cancer may be of no value and could be detrimental.

My approach to this issue is to inform men of the above facts in a non-judgmental manner. Instead of an arbitrary cutoff age, such as seventy, I try to assess their realistic health and life expectancy. If it is likely to be less than ten years, I tell them that discontinuing testing is an option thereafter.

Even after being informed of the facts, few men who have diligently followed their PSA for years will abandon screening the first time the issue comes up. Some will eventually come around with continued reinforcement each subsequent year, but some will request follow-up years after we would no longer consider treating asymptomatic cancer.

TOM'S DECISION

The screening decision for Tom was made well before I met him—the PSA was elevated. Tom and I discussed most of the above issues as they related to his situation. A case could be made either way—to biopsy or not to biopsy. His PSA (between 3 and 3.8 ng/dl, depending on which reading we used) was technically normal by historical standards, so the knee-jerk reaction was to leave it alone. However, it was abnormal for his young age, and also by the 2.5 ng/dl cutoff that many urologists currently use. The velocity was completely confusing with no clear trend. His free PSA (10 percent) and calculated complexed PSA (2.7) were both abnormal. The positive family history raised suspicion.

Despite a large amount of objective data to help us decide whether to do a biopsy, one subjective issue was also in the equation. Tom had watched his father deal with prostate cancer. The unknown was too frightening for him to tolerate. We agreed on the decision—a biopsy was in order.

KEY POINTS

- PSA is the best tumor marker ever identified. However, it is still only a tool to predict the likelihood of cancer.
- The normal level of PSA rises with aging, but most men should probably have a PSA below 2.5 to be considered normal. A level higher than that doesn't automatically require biopsy, but you should discuss it with your physician.
- A number of forms of PSA are now available to assist in the decision, including free PSA, complexed PSA, and other emerging variants.
- The American Urological Association recommends all men over age fifty with a life expectancy of at least a decade be tested with DRE and PSA annually.
- Men at increased risk—those with a family history of prostate cancer and African American men—should be evaluated beginning between the ages of forty and forty-five.
- The value of prostate cancer early detection programs is controversial, but evidence is emerging to suggest that mortality is decreased substantially in populations aggressively screened.
- No one ever died of PSA. The concern is not its level; the concern is why it is elevated.

12.
DIAGNOSING PROSTATE CANCER: TRANSRECTAL ULTRASOUND AND BIOPSY

Couldn't another place for the prostate (have) been found?
—Bert Gottlieb, in *The Men's Club*

After going through the steps discussed in the previous chapter, most men suspected of having prostate cancer that are healthy enough to benefit from treatment will undergo prostate **biopsy**. Until recently, biopsy was often an objectionable prospect. It elicited immediate thoughts of embarrassment and fear of cancer. Pain was expected, although men were usually told it didn't really hurt. Finally, biopsy missed approximately half of all cancers, so careful follow-up was necessary in order to find the rest. This chapter will depict a markedly different story.

WHAT IS A BIOPSY?

The term "**biopsy**" is defined in its verb form as removing living tissue from the body. This procedure is followed by staining the tissue with special agents that help identify abnormalities, so a pathologist can subsequently examine the tissues under the microscope. In addition, the term can be used as a noun to refer to the tissue itself.

The biopsy is obtained by a clinician (a urologist usually, although a radiologist does the procedure in a few institutions). Although surgery is still an occasional source of prostate tissue, we now usually perform a biopsy in the office by placing a needle through a transrectal ultrasound probe into the prostate.

Some physicians will allow you to see the tissue removed. I do if the patient asks, but most men have no desire to see their own tissues. The fragments are smaller than a pencil lead and are so flimsy that they may look like little smears on the paper holding them. There is rarely significant blood remaining on the sample, so they're not especially "gross." However, if you easily become nauseated by anything medical, you may choose not to look. After all, that's the pathologist's job, not yours. (A pathologist is a physician who specializes in such laboratory examinations that evaluate the presence, absence, and qualities of a disease from the biopsy.)

STICKING TO THE POINT: BIOPSY

In the early twentieth century, prostate biopsy was a major operation performed under general anesthesia. Prior to the identification of PSA, there was no way to suspect cancer unless we could feel it, so we found malignancy only when it became large enough to detect on DRE. The only other way we detected it was coincidentally when the specimen removed during a TURP might contain "occult" or unsuspected cancer in up to one-fourth of cases.

In the middle of the twentieth century, the invention of hollow needles that passed through the perineal skin to obtain a small "core" of tissue eventually allowed biopsy without major surgery. However, these initial needles were large and painful. In addition, they were difficult to master, making tissue sampling inconsistent.

Three advances converged in the late eighties to create a revolution in the diagnosis of prostate cancer. First was the identification of PSA,[1] followed by the invention of spring-loaded biopsy "guns" that allowed sampling of consistent quality cores.[2] Transrectal guidance for biopsy allowed accuracy. We learned that men with an elevated PSA had a higher risk of cancer that could not be felt by DRE, and that we could detect it earlier using a systematic *sextant* (six-core) biopsy technique, which sampled seemingly normal tissue to find cancers before they became obvious.[3] Refinements since that time have led to even greater accuracy with improved acceptability from the patient's standpoint.

PREPARING FOR THE BIOPSY: ANTIBIOTICS AND ENEMAS

The measures necessary to prepare for prostate biopsy are controversial. Although some reports indicate a lower infection rate when enemas are used, these reports may be biased and may simply reflect different patient populations or surgeon preferences.[4] The rectum is actually empty except during defecation (bowel movement), so an enema may actually increase the amount of stool present during biopsy. Moreover, an enema will potentially introduce air into the rectum, which could interfere with visualization during ultrasound. Finally, patients clearly don't relish the idea of using an enema unless it will unequivocally yield benefit, so I don't recommend them for my patients who are having a biopsy unless they suffer chronic constipation.

To be fair, many of my colleagues do recommend enemas, so there is no consensus. However, I use a general rule of thumb that unless something is clearly shown to yield benefit, I don't recommend it because it has the possibility of causing harm. This precludes a recommendation for routine enemas.

Antibiotics should be given for men undergoing biopsy, but urologists also don't all agree on which one or how many doses. A recent study showed that the recommendations are all over the map,[5] so trusting your physician's recommendation is probably best. I use an approach similar to that regarding enemas: simplicity. Since no method has been shown to be clearly better, I recommend a single dose of a drug from the *flouroquinolone* class of antibiotics for most men I biopsy. Alternatively, some urologists will use medications from almost every class of antibiotics and have good success with preventing infections. Many use extended dosing of up to seven days as well.

Additional antibiotics are especially appropriate in three circumstances. Patients who have a urinary tract infection or prostatitis need antibiotics to treat—not prevent—infection. Since infection should be treated before performing biopsy, this situation should be rare. The second situation is for men at increased risk of infection following biopsy. This would involve either a history of infection or recent catheterization or instrumentation. Immunosuppressed men are also at increased risk. Finally, the American Heart Association recommends that men with heart valve problems receive specific antibiotics before undergoing any invasive procedure, including prostate biopsy. The recommended antibiotics lessen the chance that bacteria will migrate to the heart to cause rare but serious complications. If you have been given such instruction, make sure your urologist is aware of it. He will know the protocol and intercede accordingly.

BLOOD THINNERS

Anticoagulants are medications that make bleeding less likely to stop. Although often called "blood thinners," they really don't thin the blood. For that matter, they also don't actually cause bleeding—they simply block the coagulation cascade that is supposed to stop bleeding once it starts.

A good way to understand this principle is to think of someone on an anticoagulant or "blood thinner" that cuts himself shaving. Unless the cut occurs, he will not bleed at all. The anticoagulant certainly won't cut the face by itself. However, once the skin is physically cut, the body won't be able to stop the bleeding as quickly or effectively with an anticoagulant present. Whereas bleeding might stop with a little simple pressure under normal circumstances, it may persist all morning if the man is using an anticoagulant. In addition, a little movement like a sneeze or a smile might cause the bleeding to start again more easily if the dried clot on top breaks off.

If this same man has a prostate biopsy, there is a chance of bleeding simply from a needle going into the prostate through the rectal wall. Most people have heard of hemorrhoids—dilated or enlarged veins near the rectum that can bleed, most often related to straining on them while constipated. What most people don't understand is that the hemorrhoidal veins are actually blood vessels that are normally present in the rectal wall. Therefore, even if the man doesn't clinically exhibit hemorrhoids, the veins are still there in the path of the biopsy needle, so a majority of patients will encounter minor bleeding. It usually resolves in a matter of days. However, about 1 percent of the time, bleeding requires attention.

Although we know bleeding is possible during biopsy, most anticoagulants will cause minimal increased risk. Aspirin and other medications from the NSAID category (e.g., ibuprofen, naproxen, Celebrex, Bextra, and several others) impair the ability of platelets to stop bleeding. The effect of aspirin on any given platelet is permanent, so new *platelets* must be generated. It normally takes three to seven days to replace an adequate number of inhibited platelets. The other drugs from this class have a temporary effect, so their inhibition of clotting is gone within twenty-four to forty-eight hours as the body clears the drug from its bloodstream.

Under ideal circumstances, all anticoagulants will be discontinued. However, multiple studies and our own experience at the Cleveland Clinic Foundation have shown that biopsy can be performed safely while taking aspirin or other NSAIDs if there is a risk from stopping them. The bottom line is that you should discuss this with your physician in order to assure that you make the right—and safest—decision for you.

Warfarin (*coumadin*) actually blocks clotting. You should stop taking it for several days prior to biopsy. The duration of this period should be determined by the prescribing physician and your urologist.

Some newer blood thinners, such as *Plavix* (*clopidogrel*) and *Ticlid* (*ticlopidine*) can lead to serious bleeding and should be discontinued under these circumstances. If your physician feels you need these too much to discontinue for a few days, you should ask whether you are healthy enough to benefit from biopsy as discussed above.

Also, recall that vitamin E is a blood thinner. Make sure your doctor knows you use it before you have any invasive procedure, and remember to stop taking it several days before the biopsy in order to minimize the chance of bleeding.

TRANSRECTAL ULTRASOUND: GUIDE TO THE BIOPSY

Once the decision is made to perform a biopsy, you might undergo the procedure on the day of the decision, but you will more likely be scheduled to return. A later visit is especially likely if your urologist recommends prolonged antibiotics, an enema, or discontinuation of anticoagulants. In addition, it offers time to plan for the procedure and to assure that nothing crucial is scheduled in the following twenty-four hours that would present problems if complications occur.

Someone will take you into an ultrasound room, usually located in the doctor's office. (Some physicians don't want to or can't commit the resources to invest the significant cost of a prostate ultrasound machine, so they will perform the procedure in the hospital radiology area or operating room). You will probably be asked to undress from the waist down (leaving socks on) and will be given a sheet or hospital gown.

Most urologists prefer the patient to lie on his left side with his buttocks placed on the lower corner of the examining table almost hanging off the table. This allows maneuverability of the ultrasound probe, which becomes important later in the procedure. Flexing the knees toward the chest allows access to the rectum for biopsy ease.

The ultrasound probe is placed gently through the *anal sphincter*, using a great deal of lubrication to assure that it slips in atraumatically. Most urologists will do this slowly and with care to minimize pain. Although a certain amount of discomfort is not cause for alarm, a doctor (or his technologist) who shoves it in may raise instant concern that his interest in your well-being is not as high as it should be. Once the probe is in, the prostate is quickly visualized and the urologist will look for visible abnormalities in the prostate that might indicate the possibility of cancer. The probe is shown in position in figure 12-1.

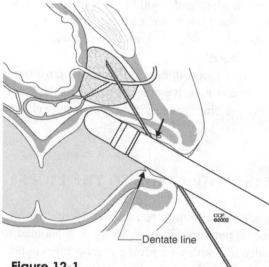

Dentate line

Figure 12-1.

Early *ultrasonographers* placed great faith in the ability of the ultrasound image to identify cancer. Initially, they thought that *hyperechoic* locations (areas that appear whiter or echo more ultrasound waves) were cancerous. They soon found that the opposite was true—that *hypoechoic* locations (areas that are darker because they reflect fewer ultrasound waves) were more likely to contain cancer. Such an abnormal-appearing area is shown in figure 12-2. The problem was that the presence of either one could not reliably identify cancer. Abnormal-appearing areas indeed were slightly more likely to contain cancer, but completely normal appearing areas could also harbor cancer. Only a minority of prostate cancers are actually visible on ultrasound. This is primarily due to the fact they are infiltrative (blending into the adjacent tissue) instead of distinct nodules. In fact, even if a nodule is palpable, we often will be unable to see it on ultrasound even when we know where to look.

This observation led Dr. Tom Stamey and his associates at Stanford in 1989 to describe the **systematic biopsy**. Instead of simply performing biopsies on areas that felt abnormal or looked abnormal on ultrasound, they performed a series of six random biopsies in all men who underwent ultrasound based on the indication of an elevated PSA. As it turns out, they found that many of the men whose prostates looked normal on ultrasound actually had significant malignancies that would have been overlooked unless the normal-appearing areas were biopsied. Because they obtained a whopping six cores (it was unheard of at the time to simply stick a needle into a normal appearing prostate for biopsy), their biopsies were called **sextant biopsies**. Their landmark publication[6] caused controversy initially for the concern of complications from performing multiple needle biopsies on prostate glands that were previously believed to be normal. The greater stir occurred when urologists realized that the systematic biopsy would allow identification of huge numbers of curable cancers previously overlooked. When this finding closely followed the identification of PSA and the invention of the spring-loaded biopsy gun, it was the final piece in the trifecta that allowed the number of prostate cancer diagnoses to explode.

Before Stamey's introduction of the systematic biopsy, most urologists would simply examine the prostate using an ultrasound on a man who had an elevated PSA. If they saw an abnormality, they would then perform a biopsy; if it appeared normal, biopsies were usually avoided. It soon became clear that *if there is a reason to perform transrectal ultrasound looking for cancer, the patient should receive a systematic biopsy no matter what the ultrasound shows.*

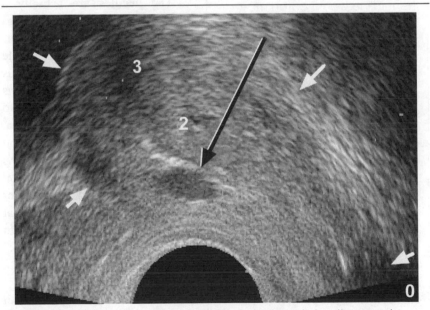

Figure 12-2. The dark zone identified during prostate ultrasound (arrow) is suspicious for malignancy. However, biopsy of this area confirmed that this was actually not a cancer. This example is common, since we know that abnorma-appearing areas are often benign, while normal-appearing areas are often malignant. Therefore, the appearance may help direct biopsy locations, but a normal appearing prostate does not rule out prostate cancer.

In medicine, it is sometimes interesting to note how a specific method arises. I asked Dr. Stamey why he chose six cores when he began doing **systematic** biopsies. He told me that his group simply recognized that routine biopsy techniques missed many of the cancers that they later identified on radical prostatectomy specimens. Therefore, if these additional cancers were missed, it was likely that many men without nodules also had cancers that were missed. They therefore decided that six samples taken in a distribution down each side of the midline would catch most cancers of any significant size.

To Dr. Stamey's credit, he recognized before anyone else that most cancers actually originated lateral to where his original biopsy sites were.[7] Thus, he found that simply moving his sextant technique laterally improved his cancer detection rate significantly. Multiple investigators, including our group at the Cleveland Clinic Foundation, have subsequently confirmed this.

Interestingly, Dr. Stamey has more recently been one of the most vocal critics of aggressive screening. He feels that we are identifying too many men with **clinically insignificant** prostate cancer and should be paring back our efforts.[8] This controversy will persist for some time until we are able to determine accurately who needs treatment and who can be safely observed.

TO THE POINT

The actual biopsy involves placing a small needle (about the size of the needle used to draw blood for the PSA) through a small channel in the ultrasound probe. It passes through the rectal wall and into the prostate tissue. The biopsy occurs very rapidly using a spring-loaded biopsy gun, an instrument that pushes in the needle in a split second so that tissue is obtained accurately even if the patient moves.

The needles are actually a fairly ingenious invention (see figures 12-3 and 12-4). An inner cutting portion protrudes out a little less than an inch. This portion has a cut-out segment on one side as shown that allows prostate tissue to fill quickly into the hollowed area. This prostate tissue will soon become the actual biopsy core. As soon as the inner cutting portion stops, an outer cylinder slides over it to shear off the tissue core that has filled in the hollowed area. In the time it takes to hear a "pop," the biopsy needle has secured a piece of prostate inside.

Because of the speed with which this occurs, the tissues samples are amazingly consistent in size and length. Unfortunately, the spring-loaded mechanism currently required to create this rapid double-action makes a loud pop-

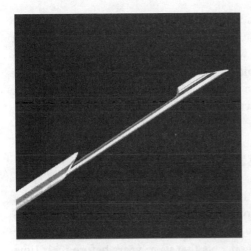

Figure 12-3. The biopsy needle has an inner cannula that springs forward into the prostate tissue. An outer sheath follows in a split second, shearing off a core of tissue that may be sent to the pathologist to examine to determine whether cancer is present. (Courtesy of Cook Urological)

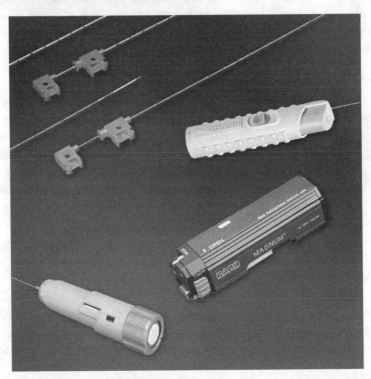

Figure 12-4. A variety of different biopsy "guns" are available. To date, all depend on a firing mechanism based on a spring-loaded force to push the inner cannula and outer sheath into the prostate in a split second. (Courtesy of Bard)

ping noise that patients find disquieting. This is no surprise, since a stranger is behind them, holding a sharp instrument inside the rectum that makes a loud noise each time it fires. Since we know how to block the pain of prostate biopsy (see below), this noise is often the most unpleasant part of having it done. We are currently working on ways to eliminate this pop, but have not yet solved the problem as of this writing.

THE MORE THE MERRIER?

Soon after Dr. Stamey described the **sextant systematic biopsy**, questions arose regarding whether the six cores obtained in the specific locations he chose were optimal. In short, they weren't. That doesn't mean Dr. Stamey was wrong—indeed he identified concepts that were years before their time regarding a systematic sampling technique. It's just that now we know that even more biopsies performed in more specifically chosen locations were required in order to find most cancers and complete the process that he started.

Multiple other investigators confirmed Dr. Stamey's finding that cancer detection is improved when biopsies are obtained laterally, but an even greater increase occurred when combining this concept with a greater numbers of cores. Common sense tells us that if we sample the prostate for cancer using a small needle, there is a real possibility that we can miss the cancer purely based on the mathematic probability of hitting a little target with a little weapon. If we shoot the weapon (needle) at the prostate more times, we have a greater chance of hitting the area of interest, which in this case is the cancer.

HOW MANY ARE ENOUGH?

Urologists do not agree on the ideal number, but those keeping up with current concepts all agree that six is not enough. Our own studies suggest that up to half or more of cancers may be missed by a single traditional sextant biopsy.[9]

As we increase the number of cores we will obviously reach diminishing returns, missing fewer and fewer cancers. The current medical literature indicates that the bare minimum is to obtain eight laterally based cores. Most urologists will perform ten to twelve cores. If biopsy did not identify cancer and there is still suspicion, many urologists will perform a **saturation biopsy**, which typically obtains twenty or more cores.[10] With this many shots, the chance of missing a cancer of any significant size appears to be small, so it may be preferable to do a saturation biopsy once instead of bringing the patient back for multiple sextant biopsies.

Saturation biopsy remains controversial because some urologists are hesitant to perform that many sticks, but we have found that complications are no higher than in traditional biopsy.[11] In addition, some urologists are concerned that we may be more likely to detect **clinically insignificant** tumors, although the likelihood of this remains debatable. Saturation biopsy is described in detail later.

DOES BIOPSY HURT? IT DEPENDS ON WHICH END OF THE NEEDLE YOU'RE ON

Before transrectal ultrasound allowed more direct access, biopsies were performed through the **perineal** skin. Urologists routinely injected local anesthetic into the tissues to block biopsy pain. However, with the introduction of transrectal ultrasound, we knew that the rectum has no sensory pain fibers. Therefore, urologists accepted that biopsy by that route was painless and local anesthesia was unnecessary. We would tell patients they would feel "a little stick" but that it would not hurt. Boy, were we wrong!

In retrospect, I was as guilty as anyone of trivializing this pain. We didn't have a good way to anesthetize the area because our understanding of pelvic nerve anatomy was poor, so we chose instead to use *okay anesthesia* ("It's okay, sir, it's okay . . ."). It wasn't okay.

That changed in 1997 when investigators from the University of California, San Francisco, described injection of local anesthetic into the nerves at the base of the prostate that blocked pain during biopsy on the injected side.[12] Even this did not have much impact on urological practice until Dr. Mark Soloway and his team at the University of Miami confirmed that it worked and began publicizing the benefits.[13] Finally, many of us (ahem, me included) saw the error of our ways and began to investigate why and how anesthetic block works. Since that time, innumerable reports have confirmed what becomes obvious to the urologist immediately upon adapting the technique: prostate biopsy hurts . . . but it doesn't have to.

Once my friend Dr. Michael Koch—chairman of urology at Indiana University—convinced me to try it, I recognized that its effectiveness was obvious on the very first patient. I immediately adapted anesthetic injection for prostate biopsy—termed **periprostatic block**.

However, I also realized that most urologists still underutilized the technique. The approach was reminiscent of the old doctor joke, "It won't hurt *me* a bit." I therefore began advocating the position that the pain involved depended on which end of the needle you're on. During my course on the subject in Chicago at the 2001 Annual Meeting of the North Central Section of the American Urological Association, a urologist who had been treated for prostate cancer told me that he'd been on both ends of the needle (presumably at different times). He said he understood from the first time he was on the sharp end why it was so much easier to convince a patient to have his first biopsy than it was to convince him to have a second biopsy if needed. That should have told us something.

How Much Does It Hurt Without Anesthesia?

The way we quantify pain in medicine is by use of a *visual analog scale (VAS)*—a ten-centimeter line drawn on a sheet of paper with the number zero on one end with a smiley face, indicating no pain and on the other end the number ten with a frowning face, indicating the worst pain the patient has ever experienced. A severe sprain might rate in the four to five range. Most studies find that patients rate the pain of prostate biopsy between four and five on that ten-point scale unless anesthesia is used. Fortunately, if we inject local anesthetic we can reliably block this pain. Our pain scores are about 1.4 on that ten-point VAS.

The most alarming report regarding the pain of prostate biopsy without anesthetic block found that 96 percent of patients said that biopsy hurt (a pretty convincing number—maybe the other 4 percent were just being tough guys?). In addition, one in five men in that study stated they would refuse another biopsy even if indicated unless they received anesthesia.[14] Other reports have shown that up to one-third of patients who had no anesthetic block will refuse the recommendation for repeat biopsy despite concern that cancer is present.[15] Fortunately, we have now changed all that.

Periprostatic Block: Prostate Anesthesia for Painless Biopsy

A single group of nerves on each side of the prostate appears to be responsible for pain sensation in the gland. We can block these nerve bundles by injecting a local anesthetic agent into the area where the *seminal vesicles* enter the prostate (see chapter 2 for a description of this anatomy). Since lido-caine works immediately, the prostate is numb from the moment of injection. We have also shown that even the longer-acting *bupivacaine* (*Marcaine*) works immediately for this purpose if a longer duration of action is desired.[16]

Figure 12-5 shows the needle placed in the proper spot for local anes-thetic injection. Since the rectum has no pain fibers at this level, the injection is virtually pain free. The urologist can easily see this location on ultrasound by visualizing a white pyramid of fat that exists in the notch between sem-inal vesicles and prostate. In order to facilitate teaching other urologists how to perform the procedure, I named this the **Mount Everest Sign** in 2001 based on the white appearance that looks like the famous snowy peak (see figure 12-6).

When local anesthetic is injected into the area as shown, you will note the dark fluid dissecting between the prostate and the rectal wall. This *ultra-sonic wheal*[17] indicates that all the branches have been blocked by the injec-tion. Although some urologists inject at several different sites on each side, I have found that allowing the fluid to migrate as shown assures adequate anesthesia without additional injections. Alternatively, some even perform a single injection in the middle, allowing the anesthetic to dissect each direc-tion. The exact technique isn't nearly as important as simply using *any* tech-nique. As long as your urologist can prevent pain, you're ahead.

Does It Work? Does It Ever!

Recall that patients typically rate the pain of prostate biopsy between four and five on a ten-point VAS without anesthesia. Indeed, our study at the Cleveland Clinic Foundation had the same results in control patients (who received no anesthesia) when we initially investigated the role of peripro-static block in 2001.[18] I had been convinced of its effectiveness from the first time I tried it, but many urologists remained skeptical. Even my own col-leagues were until we began a randomized, controlled trial where half of patients received a periprostatic block and half (the *control* patients) had their biopsy performed the traditional way, without anesthesia.

Those who received no anesthesia had a predictable average VAS of 4.5. However, those who received a periprostatic block had an amazingly low VAS of 1.4—not much more than the level of pain experienced with combing your hair. Even better, whereas a majority of patients in the control group had moderate to severe pain, only a single patient who received a block experi-enced even moderate pain. That man, with the most severe pain in the entire

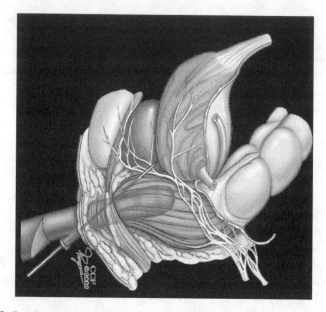

Figure 12-5. Injection of a local anesthetic into the area where the sensory nerves enter the prostate allows the urologist to perform biopsy essentially pain free. The needle is shown at the proper location at the base of the prostate.

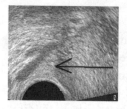

Figure 12-6. The urologist performs a periprostatic block under ultrasound guidance. This illustration shows the white pyramid recognized as the Mount Everest Sign that serves as his landmark to know that he is in the proper location. (Courtesy Bard, Inc.)

block group, had a VAS of four, still less than the *average* score for patients in the control group. My colleagues were so convinced of the results that we had to close the study early, prior to completing enrollment. No one would agree to do any more biopsies without periprostatic block, even on an investigational basis! For those involved, the days of prostate biopsy without periprostatic block had ended.

***

"I want to be put to sleep," Tom declared as we arranged an appointment for his biopsy.

Respectful of his concerns, I firmly countered, "That's not necessary, and in fact . . ."

His wife, Anne, interrupted before I could finish. "It may not be necessary, but we want it anyway. We don't want him going through the things his father did. Put him to sleep."

"That's an option," I assured, "but I'm not sure it's what you really want to do. Let's talk about it." Talk was not on their minds. "Let me at least make sure you understand the issues." I proceeded to discuss the advances in prostate biopsy techniques as noted above, emphasizing the ability to get the patient comfortably through the procedure in the office. I explained that putting Tom under general anesthesia would essentially involve a hospitalization. He would miss a day of work, and Anne would as well in order to drive him home, since he would be under the influence of strong drugs. He might become nauseated or have other lingering effects of general anesthesia. In addition, it is more difficult to adequately biopsy the prostate under anesthesia because it is harder to position the patient optimally for ultrasound probe placement. Cost was the least significant issue.

For this combination of reasons, I informed them that I hadn't performed a single biopsy in the operating room under general anesthesia for the past three and a half years. I had done hundreds of biopsies in that interval using periprostatic block. "As it turns out," I concluded, "doing the biopsy under anesthesia is actually a disadvantage for a long list of reasons."

Alternatively, Tom could work most of the day and still drive himself to the clinic for an office-based biopsy under periprostatic block. The time involvement alone was enough to make them consider the suggestion.

"Are you sure you can control the pain?"

With knowledge of the experiences described in this chapter, the response was easy. "I'm sure."

Risks of Periprostatic Block

Complications appear to be no more common in men who have a block than in those who do not. Common sense would dictate that additional needle sticks might cause more bleeding, infection, or swelling. However, multiple reports have shown that the complication rates appear to be unchanged (unless you consider pain a complication—it is far *less* likely with a block). In fact, bleeding may actually be less when a block is administered, possibly related to decreased pain.[19]

When we first began giving these blocks, some physicians (who apparently recalled experiences in a dentist's chair) gave large doses of lidocaine out of concern that smaller doses might not be effective. That led to the occasional patient becoming light-headed if too much lidocaine was absorbed into the bloodstream. Bringing the doses to more reasonable levels has allowed us to avoid this complication completely.

Another concern has been whether scarring from injection into these nerves might make it more difficult to spare the nerves at the time of prostate surgery in order to preserve potency. This has not been shown in the published literature, and has not been our experience in more than five hundred patients operated on at the Cleveland Clinic Foundation following periprostatic block.

MANAGING COMPLICATIONS OF PROSTATE BIOPSY

Minor annoyances such as limited bleeding are common with prostate biopsy, but major complications are uncommon. However, no procedure is risk free. Most men will experience some temporary bleeding into the three body fluids the needle might affect: stool, urine, and semen. The reason is obvious for urine and stool, as the needle can puncture either the lower urinary tract or rectum. Blood in the semen is the result of the needle puncturing the ducts of the prostate gland where much of the semen originates. Therefore, an ejaculation will contain this old blood when the semen is released naturally. This can occur for several weeks (and occasionally months) following prostate biopsy. It is not a sign of serious problems and, no matter how long it takes, should be left alone. The blood is not harmful to either the man or his partner (assuming he has no blood-borne diseases, which would be carried in semen anyway), so its presence is not of concern.

If blood in the semen (**hemospermia** or **hematospermia**) is alarming, a medication to cause shrinkage of the prostate, such as **finasteride** (**Proscar**) or **dutasteride** (**Avodart**), might speed up the process. However, the use of these medications for this purpose has not been adequately studied, so their value is anecdotal for now. Although antibiotics are frequently employed, there is no real reason to believe that they would speed resolution either, since the cause is not infection.

Hematuria or blood in the urine is due to the needle passing into the nearby lower urinary tract. This is not harmful unless clots form that are so large that passing them becomes difficult. If this occurs, a temporary catheter will allow the doctor to irrigate out the clot.

Rectal bleeding can occasionally be troublesome. Although minor bleeding occurs in most men, it is severe enough to require attention in only about 1 percent of patients. Most often, when a patient complains of rectal bleeding it stops by the time he returns to the office or goes to the emergency department. Infrequently, the patient requires hospital admission. Reports of transfusion requirements vary, but I have seen only one patient who received a transfusion.

The treatment for most bleeding is to place pressure on the bleeding site—not an easy task if the bleeding site is inside the rectum. Sometimes a bandage or a tampon placed into the rectum can apply pressure. I have not found this particularly helpful, but there are reports of success from some centers.

Prostatitis can occur following prostate biopsy due to rectal bacteria. This occurs about 1 percent of the time no matter how many doses or which antibiotics we give, but will be more common if no antibiotics are used. These infections can usually be treated with oral antibiotics such as Cipro or Levaquin. Rarely, the patient becomes ill enough to hospitalize for intravenous antibiotics.

Acute **urinary retention** describes the situation of not being able to empty the bladder. After a prostate biopsy, the prostate can swell. If urinary flow is already constricted, this swelling might cause the complete inability to urinate. This can be temporarily relieved with a urinary catheter until the swelling subsides. Medications to relax the prostate (such as those discussed in chapter 8) may allow quicker return to normal function.

Swelling inevitably dissipates in a matter of days to weeks. However, if a man was reaching the point where the urinary tract was about to close off anyway, this may be the final blow and he might require surgical intervention before resuming normal urination.

Interestingly, the medical literature finds that the likelihood of any of these complications occurring is relatively independent of the number of biopsy cores obtained. Although common sense would suggest that more needle sticks would cause more problems, this has not been proven to be the case statistically. The exception to this has been that bleeding is more *common* with greater numbers of sticks, but does not appear to last longer or be more *severe*.

In short, a *1 percent rule* seems pertinent when considering the risks of prostate biopsy. The three most common risks—significant bleeding, infection, and urinary retention—all occur about 1 percent of the time. Fortunately, they are almost always easily manageable.

AFTER THE BIOPSY

As soon as the biopsy is completed, you should center yourself on the table before turning onto your back. You don't want to roll off the table. Some people experience a *vasovagal response* to certain stimuli, including rectal discomfort. This lowers pulse and blood pressure and can cause you to become light-headed or faint if you sit up too quickly. Someone will be beside you as you arise to make sure you don't faint. The condition can be scary but is rarely dangerous—unless you end up on the floor!

You may want to go to the restroom to empty the bladder. This confirms that the amount of blood in the urine is low enough that clotting off is unlikely, as well as affirming that urinary retention is unlikely to follow. A bowel movement at that time is possible, and will often have some fresh blood with a few clots. This blood is almost always less than it appears; it doesn't take much of your own blood to seem a lot. Unless active bleeding persists, it is acceptable to go home, shower, and take it easy for the rest of the day.

WHAT IF SOMETHING MORE SERIOUS OCCURS?

Once home, the most significant reason you would call the doctor would be persistent bleeding for more than an hour or two that seems to be increasing. Urinary retention is a concern only if you feel bladder pain from being too full. If you cannot void but don't really feel the need to, it may simply be that the bladder is not full enough to urinate yet; until full, there is no reason for alarm. If you have bladder pain and can't empty, you might as well head to the doctor's office if still open or the emergency room if after hours. You will temporarily need a catheter to treat the problem.

Though it is tempting to go to the closest emergency room for convenience, I strongly recommend you go to a hospital where your physician has privileges to provide care. Otherwise, a stranger will end up handling your doctor's work. Moreover, if you should require hospital admission, it's an onerous task to have a patient transferred from one emergency room to another hospital, so being in the wrong place substantially slows down the amount of time it takes for you to receive appropriate care.

Fever over 101° will occasionally require hospitalization to administer IV antibiotics for a day or longer. If you feel all right and simply have a low-grade fever, the physician may try to manage it on an outpatient basis. This is reasonable, since modern antibiotics such as Cipro and Levaquin reach blood levels equal to those of IV antibiotics. Therefore, unless you are unable to take medications orally (or keep them down), you may not require hospitalization. Nevertheless, some physicians are still more comfortable managing patients with infections following biopsy as inpatients

CAN BIOPSY SPREAD CANCER CELLS?

This common question is primarily based on old wives' tales. Since metastasis occurs when cells break off and spread through the bloodstream, it makes sense that a needle placed through cancerous tissue might break off some cells. In fact, this can occur rarely with certain types of high- grade cancers.

Prostate cancer is not one of those types.

A couple of points should reassure you on this concern. First, to my knowledge there has never been a single case reported where this occurred following transrectal biopsy—not a single case in the most common cancer in man. If it were a significant risk, we would know by now. Therefore, you can relax—needle biopsy does not pose significant risk of spreading prostate cancer.

ON THE ROAD TO PATHOLOGY: WHAT HAPPENS TO THE REMOVED TISSUE?

Once the biopsy is completed, the process has actually only just begun. The urologist or his assistant will place the tiny pieces of tissue into formalin or a similar fixative. This preserves the microscopic architecture of the tissue until it can be transferred to the pathology lab and embedded in paraffin wax. The pathology technologist will slice the pieces paper thin, then place the slices on a glass slide and stain them with dyes that help distinguish specific findings. An even thinner glass coverslip seals the deal.

Once the sample is processed, the pathologist will take a preliminary review through low-power magnification. Think of it as looking through your camera with the low-power lens before zooming in for the close view you ultimately want. This allows her to focus on suspicious areas. If something catches her eye, she will quickly zoom in and sometimes the answer becomes obvious. Closer scanning allows complete assessment of the tissue on the slide. If there are suspicious areas, they might be marked so she can

The vast majority of prostate cancers are detected during biopsy. However coincidental recognition of cancer sometimes occurs following removal of prostatic tissue for other reasons. This was common two or more decades ago when TURP was common.

The most common situation in which this occurs now is when the prostate is removed during cystectomy, the operation required to take out bladder cancer. Recall that the prostate and bladder almost blend into each other at their fusion at the bladder neck. As a result, surgery to remove the bladder traditionally removes the prostate simultaneously. The reasoning is that bladder cancer may have invaded the prostate, but we also know that prostate cancer is found coincidentally in at least one-quarter of these cases. Dr. Louis Liou reviewed more than two hundred patients who had this operation at the Cleveland Clinic Foundation and 39 percent of them were found to have previously unsuspected prostate cancer.[20]

The good news was that follow-up on these men showed that their survival was determined solely by their bladder cancer—not prostate cancer. In other words, if their bladder cancer was cured, their life expectancy appeared unchanged in comparison to those cured of bladder cancer that did not also have incidental prostate cancer.

return to them later, potentially with a colleague to lend an unbiased eye. If complete assessment fails to show any malignancy, she issues a negative report.

DRUMROLL, PLEASE: GETTING THE NEWS

Urologists differ on the method of delivering the news. The most efficient is a phone call from the nurse. I prefer to deliver the news myself, especially if the biopsy is positive for cancer. If negative, the patient would usually prioritize receiving good news quickly over who gives it, so the nurse might go ahead and make the call so the man can relax.

I usually schedule a return appointment to meet with the patient when the report is available. I make an exception for those who request a phone call, often because they live out of state.

When I sit down with the patient, I quickly let him know whether it's cancer or not. If positive, we will begin a discussion of its implications. I reassure the patient that it's almost always manageable, and usually curable. We wouldn't really have a reason to screen if we couldn't take care of it.

WHEN CANCER IS THE ANSWER: UNDERSTANDING THE GLEASON SCORE

Once the diagnosis of cancer is established, the pathologist will assign a **Gleason score**. Dr. Donald Gleason is a pathologist at the University of Minnesota who designed a grading system to classify prostate cancers on a scale from 1 to 5. Gleason grade 1 cancer is low grade, meaning it is typically slow growing and unlikely to progress. Gleason grade 5 cancer is the opposite.

Because many prostate cancers have areas of varying grades, Dr. Gleason proposed a score, that can be easily confused with the Gleason grade. The difference is that the two most common *grades* of cancer identified in the biopsy specimen are added together to give the *score*. We usually list it by showing the two grades added, so it ends up looking like an elementary school math problem. An example might be when a cancer is primarily Gleason grade 4, with a smaller area of Gleason grade 3. The report for this would be shown as "Gleason score 4+3=7." If their relative percentages were reversed (more grade 3 than 4), the report would state "Gleason score 3+4=7." Notice that the numbers may add up to the same total, but their relative percentages carry different prognoses.

Note that the lowest possible Gleason score is 2 (1+1=2). Therefore, when the Gleason score is 6, it's really not more than halfway to the highest score of 10. It's actually right in the middle—3+3=6. The implications of the Gleason score are huge, and will be discussed in detail in the next chapter.

WHAT ELSE MIGHT THE BIOPSY SHOW? (*MOSTLY* GOOD NEWS)

Patients like answers in black and white—cancer or no cancer. It isn't always that straightforward. The biopsy might identify a couple of abnormalities that are neither. The most common is **prostatic intraepithelial neoplasia (PIN)**. The other is **atypical small acinar proliferation (ASAP)**.

PIN is the presence of atypical (abnormal) cells inside benign prostatic ducts. The cells may be in the early stages of abnormal growth, or may be arranged haphazardly, almost as if they are turned upside down. The condition was originally classified as either low-grade PIN or high-grade PIN, but most pathologists now regard low-grade PIN as essentially a normal variant. As such, low-grade PIN should be disregarded and omitted from biopsy reports.

At the Cleveland Clinic, Drs. *Lynn Schoenfield, Ming Zhou,* and *Cristina Magi-Galluzzi* reviewed my biopsies and found that PIN occurs in 22 percent of patients who don't have cancer.[21]

Prostatic Intraepithelial Neoplasiza: PIN

The big controversy with PIN is whether it is a precancerous condition or whether it simply exists commonly in association with cancer. Since it is impossible to show the actual progression of PIN to cancer in a given patient, we have to rely on the circumstantial evidence that men with PIN will more likely develop cancer in the coming years than will men with normal biopsies.

Knowing that sextant biopsy can miss small cancers, some urologists and pathologists believe that cancer was actually present at the time PIN was identified, but that the biopsy missed it. This is based on the fact that a repeat biopsy performed soon after finding PIN on sextant biopsy will identify cancer in up to half of such men. Therefore, if a sextant biopsy was performed, it appears cancer was simply missed in up to half of men with PIN.

In contrast, I am of the school that considers PIN potentially precancerous. A couple of facts explain this. First, we know that when men die traumatically and undergo autopsy, the likelihood that they will coincidentally be found to have PIN predates the likelihood they will be coincidentally found to have prostate cancer by about a decade. This is circumstantial evidence, but logical.

The second significant reason to believe PIN is precancerous is found in published biopsy literature. Before we began doing adequate biopsies (as discussed above), we recommended that men found to have PIN undergo repeat biopsies, sometimes on a frequent basis. At that time, we believed that probably up to half of the men would have cancer on a repeat biopsy, suggesting that the cancer was actually just coexistent with the PIN and was simply missed on the first biopsy. However, after we found out how to minimize the chance of missing cancer by taking greater numbers of laterally based cores, we found that a repeat biopsy would rarely find cancer in these men (about 2 to 3 percent of the time). This implies that PIN did not simply exist alongside undiagnosed prostate cancer.[22] However, when those same men were rebiopsied three years later, almost one-quarter of the men had biopsies positive for cancer, implying a precancerous condition had progressed to cancer.[23] This suggests that PIN developed into cancer in that percentage of men during that period.

Most urologists will recommend rebiopsy when PIN shows up. However, I do not automatically do this, for the reasons listed above. I recommend following the situation closely. If there is any suspicion of a change either on DRE or in the PSA, a repeat biopsy may be in order; for that matter, the man may simply choose "to be sure." However, we know the chance of finding cancer is low, so it's not clear that all men should automatically have a repeat biopsy.

That recommendation changes at the three-year mark, however. We know that there is about a one in four chance of developing prostate cancer in that time frame, so a repeat biopsy is in order if the man is still healthy enough to be concerned about prostate cancer.

Blocking PIN from Becoming Cancer?

If a man has a potentially precancerous condition, he obviously might think of doing something to stop it in its tracks. Logically, we might use any of the prostate cancer prevention strategies discussed previously. The only problem with this logic is that no one knows whether the die is cast, or whether we can still have an impact by this point.

Therefore, I recommend that men consider some of the prevention strategies listed elsewhere, but acknowledge that we can't be sure whether it's not too late to change the ultimate progression that might already be in place. Such strategies allow them to exert some control, or at least know they are doing everything that can be done. These strategies are consistent with a healthy lifestyle anyway, so there is no clear downside.

WORRYING ABOUT "A POTENTIALLY PRECANCEROUS CONDITION"

Many men are uncomfortable with observing PIN. My best words of reassurance relate to the time it takes for anything bad to happen. Although the man is at increased risk, our hope is that he never develops cancer.

If he does, often it will take several years to happen. If it takes twenty years to develop cancer and another twenty years to die from it, PIN doesn't seem so scary if you're already 70 years old ("Hmm. . . . 70+20+20=110 years old. I'll take my chances.") Therefore, we watch to see if it occurs earlier than that, and to make sure that if cancer develops, it's not a high-grade, serious tumor. Unless that unlikely scenario develops, most men with PIN will live long, healthy lives.

ASAP: Cancer in a Hurry?

Atypical small acinar proliferation is another finding on biopsy that may be an even more serious finding than PIN is, and is often found in association with cancer. The area is invariably very small—often around the size of a pinhead or smaller. Although a larger area might be deemed obviously malignant, the pathologist cannot be certain if only a few small glands are abnormal.

In contrast to PIN, ASAP is uncommon. Nevertheless, repeat biopsy in men with ASAP will confirm the presence of cancer around half the time, so it should proceed as soon as is convenient.

ASAP will sometimes be the interpretation used when there is not enough proof to diagnose cancer, but there are findings of concern on the slide. The first thing I do when I am referred a patient with this report on his biopsy is to ask for a reinterpretation of the slides. Sometimes, the pathologists at a major university laboratory will be able to determine that the criteria for cancer are actually present, and will make the correct diagnosis while sparing the patient a repeat biopsy.

This reinterpretation of the biopsy doesn't mean that the first pathologist was "wrong." I discuss in the next chapter why the pathologist has to be certain before declaring cancer present. Therefore, if the criteria are borderline, someone has to make a tough call. A team of specialized urological pathologists at a major university reference lab may be more prepared and confident to make that tough call.

A similar reading is, "Suspicious, but not diagnostic for cancer." This means that some findings of concern are on the slide. The pathologist usually suspects cancer is present, but there isn't enough evidence on the slide to commit. A repeat biopsy is clearly in order unless a second pathological opinion renders a definitive diagnosis.

WHEN THE BIOPSY IS NEGATIVE

This is our favorite report. When there is nothing cancerous or even suspicious on the biopsy, we know that the patient should be fine. He gets to take a deep breath and relax. Many grown men get at least a little frosty-eyed at the relief. It's okay—you deserve it.

The only thing left to discuss is follow-up. With contemporary biopsy techniques as described above, we miss very few cancers. However, if suspicion persists due to a continued elevation of the PSA or suspicious findings on DRE, it is still possible that there was a sampling error. A repeat biopsy might be required at some point to clarify the situation. However, as long as an adequate biopsy was performed initially, rest assured that it usually would take a pretty small cancer to slip through the needle "cracks." Even if follow-ups detect a small tumor, your chance of cure remains very high.

REPEAT BIOPSY

Most urologists now concede that sextant biopsy is inadequate and have made the transition to the higher yielding eight to twelve-core biopsy strategies. However, there still exists the possibility of a sampling error that could overlook small cancers. Thus, men suspected of having undiagnosed cancer should consider repeat biopsy. This most commonly occurs in men with a persistently elevated or rising PSA. Men with suspicious nodules on DRE will also raise concern. Finally, men with ASAP will usually require repeat biopsy in the coming weeks, while men with PIN will require repeat biopsy at some point. As noted, the timing of this will vary among patients.

Prior to the development of **periprostatic block**, it was difficult to convince a man he should undergo a repeat biopsy. Although it had been relatively easy to make the case before he had experienced the procedure, the second time around he knew what to expect and was less enthusiastic. (Fool me once, shame on you. Fool me twice, shame on me.) Up to one-third of men in some studies would refuse repeat biopsy without anesthesia based on their experience; this alone should have made us more alert to the pain. Fortunately, this reticence is essentially gone with the advent of periprostatic block. The only men whom we usually have a difficult time convincing at this point are those whose previous biopsy was performed without anesthesia.

When repeat biopsy is required, the number of cores needed is controversial. The old way to do it was to repeat a sextant biopsy. This made no sense. Why would we expect that cancer missed during a first sextant biopsy would be found when we put the needle back right in the same place? Interestingly, even with this glaring error in place we know that about 20 percent of men had positive repeat biopsies.[24]

Based on the information above regarding biopsy location, we now perform biopsies focusing on the lateral aspects of the prostate, especially repeat biopsies. We recently found that cancer was effectively never found in the middle of the prostate unless it was also identified in the lateral prostate when a man underwent repeat biopsy. Therefore, no matter how many cores are taken, the focus should be lateral.

The number of cores needed remains unclear, but should be at least eight. Since the patient is suspected of having cancer that has already been missed, most urologists will take at least ten. Despite concerns of increased risk with additional cores, it appears risk does not increase with biopsy schemes at least as high as fifteen,[25] and probably twenty-four.

TIME AFTER TIME

Some men will still have suspicious findings after multiple biopsies. Almost every urologist has seen men whose cancer was identified only after five or more biopsy sessions. Indeed, when we do saturation biopsies as described below, we find cancer in almost 30 percent of men even if they have been biopsied repeatedly using traditional methods.

Although cancer may be present in this setting, repeat biopsy is not automatically indicated. One reason is that we really don't want to know about small, **clinically insignificant cancer**. Missing these simply avoids worrying a man unnecessarily. Also, prostate cancer is usually a slow-growing entity. As a result, a cancer small enough to elude the needle tracks used on an adequate biopsy will usually be slow growing enough that when detected during follow-up, the patient will have plenty of time for cure.

SATURATION BIOPSY

In order to answer the question definitively, several centers now perform **saturation biopsy**. This technique examines larger numbers of tissues samples from throughout the prostate in order to minimize the chance of sampling error. Most urologists consider saturation biopsy to involve twenty cores or more.

We could obviously never put a needle into the prostate that many times prior to the advent of periprostatic block, so the original reports involved patients taken to the operating room to perform biopsy under general or regional anesthesia. Up to one-third of these patients were found to have cancer even if they had undergone multiple repeated biopsies.

In the past, the greatest disadvantage of saturation biopsies was the requirement of the operating room. Any visit to the operating room involves substantial charges over the cost in the office. There is the small but real risk of complications from general or regional anesthesia.[26] There is a substantial time commitment, as these patients must stay in the hospital or ambulatory surgery center for several hours. A family member must miss a day of work to drive the patient, who also misses a day of work. Finally, the surgeon must spend considerable time and do a stack of paperwork in order to perform the procedure in the operating room.

After we found that we could get our patients through biopsies with minimal discomfort, we began looking at the possibility of performing saturation biopsy in the office. With periprostatic block, we have been able to do *all* our saturation biopsies in the clinic as a simple office procedure.[27] Hundreds of cases later, we are pretty comfortable that the procedure is tolerable and that the hospital should be reserved for sick people.

Our original saturation biopsies involved twenty-four widely dispersed cores. Based on our finding that medial cores are almost never positive unless the lateral cores have cancer, we concluded that the medial cores add little and can be minimized without risk of missing cancer. Therefore, we have decreased the number of cores for patients undergoing repeat biopsy using a saturation technique to 20.[28] Using this technique, we have found that even following several negative biopsies, almost thirty percent of patients still harbor previously unknown malignancy.[29]

WHEN DO I QUIT WORRYING?

The short answer to this question is that most people never quit worrying when cancer is on their minds. Because of its frightening nature and the fact we can never be 100 percent sure cancer is absent, the issue may remain a concern even after repeated biopsies.

Nevertheless, risk from cancer is minimal in most men who have undergone appropriate evaluation. When it comes to slow-growing cancer, missing a small prostate tumor presents minimal peril as long as an adequate biopsy has been performed. As noted above, this usually means at least eight and preferably ten or more laterally based cores. If suspicion persists, at least one repeat biopsy is clearly indicated. Many urologists perform a repeat of their initial biopsy, but under our care, this will be a saturation biopsy with twenty laterally based cores. Finding no cancer on this combination suggests that any cancer that could be present is probably so small that it will take years to become clinically significant. More likely, there is no cancer so the worry is unnecessary.

Even in the presence of PIN, the risk is low as long as surveillance is adequate. A repeat biopsy may be required on an intermittent basis, but this is tolerable with the techniques described in this chapter. If it takes years to develop cancer, and years to progress, you may never reach a point that requires treatment.

Following several negative biopsies, you can rest assured that the chance of **clinically significant cancer** is low. You should simply put a plan in place with your physician to monitor the situation. If something changes (the PSA goes up or a nodule develops) you adjust and change your plan. If things remain stable—whether the PSA is 4 or 40—you are unlikely to get into trouble.

***

A twelve-core biopsy went well for Tom. Periprostatic block prevented him from feeling pain from a single stick. The popping noise of the biopsy gun was a little disconcerting, especially when I forgot to warn him before I took a few of the cores. He had light pink urine the first time he voided and a couple of small clots in his first bowel movement. Prewarned, he was not concerned and this resolved quickly. He conceded that he had not needed general anesthesia.

A few days later, I received the pathology report finding that Tom had several cores positive for high-grade PIN. After discussing the issues as discussed in this chapter and some possible prevention strategies as described earlier, I scheduled a repeat free and total PSA and DRE in six months. The plan was to follow him closely, and perform repeat biopsy in three years if things remained stable. Hematospermia accompanied ejaculations for the first three weeks, and recurred once about four months later. Although I had advised him that this was the most likely to linger, he still called for reassurance when his wife expressed alarm.

At the six-month visit, the PSA was 4.8 with 15 percent free. Again, a dilemma. The total PSA was worse, but the free percentage was better. After a lengthy discussion, we decided to repeat the biopsy. Neither he nor Anne even asked about an anesthetic this time. Saturation biopsy obtaining twenty cores found Gleason 3 + 4 = 7 cancer in three lateral cores from the left side. Although his prognosis appeared favorable, I recalled how anxious he was, so I wasn't looking forward to this discussion.

KEY POINTS

- Biopsy accuracy depends on whether the needle hits the tumor; a negative biopsy means there is no cancer in the specimen and is great news. However, careful surveillance should be continued until it is clear that there really is no cancer.
- Prostate biopsy doesn't have to be painful. Placing local anesthetic via periprostatic block allows the urologist to perform prostate biopsy as painlessly as the dentist can perform a procedure.
- PIN is a potentially precancerous condition that warrants careful follow-up and repeat biopsy at some point. In that circumstance, the chance of developing and serious problems is low.
- ASAP is often cancer in disguise. It should be biopsied again in a manner consistent with its acronym.
- During prostate biopsy, the bare minimum is to obtain eight laterally based cores. Most urologists will remove ten to twelve cores for men having their first biopsy.
- Only a minority of prostate cancers are actually visible on ultrasound.
- If the first biopsy fails to identify cancer and there is still suspicion, a repeat biopsy is in order. Many urologists will perform a **saturation biopsy**, which obtains typically twenty or more cores.
- A 1 percent rule seems pertinent when considering the risks of prostate biopsy. The three most common risks—significant bleeding, infection, and urinary retention—all occur about 1 percent of the time.

13.

THE BIOPSY SHOWS CANCER

I thought I knew what fear was until I heard the words, "You have cancer"

—Lance Armstrong

I was glad Tom had a follow-up appointment to discuss his biopsy results. He had been notably nervous during our previous conversations and I didn't think I could calm him over the phone. He seemed to look right into my head when I entered the room.

"You do have a small amount of cancer," I directly advised. "Fortunately, we found it early and while it is small. This should be manageable." I always try to get the facts on the table quickly; it helps avert the patient reading between the lines.

His wife, Anne, became misty-eyed. "Are you sure?" Her husband, the businessman, stood up, gazed out the window, and drew in a deep breath in a failed attempt to avoid looking terrified. Anne placed a hand on his forearm as we settled into a long discussion.

***

Even before the biopsy, each man knows there is a chance that the diagnosis is going to be cancer. If you are one of the men whose report is positive for cancer, don't panic. The diagnosis doesn't have to be devastating.

Take a deep breath. Remember why we performed a biopsy in the first place. Because prostate cancer is typically slow growing and usually diagnosed at a curable stage, the discussion with most patients starts with reassurance that things are probably going to be all right. If we couldn't manage the disease, we wouldn't really even have a reason to screen. This should let you know that we can successfully manage most cases.

As we have emphasized, a vast majority of men diagnosed with prostate cancer will eventually die of causes *other than prostate cancer*. Therefore, try to overcome the natural tendency to panic when the word "cancer" comes into the discussion so that you can focus on learning what you need to know in order to deal with the problem.

STEP ONE: DENIAL

More than thirty years ago, the late Elisabeth Kübler-Ross described the five stages humans use to deal with serious news.[1] Although she specifically described the states of dealing with death, these stages also describe the events that many people experience when dealing with a diagnosis that a number of people (incorrectly) equate with death—cancer. Predictably, the first stage is denial.

Men and their wives are often incredulous when told that the biopsy shows cancer. This is not surprising for a couple of reasons. The first reason is the defense mechanism described by Kübler-Ross. Denial is easy and doesn't cost much. Its existence allows us to deal with realities that otherwise might be insufferable. It allows us to sleep at night in a world that isn't as secure as we would like it to be. It allows us to continue playing basketball with our teenage children long after our fade-away jumper has faded away. Unfortunately, when the reality requires attention, such as when there is cancer, denial (if not overcome quickly) only impedes progress.

The second reason incredulity is predictable following the news is the fact that prostate cancer causes no symptoms in its early stages. "I feel fine, Doc," is the typical line. We expect you to feel fine, so that means nothing.

"Are you sure?"

ARE YOU SURE?

Yes, if the urologist tells you it's cancer, he's sure. Biopsy accuracy is exceedingly high when the reading is cancer for several reasons. First, most pathology departments will have more than one pathologist examine the biopsy unless the biopsy diagnosis is absolutely unquestionable. In a major academic medical center such as ours at the Cleveland Clinic Foundation, a resident and/or fellow might yield an initial impression. That is never the final answer, though. A board-certified pathologist will review it, and if he determines cancer is the reading, he will probably have a second, equally qualified colleague read the slide with him. This often occurs during a team meeting or conference involving several specialized urological pathologists. If there is a doubt, special stains may resolve the diagnosis.

Nonetheless, there is no such thing as 100 percent in medicine. As the surgeon-author Atul Gawande described it, we practice "an imperfect science." Don't let that scare you too much. I've been in medicine for over two decades and have *never* experienced a single case where the pathologist called my patient's prostate biopsy positive for cancer in error. If there's a doubt, the pathologist will give it a reading such as "Suspicious, but not diagnostic for cancer," and will recommend reinvestigation.

The realistic possible error occurs when prostate cancer is actually present but the biopsy fails to prove it—a *false negative*. The chance of a misreading is exceedingly low, but the sampling error is substantial. Recall that we are sampling a large gland with a small needle, so it is possible that a small cancer could elude the needle path. This possibility is minimized by taking adequate numbers of cores in the proper locations.

To summarize, when looking for cancer there are two possible errors. One is a *false negative*. That can happen occasionally (as discussed in the last chapter). To minimize the impact of this possibility, careful follow-up will be necessary. Because of the slow-growing nature of most prostate cancers, as long as it is detected in follow-up, it is very unlikely that the delay in diagnosis will be harmful. The second possible mistake is a false positive. The equation is skewed completely in the direction of erring on the side of caution, so the chance of giving the diagnosis of cancer in error approaches zero.

When cancer is the answer, we're sure.

HOW SERIOUS IS IT? STAGE AND GRADE

The next question involves how much and how serious it is. This is based on two factors—stage and **grade**. A stage is assigned to cancers to describe how advanced the disease is. *Low-stage* cancers are those detected early while limited to the gland. Advanced or *high-stage* cancers have progressed into nearby structures, or have spread to distant sites.

With contemporary screening techniques we can catch most cancer at an early or low stage. Table 1 shows the two major staging systems in use. The TNM (Tumor, Nodes, Metastasis) system is preferred, but some urologists still refer to the older Jewett-Whitmore system. (Note that this table is slightly simplified from those found in a medical textbook in keeping with the goals of this book to be understandable and usable by the layman. The important issues are maintained completely.)

Table 1.
The Two Main Prostate Cancer Clinical Staging Systems

TNM System	Description	Jewett-Whitmore System
T1	**Tumor found coincidentally due to surgery or elevated PSA; Patient has normal DRE**	**A**
T1a	Tumor found coincidentally in tissue removed at the time of TURP; 5 percent or less is cancerous and grade ≤ 7	A1
T1b	Tumor found coincidentally in tissue removed at the time of TURP; >5 percent is cancerous or grade > 7 T1c Tumor found on needle biopsy resulting from elevated PSA none	A2
T2	**Palpable tumor apparently confined to the prostate**	**B**
T2a	Tumor in one lobe (half of prostate) only	B1
T2b	Tumor in both lobes	B2
T3	**Tumor extends beyond prostate**	**C**
T3a	Extension beyond capsule on one side only	C1
T3b	Extension beyond capsule on both sides	C1
T3c	Extension into seminal vesicles	C1
T4	Tumor fixed to adjacent structures beyond seminal vesicles	C2
N (+)	**Tumor that has spread into lymph nodes**	**D1**
M (+)	**Tumor that has spread to distant sites**	**D2**

Let me emphasize a few issues regarding the above table. First, we rarely find stage T1a or T1b (stage A in the older system) cancers any more. This is due to two things. First, with fewer TURPs being performed, we simply won't find many cases in this manner any longer. Second, we catch most cases of prostate cancer through screening prior to TURP. My review of patients who underwent TURP in the era of PSA screening found that the risk of finding occult (previously unidentified) prostate cancer has decreased from 15.4 percent to 5.3 percent.[2] Therefore, very few people are identified at the top of the chart, so don't let the fact your cancer is lower on the list be of automatic concern.

Second, the top of the staging table—the "T1 stages"—seem to be in the wrong order in today's environment. Instead of stage T1a and T1b (tumor coincidentally identified during TURP) being listed as the earliest stages, T1c should probably be the lowest. It is now realistically the earliest stage detected in most patients since diagnosing cancer during TURP has become rare. However, it arose only after PSA came into the equation in the nineties, long after stages T1a and T1b were established. As the Johnny-come-lately, it was relegated to the next letter available, c.

Third, the TNM system was designed by the American Joint Commission on Cancer (AJCC) and is revised every few years. These revisions are attempts to adjust to advances in our understanding of prostate cancer. The hope is that improved staging will allow improved ability both to predict cancer behavior and to treat it more appropriately. Unfortunately, the more complex the systems become, the more confusing they may become as well. As a result, it appears to some investigators that the most recent revisions of 1997 actually predict prognosis worse than the 1992 version. Therefore, I would recommend that you not fixate on minor variations in stage, but rather focus on the major breakdowns as shown in bold in the table. In other words, the cancer is either confined to the prostate or extends beyond it. It is our hope that it was detected coincidentally through PSA testing or during a TURP. In these circumstances, prognosis is usually good. Even if not in these circumstances, prognosis may still be good.

Finally, the cutoff between stages T2a and T2b is sometimes described as being more than half of one lobe, depending on whether you use the 1992 or 1997 version. This is scientific nitpicking and only moderately related to prognosis, so don't waste much energy on determining the difference.

UNDERSTANDING PATHOLOGICAL STAGE VERSUS CLINICAL STAGE

The table and discussion above relate to **clinical stage**. In other words, they are based on the clinical information available at the time of diagnosis. This could change substantially if you have surgery to remove the prostate. In that setting, it could be found that the cancer has extended beyond the capsule. It also might be found in the lymph nodes at the time of surgery. This occurs a minority of the time, but you need to understand that the possibility exists.

This more accurate staging based on actually examining the removed prostate is called **pathological staging**. Patients who do not have the prostate removed and examined in its entirety (which means everyone who doesn't undergo prostatectomy) will not have as accurate staging. That makes comparison of outcomes between treatment options difficult, since we know more about cancer in men who have surgery, and less about those who underwent radiation. We may find that men who undergo surgery actually had higher-grade cancer than the biopsy showed. This limitation shouldn't play a major role in the decision process, but should be understood.

UNDERSTANDING GRADE

In addition to stage, the other thing we need in assessing the seriousness of a cancer is its **grade**. Grade refers to the degree of abnormality and aggressiveness of a cancer. A higher-grade cancer is further differentiated from normal tissue than a lower-grade cancer, so is more likely to grow uncontrollably.

The most significant part of the Gleason score is determined by the most common grade of cancer tissue. This is called the *primary Gleason grade*. The second most common area of cancer is termed the *secondary Gleason grade*. Therefore, a man with Gleason 3+4=7 cancer has fewer high-grade areas, and thus has a better prognosis than a man with Gleason 4+3=7, even though their Gleason score ends up being the same. However, the presence of even a small amount of higher-grade cancer is cause for concern.

The big break from *moderate* to *high grade* should be considered to be somewhere around seven, although not all sevens are equal as noted above. Although urologists don't agree on an absolute cutoff, most of us regard 4+3=7 cancer as the lowest score that should be considered truly high grade.

Fortunately, very rare cancers will be all grade five (5+5=10). I don't recall a single case. However, those men with Gleason 5+4=9 have very serious cancers and should consider aggressive treatment in hopes of beating their serious prognosis.

The concept of *tertiary Gleason grade* has an impact on prognosis in some men. This might involve a man with Gleason 4+3=7 cancer, determined by the two most common areas of cancer being grades four and three, respectively. However, there might be a smaller *third (tertiary)* area of Gleason grade-five cancer. Traditionally, we would not take this into account since it isn't one of the two largest areas. However, this small area of very high-grade cancer might actually be more dangerous in the long run than the larger areas of slower-growing cancer cells. Therefore, we now report a tertiary Gleason grade if such a situation occurs. This might push a man who is considering aggressive therapy to proceed because of this concerning finding. A recent trend is to count such a tertiary higher grade as the second part of the Gleason score, which most pathologists believe better reflects the aggressiveness of such cancers.

While interpreting the biopsy report it is important to be aware that we are talking about a clinical grade. If the prostate is completely removed, the grade may change because we can examine the entire cancer and may find that the actual overall score is either higher or lower than that identified during the biopsy sampling. This is called the pathological grade. It is not obtainable in men managed with any method other than prostatectomy.

The Gleason scoring system is shown in figure 13-1.

OTHER THINGS THE BIOPSY MIGHT TELL YOU

Prostate cancer is of the cell type *adenocarcinoma* in 99 percent or more of cases. Adenocarcinoma simply describes cancer that originates from glands or glandular tissue, which is the type of tissue comprising the prostate. The urologist will usually use the term *"prostate cancer,"* although some urologists will use *"adenocarcinoma"* when discussing biopsy findings. They are effectively the same thing. (Other cell types are rare enough that they are not the focus of this book. If you have another cell type, you will need to discuss its unique features with your urologist and probably a medical oncologist.)

For many years we believed that cancer's invasion of nerves found on biopsy was a finding of concern. This situation, perineural invasion, actually appears to be nowhere near as serious as we initially believed, so most urologists currently disregard the finding and certainly don't worry their patients with it.

Unlike perineural invasion, lymphovascular invasion actually does

PROSTATIC ADENOCARCINOMA
Histologic Grades

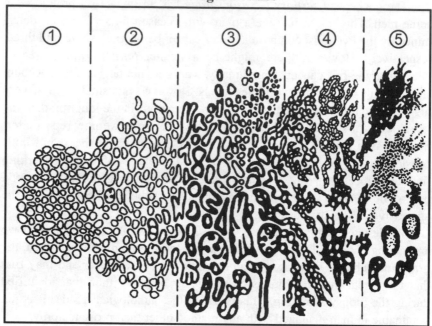

Figure 13-1. Dr. Donald Gleason developed the grading system we use to determine the severity and potential aggressiveness of prostate cancer. His system grades tumors from round, orderly cells as shown on the left (grade one) to disorderly, irregular cells as shown on the right (grade five). The two most common areas are graded and their sum added together to determine a **Gleason score**. (Gleason Scoring Chart 86–2(A), from Walsh, *Campbell's Urology* 8/e Vol. 4,© 2002 Elsevier Inc.)

appear to correlate with aggressiveness.[3] This relatively new concern may become more prominently discussed in the future as a prognostic indicator. For most men, neither of these conditions—perineural invasion or lympho-vascular invasion—will have an impact on their decision making. However, if a man is weighing the risks and benefits of aggressive therapy against those of conservative options, these findings (especially lymphovascular invasion) may provide another piece of information to push him one way or the other.

WHY DO WE HARDLY EVER SEE GLEASON SCORES LOWER THAN 6?

Patients are often confused and concerned when the discussion turns to grade or Gleason score. This is understandable for a couple of reasons. First, the scoring system is unavoidably complex because of the complexity of prostate cancer. We can't change that.

The second confusion comes when men predictably place themselves on a continuum on a scale that they perceive as being from zero to ten. All through our lives we think in terms of ranking. We are awarded class rank in school. We follow the sports polls. It is only natural that we automatically rank ourselves on the mental ten-point grading curve.

Since the highest score is bad (opposite class rank) when prostate cancer is the issue, we want to see ourselves in the lower half. It rarely happens. Dr. Gleason's system is to blame. First, the mental picture of a ten-point scale is inaccurate. Recall that two numbers must be added, so the lowest possible score is two (1+1=2.) Therefore, it is really a nine-point—not a ten-point—scale. In that light, it becomes clear that the middle score is actually six (3+3=6).

More important, the lower Gleason scores are those that we usually don't know exist. A Gleason score of five-or-lower rarely (if ever) causes an elevation in PSA or a nodule. Without raising suspicion of its existence, it usually remains unknown. Even better, it is likely to be **clinically insignificant**, meaning it doesn't matter if it's there, so it is better if we don't know it is there. Note that under one circumstance we might find these cancers; this is when men undergo TURP. This explains the stage T1a (or A1 in the older system) cancers.

As a result of the above, you could actually consider prostate cancer on a five-point scale starting at six and ending at ten. On that basis, Gleason score six is usually the lowest score of a **significant** cancer, so we are realistically talking about a five-point scale from six to ten. Try to keep that in perspective when you put yourself on the mental grading curve.

Finally, many people focus on the term *"encapsulated."* For some cancers a capsule implies they are not invading surrounding tissues, but for prostate cancer there is effectively no capsule, so this concept doesn't play a role in determining how serious the situation is.

***

Recall that Tom's biopsy found a Gleason score of 3 + 4 = 7 adenocarcinoma. The pathologist found evidence of perineural invasion but no lymphovascular invasion. This was a moderate-grade cancer that was, in all likelihood, confined to the prostate. In other words, probably curable.

Cognizant of Tom and Anne's angst, I chose each word carefully. I began exploring the issues by showing them tables of the staging and grading systems. Their interpretation of the facts was in the worst light each step of the way. Noting that the cancer was stage T1c, they fretted that it was already at the third step in the continuum (T1a-T1b-T1c). Only after the second explanation that the first two were cancers coincidentally identified during TURP did they concede that his was the earliest possible stage.

When attention turned to grade, they predictably observed that the grade seven was well above the midpoint (five) between zero and ten. Suggesting they consider true cancers as being on a scale from six to ten actually did help them see that Tom's cancer was on the lower end of the significant part of the Gleason score. Even learning the advantage of having a 3 + 4 = 7 instead of 4 + 3 = 7 struck a chord. I knew we were making progress in bringing them back into the world of the living when Tom sat back down and began to meet my eyes intermittently. "How do we know if it's contained?"

SEARCHING FOR CANCER SPREAD

Recall that most cancers will be confined to the prostate at the time of diagnosis. However, some will have spread, so we need to know when and where. When I was training in the eighties, we routinely did what is called a **metastatic workup** on every man found to have prostate cancer. Knowing that the two most common sites for cancer to spread were to the pelvic **lymph nodes** and to the bones, we would automatically order a CT scan of the pelvis and a bone scan.

CT stands for **computerized tomography**, a computerized x-ray image that pictures the body in slices, as if each slice were a playing card that you examine one by one as you go through the deck. This would theoretically find enlarged lymph nodes that indicated cancer had spread into them. Instead, we sometimes found that many men with cancer in the lymph nodes had normal CT scans, while many men with enlarged lymph nodes didn't actually have cancer in those nodes. This was because lymph nodes also enlarge in response to other foreign invasions, such as infection. Therefore, the man might have stepped on a nail when he was a child and still had an enlarged lymph node at the time of cancer diagnosis. If we had concluded that the cancer had spread, he would have worried unnecessarily. Even worse, if he gave up and decided to forgo potentially curative therapy, the consequences of this false positive examination would be obvious.

The second test we used to perform routinely was a **bone scan**. This is an imaging technique that uses injection of a **radioisotope**—a radioactive substance that accumulates anywhere there is bone damage. If a man with prostate cancer had a spot identified on a bone scan, it was assumed to be a metastasis, or spread. Therefore, it would be clear that cure was not possible by treatment aimed at the prostate alone.

Similarly, a bone scan might be falsely positive because of arthritis or an old injury the patient has forgotten. Consider this possibility—who hasn't had a backache or back injury at some point in his lifetime? Therefore, a little arthritis or an injury from falling down or another minor previous injury might be misinterpreted as metastasis. Also, some actual early metastases—about 10 percent—does not show up on bone scans at all. Therefore, the test can give a false reading either because of cancer which doesn't show up although it's there (*false negative*), or due to a reading that cancer is present when it's actually just an old injury or arthritis (*false positive*). Neither reading helps.

We now know that searching for metastasis is appropriate only in the setting when it's likely to be present. This is when the patient has either a high PSA or a high-grade cancer. The chance of finding a truly positive bone scan in men with a PSA of less than 20 is less than 1 percent.[4] If the PSA is less than 10, the chance of finding a true positive bone scan is virtually zero. Therefore, the chance that the test will be wrong (false positive or false negative) is greater than the chance it would be right! That means that a bone scan should not be done in this circumstance. The role of CT scan is similarly limited in such men with a low risk of having metastatic disease.

One might choose to do a metastatic workup on men with a very high-grade cancer (minimum Gleason score 7) as well. A conservative recommendation is that men with a PSA less than 10 and a Gleason score less than 8 should not undergo metastatic workup. Men with a PSA score between 10 and 20 are unlikely to benefit from it, but might consider it with their physicians, as might those with a Gleason score of seven or higher cancer. Most men with either a Gleason score of 8 or a PSA greater than 20 will undergo metastatic workup.

WHY NOT JUST DO IT?

Why shouldn't we just do a metastatic workup on every man with prostate cancer? Estimates show that at least $50 million can be saved yearly from the US healthcare budget by eliminating these unnecessary tests.[5] The tests take several hours' time, which might mean missing work. The CT often requires IV contrast agents—drugs that help highlight differences in tissues but carry risks of allergic reaction, shock, and occasionally death. Then, you have to wait to hear results of whether cancer has spread—even though the doctor knows up front it almost undoubtedly hasn't.

Moreover, if the test shows something abnormal, further tests are required to know more. This might include more involved imaging studies such as MRI scans. A biopsy to remove tissue from the abnormal-appearing area might be required to reach a final verdict.

After going through this cost, expense, discomfort, and anxiety, the results cannot be believed whatever the test shows in men who are inappropriate candidates for a metastatic workup, given the above. In the end your options will remain the same as they were before the charade.

That's why we shouldn't just do it.

WHEN METASTATIC WORKUP IS INDICATED

As noted, a vast majority of men will not need further investigation beyond the biopsy. However, a small minority will be at risk of having metastasis—men with PSA greater than 20 (or, more conservatively, greater than 10) and those with high-grade cancers. These men are valid candidates for a metastatic workup. Below is a more involved explanation of what to expect from studies that might be considered.

Bone Scan

The bone scan is not a radiology or x-ray procedure. Instead, it involves *nuclear medicine* imaging of the bones. A **radioisotope** or radioactive material is injected into the bloodstream through an IV puncture. You wait a few hours and then return to lie on a special table where radioactivity throughout the body can be detected. A scanner will then produce an image similar to an x-ray that looks like a skeleton, as shown in figure 13-2.

The radioisotope selectively accumulates wherever bone production occurs. Bone production is typically symmetrical except where the body attempts to repair injury—most commonly caused by trauma or cancer. Such focal areas of accumulation appear as a "hot spot" of increased activity on a bone scan (see figure 13-3). That means an old fracture may mimic a spot of cancer, so remembering where you were injured years ago is important. If your doctor cannot be sure whether it is a spot caused by cancer and if there is not a clear reason to explain it otherwise, further plain x-rays, a CT scan, or an MRI may be required to tell why it looks abnormal.

Knowing that cancer has already spread to the bones would preclude any treatment directed at the prostate alone, so if nothing else proves the diagnosis conclusively a biopsy of the area is sometimes required to answer the question definitively.

CT Scan

In this procedure, usually referred to as a CAT scan, images are taken by a camera that spirals around the patient in a matter of seconds and quickly reconstructs the images into a series of slices the that doctors can read immediately. The original scanners were unable to see small detail, but current machines can detect stones as small as one millimeter and tumors less than a centimeter (one-half inch) in size.

When CT is performed, the patient is asked to drink radiographic contrast, which usually tastes like a bad milkshake. This substance allows the radiologist to tell the difference between intestines and other tissues. When the CT is aimed at the pelvis (as is the case in prostate cancer) rectal contrast is sometimes added via enema. IV contrast is also sometimes used to help define other tissues. Each CT unit has its own protocol based on the techniques it finds most successful.

The scanner is in a lead-lined room that has a doughnut-shaped machine with a narrow bed that holds the patient. Some people become claustrophobic, but this is uncommon now that the scanners are more open in construction and the scans are performed so rapidly. You are asked to hold your breath while the machine quickly makes its spiral. It is as simple as that.

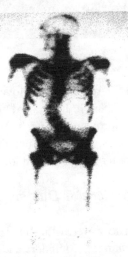

Figure 13-2. Bone scan showing widespread **metastases.** The leg bones appear relatively normal, but most of the **radioisotope** has accumulated throughout the remainder of the skeleton, as indicated by the dark areas. (Courtesy Brian Herts, MD)

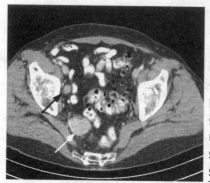

Figure 13-3. CT scan showing two enlarged lymph nodes containing **metastatic** prostate cancer on the left side of the photo (arrows), which corresponds to the right side of the patient's pelvis. Note that the two grey areas that represent lymph nodes are not matched by corresponding areas on the opposite side. (Courtesy of Brian Herts, MD)

PET Scanning

PET scanning is innovative imaging technology that identifies many types of cancer. It has failed to prove valuable in prostate cancer to date. With improvements, we hope it one day may allow imaging of microscopic cancer areas. Its greatest potential use will be to define whether an abnormal area on other imaging techniques is cancer or simply a false positive.

Molecular Diagnostics

The wave of the future diagnostically will probably be based on molecular changes. To understand this, recall that biopsy allows the pathologist to stain tissue and look at it through a microscope to find patterns associated with either **malignancy** or *benignity*. This is accurate but labor intensive.

Many tests are currently either in use or in development using changes in molecular structure (the actual chemicals that make up tissues) to yield more information than even the strongest microscope could provide. For example, we use fluorescent staining of DNA to detect bladder cancer cells in the urine with far greater accuracy than we have when looking at those same cells with a conventional microscope.[6]

Similar tests are in use for the evaluation of prostate cancer, such as the **ProstaScint** scan. It takes advantage of an *antibody* bound to a *radioisotope* (111-indium), which allows a scanner to identify abnormal areas of accumulation. Images usually are obtained at thirty minutes and at 72 to 120 hours.

When injected into the bloodstream this coupled pair goes in search of prostate cancer cells anywhere in the body. The ProstaScint will then accumulate in the prostate (unless it's already been removed) but also in lymph nodes, bones, and other sites if cancer cells are present.

Unfortunately, the ProstaScint scan has found limited use.[7] It is difficult to interpret, with the potential for false positive readings.[8] That is problematic because one will then be led to believe that cancer has advanced when it may not have done so. Therefore, I agree with most urologists that a ProstaScint should be done only very selectively. Although urologists will disagree on what that means, reasonable situations might involve circumstances when signs of cancer recurrence arise following treatment, or when a man is suspected of having metastatic disease and the ProstaScint is being used to prove it. *Systemic* treatment is preferable to localized treatment if that is the case.

The future will surely yield significant advances in the availability of molecular targeting based on similar principles. Investigators at multiple institutions, including our own at the Cleveland Clinic Foundation, are working diligently to hasten that day.

Another molecular technology you should be aware of is called RT-PCR. This blood test identifies specific RNA sequences circulating in the bloodstream. Minute amounts of such chemicals can be detected and magnified. The problem is that the test is so sensitive that many men with organ-confined prostate cancer will have a false positive RT-PCR, indicating incorrectly that the cancer has spread. Therefore, RT-PCR is not clinically useful in most patients.

The final molecule of interest is *prostatic acid phosphatase (PAP)*. It preceded PSA as the original prostate cancer tumor marker. Unlike PSA, PAP is produced in other tissues, making it an inaccurate marker. Nevertheless, an elevated PAP is suggestive of advanced prostate cancer. The older Jewett-Whitmore staging system actually had a *stage D-0*, which described an elevated PAP in the absence of demonstrable metastasis. This indicates the significance that used to be placed on this finding. Most urologists have abandoned PAP.

An interesting holdover from the days of PAP is the myth that a DRE causes an abnormal PSA. We know that PAP should not be drawn following DRE because it is elevated in the immediate aftermath. In contrast, we now know that routine DRE will not cause PSA to become abnormal (although it might go up an insignificant fraction). Therefore, there is no reason to wait on blood work to obtain a PSA following DRE. Regardless, like many old habits, this one has taken awhile to go away and many physicians still follow the habits they formed during the PAP era.

MRI

MRI or *magnetic resonance imaging* has received a lot of publicity for the evaluation and staging of prostate cancer, but few institutions have found it useful for the prostate to date. The easiest method is performed as a routine MRI, which is similar to having a CT scan inside a hollow ring. Some investigators have advocated the use of *endorectal coil MRI*. This involves use of a magnet positioned inside a smooth probe that is placed into the rectum to help show the prostate better during MRI scanning. Only a couple of institutions have found MRI helpful for this purpose, others have not followed this application. Therefore, most men do not have an MRI as part of evaluation of prostate cancer and we do not currently use MRI for this purpose at the Cleveland Clinic Foundation.

***

Initially Tom and Anne requested every possible test. Anne had undergone MRI when she ruptured her anterior cruciate ligament while running on the uneven surfaces of her sidewalk, and had already read about prostate MRI on the Internet. As an accountant, she wanted as much data as possible. She asked for a bone scan, CT scan, and RT-PCR. I wondered how the Internet search engine had allowed her to overlook PET scanning.

There was no reason to perform a metastatic workup. His cancer had been discovered early, while a clinical stage T1c. The tumor grade was moderate at 3+4=7. "Then let's do the studies just to be sure," she proposed when I first explained they were unnecessary. It took a second round of explanations to convince them. I clarified that the time-consuming tests were far more likely to be wrong than they were to be right. They cost money, even if insurance was paying. Even if they showed something, we wouldn't believe it to be real. All roads led to the same conclusion—further testing was inappropriate.

However, the accountant remained unconvinced until I related the story of another man I had met for a second opinion a few weeks earlier. This man, unknown and unnamed to Tom and Anne, had been diagnosed with a similarly favorable prostate cancer. He came to me for a second opinion because his bone scan showed a "hot spot" in his coccyx, or tailbone. He wanted to know how to treat the cancer that he had been told had spread to this site. Only after several more tests and a lot of stress did we confirm that the cause of this "hot spot" was a tumble. He had busted his backside on the Cleveland ice the winter before. This man's bone scan had been ordered inappropriately when it was more likely to have false positive findings than true positive findings. Predictably, it led to a quandary that was counterproductive to the man's care. Anne finally understood why I didn't just do it.

CONSIDERING OPTIONS

Once it is established that cancer appears to be confined to the prostate, it is time to consider options. There are several, and each man will choose one based on individual factors. The specifics of each treatment chosen are discussed in the following chapters, but let's consider the salient features of making the choice.

The Simplest Option: Watchful Waiting

Remember that most men with prostate cancer will never die of their disease. This is because it is often (to use a lay phrase that isn't really very scientific, but does accurately make the point) slow growing.

There is no definitive breakdown of cancers into two grand categories, the fast-growing and slow-growing types. There are lots of grays. However, it can be said that if you generically were forced to choose a type of cancer to have, prostate cancer might be your best bet because it is usually slow growing.

There actually is some truth that it is slower growing than most cancers. This is related to what is known as **doubling time**. Doubling time is the time it takes for a single cancer cell to divide into two cancer cells. As this happens throughout the tumor, when each cell has divided once, the tumor becomes twice as large. As this happens, some cancer cells will eventually begin to cause problems. This might be when they invade a local structure. A more serious possibility occurs when some of the cancer cells break off and begin to spread. They might travel through the bloodstream or through the *lymphatic vessels* to other sites in the body, where they establish a **metastasis**, or satellite tumor. These metastatic deposits will begin to divide in a similar manner, causing damage in their new locations.

The good news is that most prostate cancers divide more slowly (or, to rephrase, have a slower doubling time) than most other types of cancer. Particularly virulent cancers such as pancreatic cancer may have doubling times of weeks, whereas these slower-growing prostate cancers may have doubling times measured in years. That means it's almost impossible to die rapidly from prostate cancer. It also means that a rush to judgment on treatment options doesn't improve the chance of survival. So slow down and think things through. Consider a second opinion if you feel the need. There is almost always time to treat it as long as you do something within the first few months after finding it. The above facts about doubling time are why many men will be fine with or without treatment. Watchful waiting is covered in detail in chapter 14.

Get It Out! Radical Prostatectomy

Surgery to remove the cancerous prostate is called a **radical prostatectomy**, a term that unfortunately sounds scarier than it needs to. The dictionary defines "*radical*" in this setting as "making extreme changes." That means a radical operation makes a major change in the anatomy, not that it's necessarily the traumatic experience that the term might imply.

If cancer is truly confined to the prostate, its removal will assure cure. Sounds pretty straightforward that everyone with prostate cancer ought to have one, there are two problems with that thought process. First, there is no way to be absolutely sure that all cancer cells are confined to the prostate. A few microscopic cells outside the prostate or in other body areas might elude any test looking for them. Although the above tests for metastatic disease are good, they aren't perfect and never will be. Occasionally a man who appears to have organ-limited prostate cancer will actually have some microscopic cancer cells somewhere else waiting to cause a problem.

Second, recall that most men with prostate cancer will not die of their disease. Therefore, if every man with PCA has a radical prostatectomy, most of them will not benefit from their efforts. What is important is to try to determine which one needs treatment and which one doesn't.

Radiation Therapy

Radiation selectively kills living cells while they divide during growth. This principle allows us to target cancer cells—which divide more rapidly than most normal cells—while limiting damage to slower-growing cells in the surrounding tissues. Radiation therapy can be administered in two ways. The traditional method, **external beam radiation**, is to have the patient lie on a machine that focuses several radiation beams toward the prostate. Over the years, this technology has been refined greatly, using computer simulation to get more radiation to its target while minimizing harm to adjacent tissues.

A newer method, **brachytherapy**, involves surgically placing radioactive "seeds" or pellets into the prostate. These seeds emit their radioactivity into the prostate slowly over the following weeks. Eventually their energy burns out and the seeds simply sit there from that point forward. Their presence is usually innocuous.

Cryotherapy

For years doctors have destroyed tissue (including cancer) by freezing it. The role of freezing (**cryotherapy**) in the treatment of prostate cancer has been limited by complications until recently. Fortunately, the technology continues to improve.

Early versions of cryotherapy (the root, *cryo-*, means "to freeze"—think of *cryo*genics) involved placing metallic probes as large as pencils into the prostate and pumping liquid nitrogen into them to freeze "iceballs" of prostate tissue. These early versions were so large and unmanageable that the "iceballs" often froze right into adjacent organs.

Today's probes are three millimeters or less, approximately the diameter of a matchstick. Argon gas is pumped into the probes to freeze the tissue as solid as an ice cube. In order to ensure all cancer cells in the area are killed, the tissue is allowed to thaw and is then refrozen. Just like flowers die when frozen and thawed repeatedly in spring, the prostate and any cancer cells likewise swell and die in the freeze zone.

With refinements in the past decade, cryotherapy continues to emerge as a viable treatment option. Probes are more reasonable in size, and freezing techniques allow more specific targeting of the prostate while lessening damage to adjacent organs.

Hormonal Therapy

Prostate tissue—including cancerous prostate tissue—depends on the male hormone, testosterone, for its growth. Hormonal therapy for prostate cancer takes advantage of this fact by depriving the cancer of its driving force.

Blocking testosterone will block growth of prostate cancer cells no matter where they are. This makes hormonal therapy especially important for treatment of cancer after it has spread. Unfortunately, hormonal therapy only slows and doesn't actually stop or cure it, so it is employed mainly when curative local treatments such as radiation or surgery aren't possible.

Sometimes hormonal therapy can be used to treat organ-limited prostate cancer in order to slow its growth even without intent to cure. This is most often appropriate for men who have *comorbidities* that preclude them from being candidates for cure. In addition, if these men have a life expectancy of less than ten years we know that the cancer is unlikely to shorten their lives. However, many of these men will not want to go completely untreated, so hormonal therapy gives them an acceptable alternative.

High-Intensity Focused Ultrasound (HIFU)

A final interesting technology is HIFU. Just as the name implies, high-energy ultrasound waves are focused on the prostate in order to achieve cancer cell death. Because of the need for further investigation to validate its initial promising results, it will be a probably be a decade or more before it is available in the United States.

According to the chairman of urology at Indiana University, Dr. Michael Koch, it has great potential if it fulfills its early promise as a minimally invasive cure for prostate cancer.[9] However, until its safety and effectiveness are established, you should not consider going offshore to receive investigational treatments.

WHERE DO I GET INFORMATION?

As you begin to consider the above treatment options, you will be inundated with information. Well-meaning friends and family will want to put in their two cents. You will begin to notice newspaper and magazine articles. Many men will read books, sometimes by the armful. Finally, you will be tempted to go to that great cesspool of medical information—the Internet.

Be careful at this stage to avoid information overload. Although friends and family have the best of intentions, they don't know your situation. Uncle Fred who had cancer at the age of ninety during World War II doesn't have a lot in common with you as you make choices. Neither does your boss's brother-in-law with metastatic prostate cancer who is now living in Mexico taking (the fraudulent) laetrile and using coffee enemas.

But worse than any of the good intentioned advice is the morass of the Internet. A randomly timed Google search will yield almost 2 million hits using the keywords "*prostate cancer.*" Yes, there are some good Web sites. Examples are included in the back of this book, in the resources section.

However, too many Web sites are devoted to one of two malicious intents. The first is obvious as the root of all evil—money. Legions of entrepreneurs are ready to catch you at your most vulnerable moment. They will sell you supplements, advice, or anything else your credit card can stand. It should not shock you that these Web-based ancestors of the snake oil industry pioneers are better than ever at making it easy for you to let go of your money. Hold onto your cash; use it to take your wife to dinner, where you can talk about the facts instead of chasing delusions.

The second malicious intent involves those with an agenda. The Internet is the most open forum in the history of mankind. Any malcontent with a library card or two dollars for a timeslot at a Web cafe can start a Web site devoted to histrionics. You must realize that normal people don't create Web sites devoted to falsehoods and fears. Normal people live their lives and if they have problems, they deal with them constructively.

Some abnormal people devote Web pages to any number of inaccuracies. Whether they are selling, doomsaying, or criticizing, it is important for you to remember that such ramblings have zero accountability. They don't have to attribute information to research or any source. They don't have to even say who they really are. Such garbage on the Internet is no better than hate flyers you find on your windshield at the mall. Toss them.

WHERE DO I GET *GOOD* INFORMATION?

As noted, some Web sites such as those listed in the back of this book are legitimate, responsible, and helpful. Most books I have seen are written by reputable urologists. Friends or family whose situation resembles yours regarding age, stage, grade, and so forth, can *occasionally* lend insight.

Your family physician or internist will have cared for many men with prostate cancer. He may have the advantage of knowing you and your wife better than the urologist does, so he may have unique insights. In addition, as someone without direct involvement in your case regarding the cancer, he offers a relatively unbiased view.

Prostate cancer support groups such as *Man to Man* and *Us Too* (see Resources) facilitate education and networking opportunities. They meet periodically to discuss issues across the spectrum that are covered in this book. Spouses are usually welcome. Some men and their wives thrive in this environment. Those open enough to share their experiences are ideal candidates. Other men hold their cards closer to their vests and are not likely to derive satisfaction in this atmosphere. You know whether you are the type to open up in a group setting, so be honest with yourself about whether these meetings would be beneficial.

One word of caution—such groups can be diverse. You may meet patients of all ages, cancer stages and grades, walks of life, and medical perspectives. Moreover, some of the men have had the diagnosis of cancer for decades. Their experiences will be greatly different from yours, so beware drawing conclusions under such circumstances.

SECOND OPINION

It is hard to go wrong by getting a second opinion. We're talking about cancer. We're talking about complex procedures. We're talking about you. It is acceptable to seek help.

Nevertheless, there are some downsides to consider when you seek a second opinion. First, it should be a second opinion, not a tenth. Patients who bounce from doctor to doctor are known as "doctor shoppers." After two or at most three opinions, it is likely that you are simply trying to find a urologist who will say what you want to hear instead of give you the facts. This is counterproductive.

Second, the opinion should be by the right doctor—someone who routinely cares for men with prostate cancer. If you see a doctor who specializes in kidney stones, it is unlikely that he is devoted to improving the care of prostate cancer. Your family physician or internist will surely know at least one other urologist who would be appropriate. Ask his advice.

It is highly likely you will hear similar advice if you seek a second opinion from a qualified urologist. If not, it may become clear to you that one opinion makes more sense for your situation. If in doubt, a third opinion to determine who is right is reasonable, but should rarely be needed.

***

Tom did his homework, or at least Anne did it for him. I finally got them off the Internet, with the exception of valid sites as listed in the resources section of this book. He considered getting a second opinion, but decided he was comfortable with the information I had presented. More important, he was comfortable that he was informed on all the options and recognized that it was indeed his decision—not mine.

As a relatively young man with ample potential life expectancy, he wanted to maximize cancer control. Sexually active, he wanted to optimize his ability to remain so. Anxious, he wanted the cancer out. "How soon can you schedule surgery?"

KEY POINTS

- When the biopsy report shows cancer, accuracy is extremely high. Although no test (or human being, including a physician) is perfect, the likelihood that cancer is called incorrectly is almost unheard of. If you still can't believe it, a second pathological opinion can lend reassurance,, but isn't requisite.
- Stage and grade are the keys to determining prognosis. Your stage and Gleason score will probably become as familiar to you as your PSA level or social security number.
- A biopsy is just a sampling of the tumor, so the final **pathological grade** obtained when the prostate is removed will sometimes differ from the biopsy **clinical grade**.
- Although the Gleason score ranges from 2 to 10, most clinically significant cancers in actuality are graded on a scale from 6 to 10.
- Most prostate cancers are detected at stage T1c because of an elevation in PSA. Although this appears to be several steps down the staging scale, it is actually the earliest stage for practical purposes.
- A metastatic workup searching for cancer spread is rarely indicated these days unless the PSA or the Gleason score are high. In those circumstances, a bone scan and CT scan are the most likely tests to be performed.
- Men with organ-confined prostate cancer have multiple treatment options from which to choose.

14.

WATCHFUL WAITING AND COMPLEMENTARY MEDICINE: THE SIMPLEST OPTIONS

The great secret of doctors, known only to their wives, but still hidden from the public, is that most things get better by themselves; most things, in fact, are better in the morning.
—Dr. Lewis Thomas, president,
Memorial Sloan-Kettering Institute for Cancer Research

Recall that most men with prostate cancer will die of something else. Their disease progresses more slowly than the effects of time. If these men are fortunate, they will forgo unnecessary treatment.

Sometimes the treatment is worse than the disease. For men with prostate cancer, a large part of the decision involves an estimation of whether the cancer is likely to progress rapidly enough to cause problems during the patient's normal life expectancy. If this appears unlikely—and if the patient is willing to accept doing so—careful observation may be a reasonable alternative. This approach is sometimes mistakenly thought of as "doing nothing," but **watchful waiting** (sometimes also called simply *observation* or *surveillance*) actually implies *careful* monitoring. Frequent follow-up to detect disease progression are the basis of watchful waiting, and if the disease appears to be worsening at a concerning rate, the urologist will probably recommend intervention.

The dilemma is that some men will die of prostate cancer—it is the second leading cause of cancer death. Approximately one-third of men diagnosed with Gleason score 6 cancers and well over half of those with Gleason score 7 cancers will die from prostate cancer or be suffering from **metastatic**

249

disease within ten to fifteen years if not treated with curative intent. This time frame may be four or five years longer if the diagnosis is made purely through PSA testing—the most common route today—since PSA allows tumors to be recognized at an earlier stage than in the past.[1]

If only we knew at the time of diagnosis which ones would progress (**clinically significant**) and which ones would remain indolent (**clinically insignificant**)—the holy grail of prostate cancer diagnostics. Researchers around the world are working on tests they hope will do that, but it remains a dream at this point.

DOES TREATMENT ACTUALLY PREVENT PROSTATE CANCER DEATH?

Because of its slow-growing nature, it takes a long time to determine the impact of any prostate cancer treatment. Surprisingly, it is only recently that we have conclusive proof that treatment prolongs life expectancy; men who undergo prostatectomy have half the chance of dying of prostate cancer as do men who remain untreated.[2] There is a greater likelihood of treatment prolonging survival in men with high-risk disease, such as those with high Gleason scores or very high PSA levels.

The above study also looked at the quality of life in men who chose surgery compared to those who chose observation, since it is assumed that men choose observation in order to minimize the impact of treatment. Not unexpectedly, at the six-year follow-up, men who underwent surgery were more likely to have experienced impotence. However, *almost half* of those simply being observed also did.

The same study looked carefully at overall quality of life. Since it was conducted by the Scandinavian group that has long advocated watchful waiting instead of surgery, it was expected to highlight the benefits of observation. However, its conclusions were a little surprising. Despite careful use of questioning designed to detect differences in quality of life, there was no demonstrable difference overall between the two groups. Men treated with surgery seemed to have the same quality of life overall as did those who were monitored with watchful waiting.

CANDIDATES FOR WATCHFUL WAITING

Watchful waiting entails the assumption that cancer will progress more slowly than the effects of aging. Put more plainly, the person may die of something else before prostate cancer has a chance to hasten it.

Accepting that concept also involves accepting one's own eventual mortality. Even if a cancer grows slowly, it probably will not remain indolent forever. However, for most prostate cancers it may be ten, twenty, or occasionally even more years before they cause death. The good news is that most men will indeed avoid death at the hands of prostate cancer (although the bad news is that none of us escapes it permanently).

As a result of the above, candidates for watchful waiting are men with low- or intermediate-grade cancer and a life expectancy of probably no more than twenty years, who are willing to take the low risk that cancer will progress in their lifetimes. Men whose life expectancy exceeds that duration are less likely to make it through their lifetimes without eventually developing problems.

Notice that I did not mention an age at which watchful waiting is reasonable. This is because age has a limited role in life expectancy. I see healthy eighty-year-old men who will probably live another twenty years with no serious problems. Conversely, I see unhealthy fifty-year-olds with a family history of cardiac problems who continue to smoke and who could not climb a flight of stairs for free cigarettes. It is highly unlikely that such men will live long enough to die of prostate cancer no matter what happens.

Type A personalities are not usually well suited to this approach. I commonly tell patients that they are candidates for watchful waiting, but only if they will be able to tolerate the anxiety. If they are going to lay in bed awake at night, they are probably better off simply choosing one of the curative options in the following chapters. It doesn't help to survive prostate cancer but die of a stroke!

The final factor in determining candidates involves the cancer. Most prostate cancers are low grade and detected early. Short-term risk with these is low. However, some are high grade, detected later in their course, and possibly already spreading. These will become serious quickly and should not be ignored. Although urologists may never agree on which men require therapy despite age, we know risk factors for progression are a PSA greater than 10 ng/dl, a biopsy showing a Gleason score of 7 or greater, as well as involvement of multiple biopsy cores or involvement of more than half of any given core. Such men may still choose watchful waiting, but must be aware of the real potential for disease progression.

WATCHFUL WAITING: NOT BLIND IGNORING

Sometimes an assumption is falsely made that men who decline treatment initially have made a lifelong commitment to let the prostate gods determine their fate. The assumption is that they have made a bet that they will die before the cancer has time to do anything bad. Watchful waiting becomes synonymous with doing nothing in that situation.

That is a poor way to look at watchful waiting. The very term suggests this view is inaccurate. Watchfulness is an action. The doctor is still monitoring the patient, and judgment is used to decide when to intervene. A DRE is performed at least annually. PSA monitoring is usually done on the same schedule. A sudden change in either might indicate a need for more aggressive therapy.

DEFERRED THERAPY

A new concept for men who choose to decline treatment initially is **deferred therapy with curative intent**. Similar to traditional watchful waiting, deferred therapy involves an intentional strategy of observation until signs of danger arise. Instead of intending to avoid treatment altogether, deferred therapy denotes a plan to treat when PSA begins to rise to a point of concern (although this is subjective and differs among urologists) or when signs of cancer growth are detected.

Instead of sticking with the plan to withhold treatment, it may become appropriate to increase aggressiveness if clinical conditions change. In other words, therapy is deferred—not declined.

An emerging concept that we believe should play a role in men with appreciable life expectancies is the *staging* or *reevaluation biopsy*. It involves repeating a biopsy within a year after the initial diagnosis in order to determine whether progression has occurred. If there is a greater volume of cancer, and especially if the Gleason score is higher than on the initial biopsy, treatment may be in order. If there is no significant change from the initial biopsy or if the biopsy actually finds no cancer (recall from chapter 12 that biopsy is simply a sampling technique, so small cancers can be missed), the chance of problems down the road is very unlikely.[3] Progression may occur in a majority of men if a repeat biopsy shows a Gleason score of 7 or greater, more than two biopsy cores with cancer, or greater than 50 percent involvement of any core with cancer.[4] Such findings do not automatically require intervention, but make its need more likely.

Although some advocate performing a biopsy annually on men being followed with watchful waiting, my current recommendation involves a single biopsy about a year after they begin the program. Favorable findings on this biopsy lead me to reassure them that continued annual checkups with PSA and DRE are in order. Findings of the above concerning prognostic factors lead me to recommend consideration of curative therapy. If such men at risk choose to continue observation, I recommend another biopsy within the following year or two.

If and when the point is reached when therapy is required, the chance of cure still seems to be good as long as no serious warning signs have been ignored. Therefore, this may allow carefully selected men to avoid side effects of treatment for a while, but not necessarily for the rest of their lives.

COMPLEMENTARY MEDICINE

Americans spend more on complementary medical therapy ($13.7 billion) than they pay out of pocket for all hospitalizations ($12.8 billion). That indicates there is a huge amount of interest in alternative medicine. Contrary to popular opinion, the largest users are not the poor and uneducated. Quite the opposite, those spending cash on alternative medical treatments are on average more educated and have higher incomes than those who don't.[5]

Does that mean alternative therapy is a more intelligent choice? Of course not. It just means that many people have a desire for alternatives to the mainstream treatments for all conditions, including prostate cancer and BPH.

One of the basic tenets of medicine is the Latin phrase *primum non nocere*, meaning "first, do no harm." Stated in a more modern phrasing, "The treatment should not be worse than the disease." The assumption of many people is that something natural can't be harmful, while something medical has to be. Remember that tobacco is a completely natural product—grown from the soil of Mother Earth herself.

ALTERNATIVE OR COMPLEMENTARY?

Differentiating between alternative and complementary medicine involves more than semantics. The word *alternative* means that something is used *in place of* established medical care. In contrast, the word *complementary* means that something is used *in addition to* mainstream therapy. The difference is huge. Alternative therapy is more likely to be dangerous, especially if used instead of proven medical treatments to manage life-threatening conditions such as cancer or cardiovascular disease. If proven treatments are forgone for unproven alternative therapies, disastrous consequences are risked. In contrast, complementary treatment is used to assist proven medical therapies. However, since it is not adequately scientifically tested, it could also be very risky.

A good example of the difference would be when a patient has a heart attack and is prescribed aspirin and prescription medications known to decrease the chance of another, possibly fatal, heart attack. If he chooses alternative therapy, he would refuse the proven treatment and take something unknown, such as tree bark or coffee enemas. Without the prescription medications, he will have a false sense of security right up until the next (and perhaps final) heart attack. In contrast, if he chooses complementary therapy, he will take the medical treatments known to lessen the chance of death. In addition, he might make dietary changes that improve overall health. He might add vitamins and antioxidants that *might* help augment the medications. In the worst case, they at least do no harm unless he takes them in megadoses. *Primum non nocere.*

Therefore, complementary therapy may be safer than a truly alternative approach. A good example of a complementary treatment that is recommended by many urologists is the use of vitamin E and selenium for the prevention of prostate cancer. Based on observations that indicate these natural products *may* have a protective effect against the disease, I join many urologists in recommending that all men over the age of forty consider these supplements (400 IU of vitamin E and 200 micrograms of selenium daily). As noted elsewhere, this is still under investigation and there are risks to such high doses, but it is promising enough to warrant consideration.

Unfortunately, even complementary therapy has its risks as well, as some nonprescription items can affect how medications work. A good example is found in the intake of unusually large amounts of grapefruit (or its juice). Grapefruit contains a chemical that can block the liver enzyme P450, which is involved in drug metabolism. This can lead to toxic levels of many different types of medications by blocking the liver's ability to metabolize them.

Furthermore, almost three-quarters of all patients who use complementary treatments fail to tell their physicians about alternative or complementary treatments they are taking. This means that the physician is treating the patient without full information—no different than if the patient were on an undisclosed prescription drug that would interact with treatments. Therefore, complementary treatments should be discussed and taken into account by both the physician and patient in order to prevent disaster and to achieve success.

NO REGULATION

Unconventional treatments often seem to make people feel more comfortable, even when their accompanying theories are silly.
—Edward W. Campion, 1993

The most worrisome problem with alternative and complementary therapy is the lack of reliable information. Since most alternative medicine treatments are classified as food supplements instead of medications, they can make any claims they want and no one can legally refute them. Just as banana farmers could claim that eating the phallic-shaped fruit would lead to penile enlargement, the makers of *silver nitrate* or some tree bark product could fraudulently claim they cure cancer.

The reason these products aren't regulated or investigated is clear. The companies can market and sell them with any claims they want as long as they keep them in the supplements category. Compared to the millions of dollars required for research necessary to bring a prescription drug to market, these agents can be on the shelves with the minimal cost of bottling, labeling, and shipping. More to the point, if these agents were to be studied scientifically, their claims would be subject to the same rigorous standards prescription medications must meet. Since it appears likely that many of them work by the placebo effect (if they work at all), there is no way most would pass the standard.

As noted earlier, the placebo effect is a powerful tool. A placebo is something (often a sugar pill or other inactive ingredient) that is given to a patient that has no known effect on the condition being treated. About one-quarter of people will experience improvement in a medical condition purely because they've been given something. In their mind, they *are* being treated, and the mind is a powerful broker.

The placebo effect is responsible for the fact that so many unproven treatments have testimonials to their effectiveness. Therefore, in proper medical studies, some patients are given the treatment while a *control group* is given a placebo. Neither the patients nor the professionals administering the pill get to know if they are taking the drug or the placebo. If the symptoms of one-quarter of the patients in each group improve, a placebo effect is clearly the reason. However, if one-quarter of the patients in the placebo group are improved, but half of the patients receiving the tested substance are improved, the tested substance is clearly helpful for the symptoms in some patients with that condition.

A good example can be found in the studies on Viagra. The trials used to obtain FDA approval found that 25 percent of patients taking the placebo reported improvement in erections, while about 80 percent of those taking Viagra reported improvement. Therefore, the FDA agreed that the studies showed a clear benefit to Viagra in treating erectile dysfunction, so it was approved for use in the United States.

WHAT DOSE DID I GET?

Even if we did have evidence that alternative medications worked, the lack of regulation would still mean we have no idea how to use them. Manufacturers can label them as having an active ingredient without any quantification of the amount that is present. For example, the most popular alternative medicine treatment for prostate problems is *saw palmetto*, made from the bark of the small palm tree, genus *Serenoa repens*. This bushy plant was known for centuries as a "trash tree" that farmers tried to kill in order to keep it out of their fields. That all changed when it became popular as a prostate cure-all. With a mixture of traditional Native American medicine and the marketing machine of the complementary medicine industry, it has become perhaps the most widely used agent for prostate problems—prescription or not—in the world.

As it happens, the active agent in saw palmetto appears to have some effect that may actually help shrink the prostate. The problem is that the versions on the market have no clearly defined amount of active agent. When tested scientifically, the amounts in various brands are all over the map. Some brands have several times as much concentration as others, although when you are buying pills on the Internet they all sound alike. Some brands barely have enough saw palmetto in them to justify the label. Patients taking those brands clearly receive a placebo effect only, as they hardly have any of the active ingredient at all.

If this only meant that we don't know whether an alternative treatment works or not, the only risk would be the waste of money for something that didn't work. Unfortunately, the risk is much greater, since these agents aren't inert at all. Many that seem benign, such as grapefruit juice, interact with prescription medications to cause untoward effects. Many more have an effect on the cardiovascular or other body systems. Some may even trigger the risk of death.

And none of them is regulated.

PC-SPES: COMPLEMENTARY THERAPY TURNS DEADLY

> *The whole concept that a natural herbal substance can cure advanced prostate cancer has been shattered.*
> —Patrick C. Walsh, MD

A recent example of the risk of alternative medicines was evidenced in the recall in 2002 of *PC-SPES*, a benign-sounding Chinese herbal product. PC-SPES is a "natural" product that appeared to cause regression of prostate cancer. So optimistic was the maker, BotanicLab, that it took the unusual step of having its product scientifically investigated by the University of California, San Francisco.[6]

Researchers were motivated to investigate PC-SPES based on the theory that its ingredients might have chemical activities similar to hormonal treatments already approved for prostate cancer. Early noncontrolled trials showed impressive results. As discussed above, the next step in figuring out whether these results were real or just caused by the placebo effect was to begin a double-blind, placebo-controlled trial.

Early in that trial, the California-based manufacturer voluntarily recalled the medication and closed shop. According to the July 1, 2002, edition of *Urology Times*, the product had been found to contain not only herbs, but also the blood thinner *warfarin*. Yes, the same warfarin that is used as a rat poison by farmers all over the world. Its blood-thinning capability is well known and has long been used as a prescription treatment for patients at risk of stroke or blood clots. However, it is such a dangerous drug that patients who use it must be monitored closely. These patients must have a blood test monthly to assure its level remains *therapeutic* (in the proper range). If the level goes too high, a fatal bleeding episode or stroke could occur. If too low, it might not prevent the problems it is prescribed for. Patients receiving warfarin in PC-

SPES neither knew they were receiving it nor were they monitored for appropriate dosing (of a drug they actually didn't need anyway).

In addition, several lots of the product were found to contain *diethylstilbestrol* (*DES*), the same hormone reviled in the sixties because it caused *feminization* of male fetuses born to mothers who took it during pregnancy. This feminization made them develop female characteristics such as small penises, undescended testicles, and breast enlargement. Its effect on female offspring was even more alarming, as it caused a rare form of vaginal cancer when those babies reached adulthood—a long-term legacy.

DES itself is known to be an effective treatment for prostate cancer. Unfortunately, its side effects of stroke, blood clots, and other catastrophic cardiovascular problems have limited its usefulness, resulting in its being unavailable in the United States. Patients receiving DES in PC-SPES were therefore taking a cancer treatment with proven potentially fatal side effects without knowing enough to make an informed decision. The irony is that warfarin is sometimes prescribed in order to prevent blood clots in patients taking DES. In a strange twist of fate, one of the two drugs contained in PC-SPES actually might have kept the other's potentially fatal side effects in check.

A sister product, *SPES*, was marketed by BotanicLab as an immune system enhancer. It sounded benign enough in the ads—until the FDA warned that it contained *alprazolam*.[7] You might recognize that as the generic name of the prescription medication *Xanax*. It is one of the most effective tranquilizers on the market. In addition, samples were found to contain *indomethacin*, an anti-inflammatory drug used in humans and horses to treat arthritis.

The greatest danger of these drugs (warfarin, DES, alprazolam, indomethacin, and reportedly a couple of other medications) is that the recipients were taking something that they believed to be safe and "natural," when in actuality they were taking prescription medications masquerading as nutritional supplements. BotanicLab closed up shop and disappeared.

IS THERE A ROLE FOR COMPLEMENTARY THERAPY?

Urologists believe several things may decrease your risk of prostate cancer, as detailed in chapter 5. Although it is logical these will also inhibit cancer growth following diagnosis, there are no data to support that idea. Therefore, we must assume that a healthy lifestyle and exercise will enhance your overall health, but we cannot know the role of complementary medicine until much-needed research is done.

KEY POINTS

- The slow-growing nature of most prostate cancers allows that the simplest approach to localized prostate cancer involves watchful waiting. This means accepting the small risk that cancer might progress rapidly despite careful surveillance.
- Men with limited life expectancies (usually less than ten to twenty years) are candidates for watchful waiting.
- Watchful waiting does not mean ignoring. Careful surveillance with PSA, DRE, and potentially repeat biopsy are needed to determine the need for deferred treatment.
- Men with aggressive tumors (Gleason grade seven or higher, advanced disease, or PSA greater than the 10–20 ng/dl range) may be better off being treated even with limited life expectancy.
- Complementary medicine might have an impact on prostate cancer, but it is not well studied.
- Alternative therapy used in lieu of proven treatment is dangerous.

15.

RADICAL PROSTATECTOMY

I win.

—Scott Hamilton, urological cancer survivor
and 1984 Olympic gold medalist in figure skating

*"I want it out." Al was adamant and didn't want to hear about other choices.
"My father had radiation and died. I'm not taking any chances."*

*This made no sense to me. As discussed throughout this book, prostate
cancer is rarely fatal in a short period of time. Most men live for years even
after the cancer has spread. Could Al's father have been one of the rare cases
of very aggressive prostate cancer? "I can't understand how that would
happen," I respectfully conveyed. "That's almost unheard of with prostate
cancer. Is it possible he had some other type of cancer?"*

*"No, it was prostate cancer." He gave a pretty convincing story. "They
found it when he had a TURP. That was the only surgery he had. Then he had
radiation and died in less than a month."*

*This story was most disconcerting to me. There are always exceptions,
but this was so unusual I couldn't let it rest. Al's father had been a patient at
our hospital, so I placed a request for his records. It had been more than a
decade since his death, so they were stored in an off-site location.*

*A week later the records arrived. The pathology report was the first thing
I reviewed. No confusion there—the specimen from his TURP showed
Gleason score $5 + 4 = 9$ adenocarcinoma prostate, a high-grade tumor. How-
ever, even a tumor this high grade rarely is fatal in less than a month.*

Only after complete review did the story become more comprehensible.

*The **metastatic workup** had shown diffuse spread of cancer. At the time of diagnosis, Al's father had cancer throughout the skeleton and in multiple other sites. The radiation had been administered to his lower spine due to painful bony metastases, not to the prostate. Its intent had been palliation—improvement of symptoms—not cure. By the time cancer was identified, cure was no longer an option. Radiation achieved its goal of ending the bone pain, but had never been intended for cure. Al's impression was mistaken.*

I explained the difference in Al's situation from his father's. Only then did he weigh the curative options for a sexually active man fifty-one years old—surgery versus radiation.

***

Surgical removal of the prostate is described by the unfriendly term "**radical prostatectomy**." The very language is unfortunate. Belying its name, it is neither big, bad, nor political. Its origin is in the surgical tradition of naming operations. Removing an organ is described with the suffix "-ectomy." If the organ alone is removed, it's called a *simple* (in this case) *prostatectomy*. If adjacent tissues are removed, it's called a *radical prostatectomy*. Since at least part of each *seminal vesicle* is removed with the prostate, we're stuck with that intimidating name.

As usual, there is good news and bad. The good news is that prostatectomy will cure most patients with **organ-confined** prostate cancer. The bad news—major surgery is required.

OPTIONS TO REMOVE THE PROSTATE

The incisions are small with each of the three surgical options described in this chapter, but the work done through them is anything but minor. A number of surgical paths to the prostate are available. The first, **transurethral**, was described in chapter 8. Unlike the radical approaches discussed in this chapter, the transurethral route (TURP) is used to remove only the central portion of the gland in order to open a channel adequate for voiding. In this chapter, we will consider approaches that allow complete removal.

The first radical prostatectomy was performed in April 1904 by the father of modern urology, Dr. Hugh Hampton Young. He made an incision in the **perineum** between the scrotum and anus. By dissecting only an inch or two, he was able to remove the prostate without opening the patient's abdomen. Because of its approach through the perineum, this is called a **perineal prostatectomy**. Predictably, his initial patients didn't fare particularly well. This was the era before antibiotics. Moreover, his patients had advanced disease prior to undergoing therapy. Nevertheless, he proved that the procedure could be accomplished, leading to a century of improvements that have brought us to the successful point where we are today.

Dr. Terrance Millin performed the first abdominal approach in 1947 in the United Kingdom. By dissecting down the posterior (back side) of the pubic bone he was able to obtain better access, but the **dorsal vein complex** overlying the prostate formed a bloody barrier that kept most urologists from following in his footsteps until the eighties. Since this operation is performed behind (*retro*) the *pubic bone*, it is called a radical retropubic prostatectomy (RRP).

Experience with excessive bleeding limited adoption of RRP until the latter decades of the twentieth century. At that time, Dr. Patrick Walsh spent hours in the anatomy lab and at the operating room table delineating the steps necessary to safely remove the prostate via the abdomen. Combining a better understanding of the venous anatomy with an understanding of the location of the nerves necessary to preserve sexual function, his *anatomical* approach finally allowed great numbers of urologists to follow his lead. Hence, the name *anatomical prostatectomy*.

The most recent modification involves the use of laparoscopy. This operation, called a **laparoscopic radical prostatectomy**, takes advantage of optical or digital lenses that allow the surgeon to perform the procedure through small incisions. Its newest embodiment is the highly publicized **robotic prostatectomy**. This is essentially the same operation performed using different technological advances.

All three options involve the same basic steps performed via different approaches. The first two options are considered "open" operations, since an actual incision is used. This is in contrast to a "laparoscopic" technique, which includes either traditional or robotic laparoscopic prostatectomy. This chapter will explore the routes and experiences you could expect from these operations.

NERVE SPARING VERSUS NONNERVE SPARING

Most sexually active men wish to remain so. However, before we understood that the **neurovascular bundles** containing the penile nerves were adjacent to the prostate instead of running through it, impotence inevitably followed a prostatectomy. Because we didn't know where these microscopic-sized nerves were, both bundles were cut during almost every radical prostatectomy.

Removing the prostate while leaving the responsible nerves intact is called a **nerve-sparing prostatectomy**. This term leads to a lot of confusion. First, the prostate is removed during either a nerve-sparing or a nonnerve-sparing operation. The only difference is whether the penile nerves are removed along with it or not. Sparing the nerves requires considerably more skill in order to take the intended target (prostate) while leaving intact the nerves that course along either side.

The second source of confusion is in regard to potency following nerve-sparing prostatectomy. Many men assume that sparing the nerves should guarantee potency. If only it were that simple. Even if the nerves are left intact, they may be damaged by pulling them away from the prostate, an electrical current from cautery used to control bleeding, or swelling in the postoperative period.

I explain this concept as it relates to the wiring in my eighty-year-old home. If I work on a lighting fixture, sometimes the wires crumble and become damaged even if I don't cut them. Similarly, the neurovascular bundles in a sixty-year-old man are, by definition, sixty years old. Even if they are not cut, they may be damaged simply from the manipulation of major cancer surgery, so their function can be affected.

Reviewing the anatomy described in chapter 2, you can see that there is a distance of only a few millimeters between prostate and nerves. The surgeon must divide the tissue just between the prostate and these nerves. Being a little bit off in one direction might leave some of the prostate behind. A cut in the other direction could nick one or both nerve bundles, which might cause damage to the patient's ability to have an erection. Hence the degree of difficulty for nerve-sparing prostatectomy. The proximity is demonstrated in figure 15-1.

Because of the technical challenge, some surgeons do not perform nerve-sparing prostatectomy. Their patients will not be able to have spontaneous erections following surgery, and will require correction of this problem by using one of the options for erectile dysfunction (described in chapter 19) if they wish to remain sexually active.

If a man already has erectile dysfunction, or is not sexually active, a non-nerve-sparing prostatectomy will be acceptable. Most men will desire the possibility of spontaneous erections, so they will opt for nerve sparing. If you assume the surgeon is skilled at nerve sparing, success depends mainly on your preoperative status. If you are under age fifty and have absolutely normal erections, the risk of impotence is low with one report as low as 10 percent.[1] This is probably optimistic, and most urologists will simply predict that a majority of such healthy men will be naturally potent following recovery. Men older than that or those having mild erectile dysfunction already will be less likely to maintain natural potency, although they can be successfully treated.

OTHER REASONS TO PERFORM NERVE SPARING

There may be other reasons to spare the neurovascular bundles even if a man is impotent preoperatively. First, recall that the nerve-sparing prostatectomy is also known as the *anatomic prostatectomy*. Therefore, performing this operation is considered to be more true to the anatomy. It may be difficult for the layman to understand, but as a surgeon there are few pleasures to match that of an operation that plays out in a nice, anatomic fashion. Like an artist who fashions marble into sculpture, a surgeon takes great pride in removing a cancer from a patient and making the anatomy look like a picture from a textbook. A good result is likely to follow.

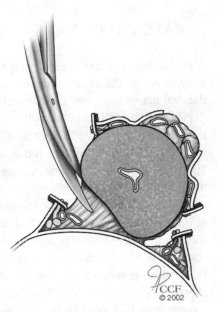

On a less esoteric level, the neurovascular bundles also appear to stimulate constriction of the *urinary rhabdosphincter*. Many surgeons have found that leaving them intact may enhance continence. There is debate on whether improved continence is actually related to the nerves or simply to having performed a more anatomic dissection, but the results may be better whatever the reason.

Figure 15-1. Scissors cut between the prostate (large round structure) and the **neurovascular bundle** (small circular areas on other side of scissors, shown in cross-section).

NERVE SPARING OR CANCER SPARING?

When we first began performing nerve-sparing prostatectomy, many surgeons were concerned that cutting so close to the prostate risked leaving cancer behind. As experience grew and more centers began performing the procedure, we found that this is not the case. The risk of cancer recurrence appears to be no higher in men who undergo nerve-sparing than it is for those who undergo traditional prostatectomy.

One caveat to the above statement: We palpate, or feel, the nerve bundles at the time of surgery if we are concerned that cancer might be extending into them. If cancer is in one of the bundles, it can be removed intentionally in order to maximize the chance of cure. Removing one bundle decreases the chance of potency, but up to one-third of men will be able to remain sexually active even with one intact nerve.[2]

SURAL NERVE GRAFT

A recent development, creating hope for potency if nerve sparing is not feasible, involves the use of a nerve harvested from the leg interposed between the two cut ends of the neurovascular bundle. The sural nerve is a sensory nerve from the calf that is not vital. Its large caliber makes it possible to sew in place of the removed segment of neurovascular bundle through magnification. Although removal of the neurovascular bundles theoretically yields 100 percent impotence, some centers have reported significant potency rates using sural nerve grafting.

Sural nerve graft was conceived by Drs. Peter Scardino and Rahul Nath at Baylor Medical Center. (Dr. Scardino has since moved to Memorial Sloan Kettering Cancer Center in New York.) They perform their procedure during standard retropubic prostatectomy. Dr. Jihad Kaouk at the Cleveland Clinic Foundation pioneered the use of nerve interposition during laparoscopic/robotic prostatectomy as well, taking advantage of the magnification and fine motor control afforded by the robotic systems.

The most significant disadvantage is the additional operative time required, which could be an hour or more. Dressing care for the leg donor site is minor. However, the technique remains controversial and has been accepted at only a few centers. Its value will become clear in the coming years only if widespread experience yields success.

PELVIC LYMPHADENECTOMY

In the era prior to PSA screening (around 1990), half of all patients already had **metastases** or cancer spread at the time of diagnosis. The pelvic lymph nodes are often the first place that prostate cancer spreads. As a result, they were traditionally removed at the beginning of RRP in a staging operation called **pelvic lymphadenectomy**. Their removal was considered a vital and final part of *staging*.

Because these nodes are readily accessible to the prostate surgeon based on their location nearby, they can be easily removed in a matter of minutes. Urologists would routinely wait for the pathologist to freeze the removed lymph nodes in order to perform a rapid biopsy view, called a *frozen section*, prior to proceeding with the prostatectomy. If the frozen section identified metastatic cancer, the operation was aborted and the patient was told it was too late to cure his cancer. Men awoke with their own variations of one question in mind: Did it spread to the lymph nodes, or were they able to remove the cancerous prostate?

The need for pelvic lymphadenectomy was a major disadvantage to treating prostate cancer with either radiation or perineal prostatectomy (laparoscopic/robotic prostatectomy had not even been envisioned at the time). Those options did not involve exposure of the pelvic lymph nodes, so staging was felt to be incomplete if pelvic lymphadenectomy was omitted. The importance placed on adequate staging was so great that men sometimes underwent surgery solely to remove the lymph nodes. When their negative status was confirmed, definitive treatment with either radiation or perineal prostatectomy ensued. In fact, the initial foray of laparoscopy into urological practice was to perform pelvic lymphadenectomy via a laparoscopic approach in order to stage such patients.

Things have *really* changed. Most cancers are now found early in their course. Whereas positive lymph nodes were found commonly just a few decades ago, it is now uncommon to do so.

Therefore, few men with prostate cancer currently require pelvic lymphadenectomy. However, some men will undergo the procedure if the risk of positive nodes is substantial, in a manner as defined in the previous chapter; this would indicate the need for staging **bone scans** and **CT scans**. This decision is typically made when the PSA is elevated to at least 10 and probably 20, or when the Gleason score is at least seven. Using these criteria, a study from the Cleveland Clinic showed that such low-risk patients did as well without performing pelvic lymphadenectomy, so it could be safely omitted in their cases.[3]

If the pelvis is already opened in anticipation of prostatectomy, removal of the pelvic lymph nodes takes a matter of minutes. Risk is minimal, although there are large blood vessels in the area that could be damaged. Very rarely the *obturator nerve* can be injured, leading to leg weakness.

It is also fairly straightforward to perform pelvic lymphadenectomy at the beginning of laparoscopic/robotic prostatectomy. The option does not exist during perineal prostatectomy, although the nodes could be removed using either a second incision or a laparoscope.

It now appears that removing cancerous nodes may allow long-term survival or even cure in some men previously thought incurable. In addition, many men are more comfortable knowing that the lymph nodes have been removed and confirmed negative. If you feel that way you should discuss this issue with your surgeon.

Several urologists have recently claimed that the cure rate might actually be higher if even more lymph nodes are removed at the time of surgery. Whether this is true remains under investigation.[4]

OPTION ONE: RADICAL RETROPUBIC PROSTATECTOMY (RRP)—THE GOLD STANDARD

Although it is sometimes portrayed as being the "biggest" alternative of the three because of the lower abdominal incision used, RRP is the gold standard. It offers direct visualization of the entire surgical field and relatively unimpeded access to the surgical site. Experience is vast and enduring for the past few decades.

After the patient is placed under epidural or general anesthesia (as described later in this chapter), the skin is sterilized. Drapes cover everything except the lower abdomen and genitals. An incision extends from the *umbilicus* (belly button) to the pubic bone, and retractors hold abdominal muscles apart to expose the prostate. The surgeon may remove lymph nodes if there is concern that cancer has spread to them, as discussed above.

The surgeon opens a layer called *endopelvic fascia*, places a suture around the dorsal vein complex, and then divides it to expose the prostate. Prostatic attachments can be dissected away. The **neurovascular bundles** responsible for erections fall away safely if the operation is nerve sparing.

The blood supply to each side of the prostate is controlled with sutures, metallic clips, or cautery. Special care must be taken with all three in order to avoid injuring the neurovascular bundles if attempting nerve sparing.

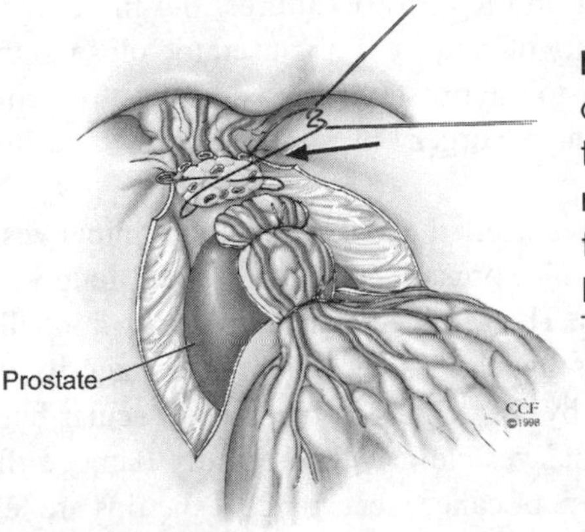

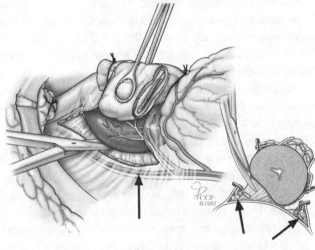

Prostate

Figure 15-2. The surgeon has divided the **dorsal vein complex** to expose the prostate underneath. A suture is placed over this open vein to control bleeding (arrow).

Figure 15-3. As demonstrated in two views, the surgeon has separated the prostate from the neurovascular bundles. Rolling the prostate to the side allows the nerves to fall away to the side in order to preserve their innervation of the penis.

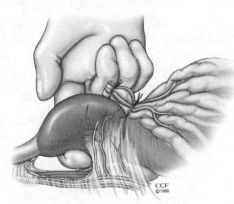

Figure 15-4. Once both neurovascular bundles are released and allowed to fall away from the prostate, the surgeon can lift the prostate away from the rectum as shown (during retropubic prostatectomy only). This allows him to protect the nerves while separating the prostate from the urethra and bladder neck.

The nerves may become entrapped in the clips or sutures, but more commonly are damaged by the electricity of cautery if it is used too close to the nerves. Because of their proximity to the prostate, this is difficult to avoid and is a major reason you should have surgery by someone who is skilled in prostatectomy.

After the main blood supply is controlled and divided, the seminal vesicles and vasi deferentia are divided. The prostate is then removed along with at least half of the seminal vesicles. The seminal vesicles were traditionally removed in their entirety, but this appears unnecessary in a majority of patients. Their tips are surrounded by the origins of the neurovascular bundles, so removing the entire seminal vesicle can theoretically damage the nerves. It appears that there is no risk of cancer recurrence if the tips are left intact,[5] and continence may be better as well.[6] Nevertheless, many surgeons still remove the entire seminal vesicles based on personal preference and long-standing teaching. The bladder neck is separated from the prostate at the point where they are essentially fused. Sometimes the opening into the bladder neck is large enough that it must be reconstructed back to the size of the urethra that it must be sewn to.

Once the prostate is out of the way, the surgeon will ensure that all blood vessels are adequately secured (with either sutures, metallic staples, or cautery). Sewing the bladder neck to the urethra completes the reconstruction. The site where they are attached is called the **anastomosis**. The sutures are tied down over a catheter that runs through the middle to hold things open until healed. One or two drains are left in place to remove any extra fluid, including urine that might seep out of the suture lines. Sutures close the abdominal wall and sutures or staples close the deal.

Different surgeons may alter many of the steps above based on experience, including changing the order. As long as all steps are completed, it is likely a good outcome will follow when the operation is performed by an experienced prostatectomist.

A final issue regarding RRP has arisen with the advent of laparoscopic hernia repair. This operation often involves placement of a large sheet of mesh to obliterate the space a hernia would occupy. Scarring from this mesh makes RRP difficult to perform (as discussed later in this book).

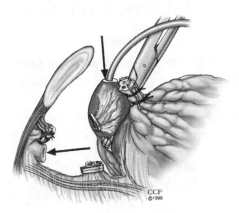

Figure 15-5. The surgeon has divided the urethra and is using the catheter to pull the prostate upward. The lower arrow shows the cut end of the urethra that is underneath the external urinary **sphincter**. The upper arrow shows the other end of the urethra (containing a catheter) as it exits the prostatic apex.

Figure 15-6. The bladder neck has been separated from the prostate and the scissors are cutting the remaining attachments away from the prostate and seminal vesical (arrow).

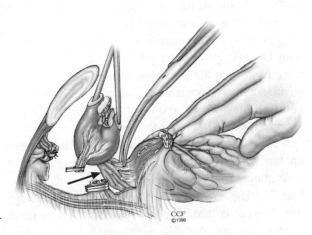

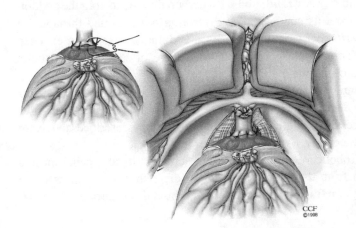

Figure 15-7. Sutures have attached the bladder neck to the urethra to form an **anastomosis**.

OPTION TWO: LAPAROSCOPIC/ROBOTIC RADICAL PROSTATECTOMY

The newest entry into the field has been the focus of much publicity. In the nineties, Dr. William Schuessler pioneered the first laparoscopic radical prostatectomy. He and his colleagues performed nine such operations, each lasting essentially an entire workday. They concluded that the operation was feasible, but not a realistic option at that time. I attended Dr. Schuessler's initial discussion of the first patients during an American Urological Association annual meeting. His conclusion was something on the order of, "Don't even think about it!"

Things have changed.

Laparoscopic prostatectomy has taken the urological world by storm. Its most technologically advanced version—robotic prostatectomy—has allowed surgeons who previously were uncomfortable with laparoscopic surgery to master the operation in a matter of months. The only thing lacking with laparoscopic/robotic prostatectomy is a good body of evidence of its effectiveness in the published urological literature—the standard by which all medical developments are measured. If eventual results prove to be as good as they are in retropubic prostatectomy, the newer operation will become a standard option for most men.

The patient is positioned so that the intestines will fall away from the operative site in order to improve visibility and to minimize the chance of their injury. That means his head must be much lower than his midsection or feet. The legs are separated and held in place using stirrups. After sterilization, five or six laparoscopic "ports" (hollow cylinders that camera lenses or instruments pass through) are placed into the abdomen in a fan-shaped pattern. The abdominal cavity is inflated with carbon dioxide to hold the abdominal wall away from its contents. The dissection is performed through the abdominal or *peritoneal* cavity, so the intra-abdominal organs are exposed and pulled on. This is one potential disadvantage of laparoscopic/robotic prostatectomy in occasional patients.

Surgeons employ a variety of approaches to remove the prostate at this point, using too many different techniques to describe in detail. All involve removing the prostate using essentially the same steps described above for retropubic prostatectomy, although the order may differ.

During the robotic version, the surgeon actually sits at a panel located across the room from the patient in order to drive the robot. An assistant holds laparoscopic retractors and puts sutures in and out through the ports while the surgeon sits in regular clothing and drives the robot by placing his hands inside controls attached electronically to ports inside the patient. It should be noted that the term "robotic" is something of a misnomer. Instead of a true robot, this operation involves a machine that is used to actually duplicate the movement of a surgeons hand inside the patient. He drives the robot's parts, making it essentially an extension of himself. Therefore, the term *robotic assisted* is more apt.

The most significant difference in procedures involves the technique used to sew the bladder neck to the urethra. For the "open" operations a series of somewhere between four and twelve sutures (depending on the surgeon's preference, usually six or less) are used to create the **anastomosis**. Laparoscopic/robotic surgeons use a "running" or continuous suture line. One suture goes from urethra to bladder neck and back repeatedly until the tissues are together.

OPTION THREE: RADICAL PERINEAL PROSTATECTOMY

Despite the fact that the initial prostatectomies were perineal, few American urologists continue to use this approach. However, some pockets of excellent surgeons continue to obtain their best results with perineal prostatectomy.

Patient position is vital to perineal prostatectomy. The incision is between the scrotum and rectum, so the patient is positioned with his legs held up by stirrups in a manner similar to a pelvic examination in women. This positioning requires that most patients be placed under general anesthesia. The combination of positioning and access away from the lymph nodes also precludes **pelvic lymphadenectomy** during perineal prostatectomy.

After sterilization as described for RRP, a curved incision extends between the two bones at the lower end of the pelvis—the same two bones you feel when sitting too long on a hard bench or bleacher. The curve looks like a frown, but its extra length facilitates exposure. The surgeon dissects along the anterior rectum until he reaches the prostatic apex. It is cut away from the urethra just as in retropubic prostatectomy. Special instruments then allow the surgeon to manipulate the prostate back and forth until all attachments and blood vessels are freed, and the prostate is separated from the bladder neck. The seminal vesicles and vasi are cut and the prostate is removed. An anastomosis is created in a manner similar to that described above.

Nerve sparing during perineal prostatectomy is more difficult because the neurovascular bundles lie slightly behind each side of the prostate. This anatomy allows the surgeon to release them to fall away during retropubic prostatectomy, but makes it more difficult for him to reach the prostate when approached posteriorly, as required during the perineal approach. In addition, large prostates can be difficult to remove through the limited space of a perineal incision.

HOW DO I DECIDE WHICH OPERATION?

The best advice I have heard on this question comes from my mentor, Dr. Joseph Smith. As chairman of urology at Vanderbilt University, he is a master of all three versions and taught me much of what I still use when performing a radical prostatectomy. Dr. Smith states that you should "choose your surgeon, not your operation." This is good advice.

I had the great privilege of serving on the faculty of the First World Summit on Radical Prostatectomy in 2002 with a distinguished panel of surgeons, many of whose work is described in this chapter. All the alternatives were explored, and it was clear to me that there are surgeons doing an excellent job using all three techniques. There are differences, and urologists debate their significance.

The most visible difference is the incision. RRP appears to have the seemingly larger incision, reaching from umbilicus (belly button) to pubic bone. The hole is deeper because that is where the prostate lies. Perineal prostatectomy incisions are more hidden below the scrotum, but their actual length is about the same as for RRP. Laparoscopic/robotic prostatectomy involves five or six separate small incisions. However, their combined length ends up being about the same as the total length of retropubic or perineal incisions.

The conventional wisdom has been that nerve sparing is better with the retropubic approach. This has been challenged by recent reports of significant potency rates following laparoscopic/robotic prostatectomy.[7] Such data are scarce, however, and must be confirmed before we know the expected potency rate as the procedure spreads through the urological community. Until multiple centers demonstrate the ability to preserve potency, this will remain controversial. The same concern arises regarding continence, as data have been slow in coming. Based on the posterior location of the penile nerves, preserving potency via perineal prostatectomy is challenging, although some surgeons report good results.

Blood loss is usually highest during retropubic prostatectomy, although it is less now than ever based on continued improvements in surgical technique and experience. Performing the operation under **epidural anesthesia** instead of general anesthesia also lessens blood loss as discussed below. Transfusion rates with any of the three should be less than 20 percent, and probably less than 10 percent in the current era.

Some centers report lower duration of hospitalization, or *length of stay*, following perineal or laparoscopic/robotic surgery as opposed to retropubic prostatectomy. However, this is a vague parameter and based more on surgeon preference than on a true difference in outcomes. For instance, during my residency in the eighties and early nineties we routinely kept patients in the hospital for about five days. I now routinely discharge patients from the hospital the day after RRP, and will sometimes perform the operation as a true outpatient procedure in properly selected patients.

It does appear that patients may return to work earlier following laparoscopic/robotic prostatectomy, probably based on less disturbance of the abdominal wall (or pelvic floor in the case of perineal prostatectomy) muscles. This must be weighed against a couple of disadvantages. On the downside, laparoscopic/robotic surgery requires general anesthesia instead of regional, as discussed below. The instruments go through the abdominal cavity. Most urologists are more experienced and skilled with open prostatectomy. The final limitation of laparoscopic/robotic surgery involves the loss of tactile sensation. In open surgery we occasionally determine if the nerves may safely be spared based on their proximity to a palpable cancer (although most cannot be felt). Laparoscopic/robotic surgery does not include such feeling, although the use of color doppler ultrasound may allow the surgeon to see this area better in order to know where to cut. Whether this risks either nerve damage or loss of cancer control remains to be seen, but it is unlikely this will be the case.

Finally, some surgeons tout an advantage of robotic instead of standard laparoscopic prostatectomy. This is especially enticing in marketing materials. Technically, they are the same operation but with the robot holding the surgical instruments while the surgeon commands the robot with joysticks. The robot helps surgeons learn laparoscopic techniques more quickly by simplifying suturing inside the patient's body, but otherwise the principles remain the same. Drs. Inderbir Gill and Jihad Kaouk at the Cleveland Clinic are highly skilled laparoscopic prostate surgeons who are so comfortable with the pure laparoscopic techniques that they find no significant improvement in the surgical outcome when using the robot. Therefore, it is basically a patient and physician preference to choose between laparoscopic and robotic-assisted prostatectomy.

HOW DO I CHOOSE A SURGEON?

> *Choose the very best doctors you can and trust the hell out of them.*
>
> —Lance Armstrong

A urologist performed the biopsy and informed you of the diagnosis in all likelihood. He is your first and most likely option. You know him and have already trusted your health to him, so at least consider his qualifications.

A second opinion is always reasonable for a diagnosis as serious as cancer. This can help not only in choosing a form of treatment, but also in finding a qualified alternative. Don't skimp. Seek someone who is dedicated to prostate cancer treatment. The surgeon should be experienced, having performed hundreds of prostatectomies. The incidence of prostate cancer is decreasing; since fewer of these operations are needed these days, he should still perform prostatectomy on a "regular basis." Though no one agrees on what that means, it would probably mean at least twenty a year. Some reports show success is greater with more than forty cases a year.[8] The difference in complication rates can vary from 5 to 18 percent, depending on whether the surgeon has done over fifteen hundred or under five hundred.[9]

A young surgeon just out of training should not automatically be dismissed. He is probably up on the latest techniques, which may help compensate for inexperience. If choosing a young surgeon (in his first one to five years of practice), you should confirm that he trained at a program where prostate cancer surgery was performed on a high-volume basis. If he didn't participate in the operation in at least fifty cases during training, you might consider letting him gain a little more experience on someone else. If he received additional training through an oncology fellowship following residency, this usually obviates concerns of inexperience.

The other question is whether your surgeon is a teaching or nonteaching surgeon. There are advantages to both. A surgeon at a teaching hospital is held to a high standard. Someone is always watching over the shoulders—a mighty quality control. Residents scrub on his cases. Visiting physicians watch to learn, often during live surgical feeds for educational forums. Observers expect him to be good, or they wouldn't be there to watch.

Postoperative care is intense with some assortment of residents, fellows, and medical students crossing every *T* and dotting every *I*. Mistakes are ruminated at a "morbidity and mortality conference," as a definitive quality control. Most nationally or internationally known physicians practice in academic settings.

Potential disadvantages of an academic center are bureaucratic. Things move more slowly. Tradition can be stifling. Doctors in various levels of training participate in each patient's care, and will typically assist during surgery.

Nonteaching surgeons operate more independently. At most, a partner assists during the complex part of the operation or covers his practice on call. The requirements for quality assurance are less defined. However, many excellent surgeons perform prostatectomy in this setting and achieve first-rate results. Many of them were trained at the programs alluded to above, and maintain their skills and knowledge through ongoing medical education.

Your choice regarding teaching is a personal one. You should decide if you prefer the higher-profile setting of an academic medical center or the low-key environment of a community hospital. Are you comfortable with physicians in training assisting in your care? Do you desire the increased intensity of care they offer?

A long-standing secret in the healthcare system is that the best source of information on a surgeon comes from those who watch him in action. Scrub techs, nurses, anesthetists, anesthesiologists, and residents on his team in the operating room know his work inside out. They know if he maintains his cool during challenging parts of operations. They know his each and every move—and whether they would send their family members to him. If you have such connections, this information can be more valuable than any other source.

RESIDENT INVOLVEMENT

Patients often ask about the role of residents and fellows during surgery and their postoperative care. Let's face it—no surgeon can do it all alone; someone must cut, tie, or help perform various other steps required for prostatectomy. Whether resident, nurse, or physician's assistant serves these functions, a team is required to perform complex maneuvers that often take more than two hands.

It is difficult to quantify the effect of resident involvement, but it has been shown that operative success is as good when a resident actively assists during an operation under the watchful eye of the attending surgeon as when the attending surgeon places every stitch himself.[10] The reputations of the top academic centers is based on the synergy of physicians at various skill and experience levels working together to provide optimal outcomes. In addition, the redundancy of care increases the intensity of observation and attention to detail in a way that a single surgeon cannot physically achieve. Residents available in-house through the night can yield immediate postoperative care.

Thus, resident involvement is an important part of care in academic medical centers, and they are an integral part of the care team. You will benefit from their participation.

WHY NOT JUST TAKE OUT THE CANCEROUS PART?

No matter which route is taken, the entire prostate is removed in order to cure the cancer. Patients often suggest taking out just the cancer and leaving in the remainder of the gland. This isn't feasible for a couple of reasons.

The first is that prostate cancer is what we call a "field change" disease. That means that the entire "field" of similar cells or tissue—the prostate gland tissue in this circumstance —is at risk of developing the same malignant changes that have already occurred in the tumor. If the remainder of the tissue is untreated and left in place, the die may already be cast that these tissues will become cancerous as well.

As a result of this field change, prostate cancers tend to be *multifocal* or occur in clusters of small tumors located throughout the gland. It is common to find one or more unsuspected *satellite tumors* in locations secluded from the primary tumor when the pathologist examines the gland following radical prostatectomy. If only the main tumor had been removed, another cancer would remain ready to do harm. **Prostatic intraepithelial neoplasia (PIN)** is commonly found in association with prostate cancer. If not removed, this cancer precursor can become malignant in follow-up.

Even if field change wasn't an issue, another problem is determining exactly which part of the prostate is cancerous. We know that one of the world's premier urological pathologists couldn't see or feel one-quarter of cancers even with the sliced prostate in his hand.[11] Therefore, a urologist operating inside the body would never be able to tell beyond doubt which part was cancerous. For these reasons, the entire cancerous prostate is removed during radical prostatectomy.

PREPARING FOR SURGERY

In the weeks prior to the operation, you will want to become mentally prepared for the experience. Clear your schedule as much as possible. Pay all bills. Arrange for coverage at work. Set limits on social responsibilities, and try to minimize the amount of drudgery that will require your attention during recovery. The last things you need are unnecessary distractions draining energy that should be directed at recovery.

It is unlikely that you need to make any major adjustments to your living space. Still, it seems a majority of patients are convinced otherwise. Believe it or not, *stairs are not a problem* (even if you had a sural nerve graft). Although safe, you may find yourself minimizing unnecessary trips up and down simply for comfort's sake. There is no need for a special bed or other change in furnishings.

Stocking up on routine items and groceries makes sense. In regard to groceries, simply have available what you like. You will be eating regular food upon hospital discharge. Your appetite may be subdued for a time, so try to be conservative in choosing foods you consistently like. It may not be a good time to try that new raw seafood dish.

You should purchase at least two packages of incontinence pads to deal with what is usually temporary difficulty with bladder control. Patients often ask which pads are best, and I never have a straightforward answer. Instead, I recommend that you visit any pharmacy and consider the options in their incontinence products section. Look at the various types and consider how you would feel about wearing the styles on a temporary basis. Some men prefer a more cup-shaped form, while others want something flat that will lie inside the shorts. Having more than one type on hand will allow experimentation to find the best way to manage this annoyance until your bladder control recovers fully.

I have found mail-order services useful because they provide incontinence products direct to your home. This lets you consider a number of products with minimal effort, and then allows you to avoid the hassle or potential embarrassment of shopping for them. The service I use is Home and Health Solutions (see Resources), although I am sure there are other companies that provide similar services.

Avoid the natural tendency to fret and worry. Stress only impairs the body's ability to handle major surgery. Don't feel the need to explain every detail to everyone you know. The mailman will get over it if you fail to elaborate on your Gleason score. Energy can better be spent on enjoying your usual activities. Even better, take any chance you get to do some things prior to surgery that you usually put off because you're too busy. You deserve it.

THE FINAL COUNTDOWN

Any blood thinners, including aspirin, ibuprofen, vitamin E, or any other pre-scribed medications should be discontinued on your doctor's advice. Most should be halted at least five days prior to surgery.

Your last meal for a day or two must be completed before midnight of the final preoperative day. (Some surgeons also recommend clear liquids and/or medications to evacuate your intestines the day before.) Patients are often asked to shower in Hibiclens or some other antimicrobial soap, with special attention to vigorously cleaning the abdomen and groin area. This decreases bacteria that might cause infection. As an added precaution, antibi-otics are given intravenously immediately before the operation so they go directly into the blood stream to kill any bacteria. In addition, some surgeons recommend antibiotics and enemas to empty the intestinal tract. This is espe-cially likely if perineal prostatectomy is planned.

All the skin in the area is shaved immediately prior to the operation. Shaving earlier than that may cause small scratches in the skin that bacteria can grow into overnight. The skin is then sterilized with a solution in order to kill as many bacteria as possible. While this occurs, members of the surgical team scrub their hands with similar solutions. Sterile surgical drapes (sheets) are then placed over everything except the actual operative site—in this case the lower abdomen and genitals. Some surgeons cover the entire area with a sticky sheet of clear plastic to seal off everything except the actual incision. The sur-gical team will wear sterile gowns and gloves as a final barrier to infection.

ANESTHETIC OPTIONS

In the operating room the patient is placed under anesthesia. This can be done using either *general anesthesia* (the patient is "completely out") or *regional anesthesia* (the lower half of the body is anesthetized). Regional anesthesia is usually done by **epidural**, where a long needle in inserted through the skin of the back into the spinal column. A small catheter is then placed over the needle and left in the epidural space, a potential cavity surrounding the nerves to the surgical area where they exit the spinal canal. The needle is then removed. Through this catheter, a local anesthetic similar to that given by dentists can be continuously injected to block sensation through the operation and in the postoperative period. Narcotics may supplement the local anesthetic.

Your form of anesthetic will largely be determined by whichever method works well in the experience of the urologist and his usual anesthesiologists. Although many prefer general anesthesia, surgeons at several high-volume prostate cancer centers such as the Cleveland Clinic are most pleased with outcomes from epidural anesthesia. The only common disadvantage is that it takes more time to administer. It poses an exceedingly low risk of nerve damage—so rare that I have never seen it occur. Nevertheless, some men prefer to be "completely out" and unaware of what is occurring in their surroundings (surgeons sometimes agree, or don't want the distraction of the patient talking to them during surgery).

The advantages of epidural anesthesia easily outweigh these minor disadvantages. Sedation can easily be administered if you prefer. Moreover, blood loss is lessened when the patient avoids *positive pressure breathing* caused by being on a respirator during general anesthesia. The ventilator places pressure into the chest cavity, raising pressure in the venous system so veins bleed more when transected.

Furthermore, the most effective way to control pain is to avoid it in the first place. Therefore, if the epidural is dosed prior to making the incision, the pain threshold is never crossed so postoperative pain control becomes easier. The impact on postoperative recovery is obvious, and the benefits of less pain trauma to the body during the operation appear to be equally substantial.

Despite these factors, many hospitals continue to use general anesthesia successfully as their preferred method for a variety of reasons. For one, epidural anesthesia will not adequately control pain during laparoscopic prostatectomy because it cannot block pain caused by distending the entire abdomen with carbon dioxide, as discussed above. In addition, sometimes the anesthesiologist simply cannot achieve an adequate block with an epidural so a general anesthetic will be required in order to proceed with surgery even if an epidural was planned.

BLOOD ISSUES

Recall that radical prostatectomy was an operation routinely associated with significant blood loss until the last two or three decades. Currently, fewer than 10 percent of men will require transfusion if surgery is performed in most high-volume cancer centers.[12]

Transfusion was a scary experience in the eighties and early nineties. AIDS was emerging and our ability to detect infected blood was poor. We routinely required men scheduled for major surgery to donate two or three units of their own blood in the weeks prior to surgery.

Such donation is done at the Red Cross or other blood banks. The blood is tested, processed, frozen, and stored until it is delivered to the operating room at the time of surgery. This is called **autologous blood donation**.

Despite improvements in surgical technique, some prostatectomies will still involve enough blood loss to require transfusion. For this reason, some urologists continue to routinely recommend autologous donation. Many urologists (including me) no longer routinely recommend it for a number of reasons. First, it is usually unnecessary since most men don't need a transfusion. Second, the blood supply is markedly safer now that we know how to detect AIDS.

Finally, there is no scientific evidence that donation lessens risk. It seems logical that it would, but there are several reasons it may not. There is always a minute chance of your blood becoming mislabeled and mixed up with that of another person. That person might have infected blood. Your own blood units could become infected with contaminating bacteria, or you could experience a reaction to some component used in processing. These risks may be as high as the risk of AIDS missed by a *false negative* test.

It now appears the chance of developing AIDS from a transfusion is about one in somewhere between 1 and 2 million, according to the American Red Cross.[13] Combined with the infrequency of transfusion with modern prostatectomy, your chance is therefore less than that of being struck by lightning in the hospital parking lot.

The greatest risks of receiving donor blood are actually not related to AIDS. The first is a transfusion reaction. Think of this as an allergy to someone else's blood. Transfusion reactions can occasionally, but rarely, be serious. Moreover, the most common transfusion risk is hepatitis. Several different viruses cause hepatitis, and they may be missed by routine testing. Therefore, although the blood supply is the safest that it has ever been, transfusion—like everything else in medicine—will never be risk free. Nonetheless, saving your own blood is not either for the reasons above, so the value of autologous blood donation is unclear. You should discuss this with your doctor prior to surgery.

METHODS TO MINIMIZE THE CHANCE OF NEEDING A TRANSFUSION

The most effective way to avoid transfusion is to avoid blood loss. The first step is having surgery in a high-volume institution performed by a surgeon experienced in radical prostatectomy. Many studies have shown this to be the case. Experienced surgeons will have a good feel for how low your blood count can safely go. The level to trigger a transfusion is subjective, so you want to know that your surgeon will only follow this course if absolutely necessary.

Epidural anesthesia is associated with less blood loss. As noted, we believe this is because the respirator used during general anesthesia creates pressure inside the veins, pushing more blood out of any veins that are cut. The pressure created inside the abdomen opposes this venous oozing, so laparoscopic/robotic prostatectomy also appears to be associated with less blood loss. Bleeding may also be limited during perineal prostatectomy because the dorsal vein complex may be avoided.

A device called a cell saver can collect blood from the operative field so that it can be returned to the patient during or after surgery. Studies have clearly

JEHOVAH'S WITNESSES

[T]hat they abstain from pollutions of idols, and from fornication, and from things strangled, and from blood.
—Acts 15:20

Religious beliefs prevent most Jehovah's Witnesses from receiving transfusions based on their interpretation of scripture. This presents a special challenge, since these patients could die during or after surgery if major blood loss occurs.

For this reason, many surgeons will decline to operate on these men. This is understandable, since surgeons are committed to keeping people alive. To watch a patient bleed to death would be unbearable. However, the surgeon is legally bound to respect the wishes of the patient despite his clinical judgment to the contrary.

Depending on their own interpretation of the scriptures, some Witnesses will consent to the use of the cell saver, which significantly improves the surgeon's comfort level in these cases. However, some Witnesses take a literal view. Most refuse autologous donation, and some decline cell saver or any other form of blood once it has left their vascular system.

I take the approach that men of the Jehovah's Witness faith have every right to stand for their beliefs. This should not preclude them from having the operation they need. Although I must admit a little higher level of anxiety during their operations than any other, because of the risk of bleeding to death, I have fortunately operated on many but have never seen a Witness experience severe blood loss (although it certainly is possible).

shown that the filters prevent recycling of cancer cells, and that patients who have the benefit of the cell saver during radical prostatectomy have no greater risk of cancer recurrence than other patients.[14]

IN THE HOSPITAL

Immediately following surgery you will go to the recovery room. If your surgery was performed under epidural anesthesia, you may be the most alert patient in the ward. If general anesthesia or sedation were administered, you will become progressively less groggy.

Nurses record vital signs and assure that your catheter, drain, IV lines, and any other appliances are in working order. They will ask you to breathe deeply in order to maintain good oxygenation and to keep the lungs open. Ice chips may be on the recovery room menu, but most physicians withhold oral intake.

You will be taken to a hospital room when the nurse and anesthesiologist confirm you are ready. If lucky, you will be alone there with your family. More likely, another patient recovering from surgery will be your roommate. Over the next one to three days you will begin drinking, eating, moving around, and eventually walking out the door to go home. The timetable will be an amalgam of how quickly you bounce back and your surgeon's preferences.

CATHETER CARE

Most men's least favorite part of recovering from prostatectomy is the catheter. It is a soft rubber tube with an inflated balloon on the inside end that holds it in place until the bladder neck heals back to the urethra.

There is no denying that the catheter is uncomfortable. However, it is tolerable. Keep the end of the penis well lubricated where the catheter exits the urethra so it slides easily as you move. Neosporin ointment is the most common recommendation since it contains an antibiotic. Despite the bias of the women in my life, the importance of the antibiotic is unclear, so any petroleum jelly can substitute.

The catheter will not fall out. The inflated balloon serves as an anchor until deflated in the office when its work is done. The other end of the catheter has an opening to connect to a plastic collection bag. This is a plastic

BEWARE CATHETER DURATION CLAIMS

In the eighties, we all left catheters in for three weeks when anatomical prostatectomy became widespread. This was empirically chosen as the duration required for complete healing. As experience grew, many urologists became adventurous in shortening this duration in an effort to improve patient comfort. In recent years several centers have reported durations as short as three days, with anecdotal reports of one-day catheterizations.

This trend accelerated with the introduction of laparoscopic/robotic prostatectomy. Advocates theorized that the running suture line was more watertight so there was no reason to wait for complete healing. This soon became another selling point for such surgery.

The problem with such decreases in catheter duration is that some men will go into urinary retention, presumably from swelling. I gave up when I reached one week. The first time a patient reported urinary retention I didn't believe him when he called. "Impossible," I claimed on the phone. "You just had a radical prostatectomy. Your problem will be urine loss—not an inability to pass it."

I fortunately had the patient return urgently to the office and found that indeed (as is not uncommon!) he was right—he was in urinary retention. I gingerly replaced a catheter and recommended he keep it for awhile. He voided fine when I removed it a few days later. This occurred in a few more patients in the coming months until I conceded that a week seemed to be too short.

Other surgeons have experienced the same thing for both open and laparoscopic/robotic prostatectomy. In addition, an x-ray called a cystogram is usually performed in order to check for leaks prior to making this bold move. If leakage persists, the catheter is left in place.

At this time, catheterization duration is controversial. I have gone back to approximately ten days as a routine and have never since experienced urinary retention. Weighing a few days extra discomfort against the need for cystograms and the risk of urinary retention involves a difficult decision, but this duration seems to work best for me. Your doctor will have his own experience, and may leave the catheter in for either shorter or longer durations.

container that either attaches to the patient's leg (called a **leg bag**) or can be laid on the floor, hung from the bedrails, or carried around (called a **bedside bag**). Most men will use the leg bag while walking around during the day and the larger bedside bag at night in order to extend time for the bag to fill.

Some men worry about the bag overfilling. This is not the end of the world, although there is a small chance it could create leakage from the anastomosis and add to healing time. If the bag becomes full, the bladder still has the ability to hold several ounces more. Don't panic, but empty the bag as soon as you notice this occurrence.

Leg bags may be uncomfortable because of the rubber straps that usually hold them onto the leg. These straps are less than an inch in width and can easily roll or pull hair. Some men are happier using elastic straps that can be purchased from most drug stores. They cost only a few dollars and can make the time wearing the catheter more comfortable.

DRAINAGE ISSUES

A small plastic drain tube will be placed near the **anastomosis** at the end of the operation. It exits the body somewhere near the incision (or through one of the port sites if the operation is laparoscopic/robotic) and drains into a plastic bulb, often called a "grenade" based on its shape. This bulb is compressed and capped. As it attempts to reexpand to its natural spherical shape, it creates a mild suction that pulls urine or other body fluid away from the surgical site. This type of drain is called a *closed suction drain*. Your care providers may also refer to it as a *JP* or *Jackson-Pratt drain*, based on a common brand name. Some surgeons use two separate drains.

The drain may also be made of softer rubber that serves as a wick, often called a *Penrose drain*. This type is more commonly used following perineal prostatectomy, since the softness helps make sitting on the site more tolerable.

Drains are usually removed within a day or two following surgery, when the amount of fluid decreases to a manageable volume. This doesn't hurt as much as you would suspect, and patients routinely state they worried unnecessarily about pain from drain removal.

Excessive drainage sometimes requires that the drain be left in place for several days, and it may be removed during the postoperative visit if this is the case. Rarely will the drainage persist long enough that the drain must be repositioned to allow the leak to close.

BLOOD CLOTS

One of the few serious situations arises when a patient develops a blood clot because of slow venous blood flow following pelvic surgery. When this occurs in the legs it is called *deep venous thrombosis* (*DVT*). The real danger occurs when the clot breaks off and goes to the lungs, called a *pulmonary embolus* (*PE*). This can block blood flow exiting the heart.

PE was common in the past, but we can now prevent most cases. Compression stockings inflate intermittently during and after surgery to "milk" blood out of the leg veins before clots can form. Some centers also give blood thinners such as *heparin* to prevent clots.

DVT becomes evident when one leg swells more than the other, and may become tender and red. Notify your doctor or nurse if this occurs postoperatively. PE occurs when the clot breaks off; though uncommon, it typically occurs during activity or while straining to have a bowel movement.

Don't let this concern limit your activity—exercise is actually the most important thing you can do to prevent clots. The body's natural prevention is the milking action of calf muscles during walking. This is the most important reason to become ambulatory even on the evening of surgery if possible.

GOING HOME

For some strange reason, an almost universally held belief among the public is that hospital discharge is impossible without having a bowel movement. Contrary to popular belief (and fortunately for healthcare workers completing long workdays), it is possible to exit through a hospital door even if you haven't had a bowel movement.

The bowel movement myth comes from the days when surgical patients remained hospitalized until fully recovered. Wounds were almost completely healed. Hospital stays are shorter in the modern era. Despite protests that insurers have ruined lives by encouraging this trend, it may be one of the most productive by-products of insurance initiatives. Hospitals are for sick people—those who need assistance breathing, receiving nutrition, or receiving treatment unachievable at home. Simply living in the days following elective surgery doesn't qualify as such.

Moreover, many surgical patients are more comfortable at home in their own beds. The food is better, the bed softer, and the surroundings usually quieter. Pain pills work as well as injections for most people within a day or two following prostatectomy. Walking around the familiar layout of your own home can be much more comfortable than maneuvering the obstacles of hospital rooms and hallways. Exposing your backside is less likely wearing your own clothes around the house than it is in a hospital gown on the urology ward.

In addition to the above comfort issues, there are medical reasons patients may be better off at home than in a hospital. Remember that hospitals *are for sick people*. Some of those people have infections that *you* don't need while recovering from surgery. Many of those infections have been treated with multiple antibiotics, so their germs may be resistant to multiple drugs. Healthcare workers are potential vectors to carry infection between the sick people and those simply recovering from surgery. You may not want to be there.

Therefore, don't assume that decreasing lengths of stay are the result of insurers limiting payments (although this has happened on occasion). Stay in the hospital as long as you and your surgeon feel that you need something that the hospital can provide that you cannot get at home. After that time, go home where you can get lots of things the hospital cannot provide.

BLADDER SPASMS

The bladder doesn't like having a catheter inside. The balloon can be irritating. Its response is sometimes a muscle contraction called a *bladder spasm*. It translates into the sensation of needing to urinate. The bladder contraction can occasionally be so powerful that it overwhelms the catheter's capacity to handle the volume of urine that is attempting to pass, so urine can come around the catheter. Some patients assume the catheter must be clogged or dislodged when they experience bladder spasm, but this is rarely the case.

Medications can control bladder spasms, although the ultimate treatment is catheter removal. Tolteridine (Detrol LA), oxybutinin (Ditropan or Ditropan XL) or new medications in the pharmaceutical pipeline can block these bladder contractions when taken orally. Faster relief comes from physician prescribed *belladonna and opiod (B&O) suppositories*, although they must obviously be placed rectally. Bladder spasms do not occur in all patients, and usually resolve within hours of catheter removal.

WHEN TO BE CONCERNED

Call your doctor if the catheter becomes obstructed and fails to drain for more than two hours. Shorter durations without urinary output may simply occur when the small opening on the catheter tip becomes occluded from lying against the bladder wall. When the bladder expands, its walls will move away from the hole, allowing drainage to resume.

Occasionally a small blood clot can obstruct the catheter, so the flow of urine will remain obstructed even after the bladder begins to fill. Unless the doctor gave you a syringe and fluid intended to irrigate at home, you will need to go to his clinic or the emergency room.

Low-grade fevers in the postoperative period are commonly associated with collapse of *alveoli*, or small air sacs in the lungs. This is called *atelectasis*. Deep breathing helps reexpand these sacs, and patients are often instructed to use a device called an incentive spirometer that simply measures breath intake to assure adequate filling. Its use begins in the hospital. You can achieve the same goal by simply forcing yourself to take deep in-and-out breaths.

Blood clots can occur even after discharge, although the mobility associated with being out of the hospital minimizes the risk. However, contact your doctor immediately if you experience one-sided leg swelling and redness. Call an ambulance if you experience severe chest pain or shortness of breath.

THE FOLLOW-UP VISIT

The purpose of your first office visit postoperatively will usually be catheter removal. Skin staples are also removed unless wound closure was via absorbable sutures. Bring a pad to this visit, as bladder control will usually return slowly. Loose pants and jockey shorts to hold the pad in place help logistically. The doctor will lay out a plan for follow-up. Each urologist uses his own intervals, but expect visits at least after successive intervals of one, three, six, and eventually twelve months.

GETTING THE PATHOLOGY REPORT

The urologist will be able to give an assessment of the likelihood of cure when your pathology report is complete, often at the first postoperative visit.

He will be most concerned with the same issues as those on the initial biopsy—stage and grade (see chapter 13).

Unlike the **clinical stage** and **grade** assigned following the biopsy and any staging tests used, he will now know the **pathological stage** and **grade**. This is much more accurate prognostic information. Without the sampling limitations of biopsy, he will know exactly what Gleason score the entire cancer comprises. The Gleason score can change once the entire tumor is examined, as there may be higher-grade tissue than appreciated on needle biopsy. Such *upgrading* occurs somewhere around 20 to 30 percent of the time. *Downgrading* is less common but occurs occasionally.

The urologist will know if the cancer was **organ confined** or whether it has extended beyond the gland. Extension beyond the prostatic capsule is termed **extracapsular extension**, which implies that the cancer *may be* more likely to progress. He will also know if the cancer has extended to the margin or edge of the tissue removed. If he finds the cancer is **margin positive** (present at the margin of removed tissue), there is a possibility the cancer was cut across, so there could be cancer cells remaining on the other side of the incision. It is unclear how often this occurs as reports range as great as 5 to 53 percent of the time, but most urologists expect to find positive margins in around 15 to 20 percent of cases.[15]

The implications of margin-positive status are unclear. Most men with this situation never develop cancer recurrence. The most common reason is that the margin may reveal findings that are false positive. This occurs most commonly when overlying tissue, including the **dorsal vein complex**, is divided and retracts back away from the prostate. Whereas it covered all cancer prior to being cut, its retraction can expose cancer cells that were not truly at the margin.

For this reason, most urologists will not automatically recommend further treatment. Instead, the recommendation may be simply to follow the patient closely with DRE and PSA. If there are signs of cancer recurrence using either at any point, further treatment might be in order.

VANISHING CANCER PHENOMENON

On rare occasions the pathologist will be unable to identify cancer in the radical prostatectomy specimen. When the pathologist fails to find cancer in the prostatectomy specimen, the first thing he does is review the original biopsy slides to assure a mistake did not occur. This is *exceedingly* rare.

There is the theoretical possibility that the cancer was so small that the biopsy needle removed a small tumor in its entirety. As you can imagine, this would be very unlikely; instead, it appears that the cancer was so small that finding its remainder is like finding a needle in a haystack. In a prostate composed of millions of cells, finding a few malignant ones might be a difficult task if the tumor is tiny.

Fortunately, we know that cancers that small are inevitably confined to the prostate. It is unheard of for a man to develop metastasis in this situation. Therefore, an exhaustive search to find the small tumor is a poor use of time or resources, so we can report an excellent prognosis and reassure the man that the cancer is gone.

A urological pathologist has named this situation the *vanishing cancer phenomenon*.[16] I have personally seen only two cases (which I was comforted to confirm were correctly reported on the original biopsy each time), and it is rare enough that many urologists may never confront such.

AL'S DECISION FOR SURGERY

Originally, Al expressed a desire for surgery for the wrong reasons. After exploring his options he still chose surgical removal, but this time for the right reasons. His wife, Janet, was in agreement.

Al was relatively young—fifty-one years old—and healthy. His cancer was detected while stage T1c because of a minimally elevated PSA of 3.8 ng/dl. His grade, however, was higher than most. With a Gleason score of 4 + 4 = 8, his cancer was potentially as dangerous as that of his father.

One thing made Al's situation different from his father's. Although as potentially dangerous as his father's, Al's cancer was apparently caught in time. He was right to have it removed. If the cancer was contained to the prostate, there was a good chance of cure.

We discussed which approach best met Al's needs. With some of the world's premier laparoscopic prostate surgeons right down the hall, he seriously considered this option. The robotic version sounded good and I informed him we had a couple of robots cranked up and ready if he was interested. After fully exploring the options, he opted for the time-honored approach—radical retropubic prostatectomy.

The day of surgery started early. Janet drove and pulled through an all-night drive-through on the way to the hospital. While she picked at a breakfast sandwich as daybreak approached, Al simply salivated and followed my directive to eat or drink nothing after midnight.

As a "first-round" case, he was taken immediately to the preop area for placement of a wristband with his name and identifying information, hospital cap, booties, gown (complete with the dilemma of figuring out which part was front and which was back), and IV. He kissed Janet wistfully as an orderly wheeled his cart out the door and down the hall to the holding area, where all information was reverified. Only then did the anesthesiologist place an epidural catheter.

Once all was set, another orderly rolled the cart down the hall to the door of operating room 21. A nurse rechecked accuracy of his name, blood type, and allergies. She asked him to confirm his surgeon's name (Jones) and his understanding in layman's terms of what was to happen that day ("remove my prostate"), then pulled the cart into the room and locked the wheels to hold it in place beside an operating room table wide enough for one person with no room to spare. He moved over and looked up to get an upside down view of the nurse anesthetist's face leaning over him as she placed EKG sticky pads onto his chest for monitoring during the operation. A blood pressure cuff confirmed that his pressure was up about ten points—expected from natural anxieties in such unfamiliar and dynamic surroundings. An oximeter to measure blood oxygenation, and nasal oxygen tubing placed almost simultaneously completed the preparatory phase.

A John Mellencamp CD was playing. The resident warned Al that he might feel the coolness of the skin prep kit he was about to use in order to sterilize the skin of the lower abdomen, upper legs, and everything in between. The team called for a "time-out," at which time the nurse and I stated the name of the patient, surgeon, and the operation planned as a final confirmation to minimize the chance of making an error. Sterile surgical towels and sheets covered everything except the operative area; the operation began.

The next couple of hours were a blur for Al. A few times he fell asleep. This was partly the result of the combination of an early awakening and coffee withdrawal (he rarely made it to 9:00 AM without a stop at Starbucks). The sedative administered through the IV to keep him calm also contributed to the effect. He felt some tugging and listened intermittently to the conversation, but such exciting dialogue as "stitch, please" couldn't hold his attention.

I startled him when I pulled the sterile drapes back to let him know the operation was over. "Everything went well—very routine."

"Did you get it all?"

"Everything I could see," I reassured, "but we have to wait on the final pathology reading to know if things look as good as I think."

A few days later I was able to tell him honestly that they did.

KEY POINTS

- Three options exist for surgical removal of the prostate—radical retropubic, radical perineal, and radical laparoscopic/robotic.
- The primary difference in the three options involves the route taken to the prostate. All usually have good outcomes.
- Prostatectomy may be nerve sparing or nonnerve sparing, depending on whether the neurovascular bundles supplying erection stimulus to the penis are resected. Nerve sparing is necessary to protect spontaneous erections, but doesn't ensure them.
- Pelvic lymphadenectomy is the final staging procedure for some patients. Its role varies among surgeons, but it may not be necessary for most patients diagnosed with prostate cancer.
- The best advice regarding surgical options is that you should choose a surgeon, not an operation. The surgeon should perform whichever operation he can assure you will yield the best results.
- Retropubic prostatectomy may be performed under epidural or general anesthesia. Epidural lessens blood loss and appears to speed recovery in the days following surgery. Since some patients do not want to be alert during surgery, sedation can address this concern. General anesthesia is required for laparoscopic/robotic prostatectomy, and usually for perineal prostatectomy.
- Deep venous thrombosis and pulmonary embolism are currently rare. Don't overworry about the risks—just stay active to minimize them.
- Stairs are not a problem.

16.

RADIATION THERAPY: TWO OPTIONS FOR ONE TREATMENT

If my best friend had this disease, my advice to him would be: Investigate, choose, and do—and do it quickly. Be aggressive now. Don't save the best for later.
—Andy Grove, former CEO of Intel Corp, treated (apparently successfully) with radiation for prostate cancer

Cancer treatment depends on the destruction of malignant cells while protecting the rest of the patient's body. In surgery the strategy is obvious—cut out the cancer or cancerous organ and leave in the rest. The same principle applies for radiation. Radioactive waves target cancer while the radiation oncologist tries to minimize damage to surrounding structures.

Radiation energy selectively kills growing cells. The very nature of cancer is to grow uncontrollably and faster than normal tissues, so radiation can target cancer while having less effect on nearby tissues. This approach has been used for decades to treat prostate cancer, and we continue to see higher cure rates and lower side effects as further improvements are made.

Radiation is delivered by two primary routes. The traditional one—**external beam radiation**—aims radioactive energy into the body. A newer alternative—**brachytherapy**—involves placing the radioactive substance inside the body and letting it release its energy outward.

EXTERNAL BEAM RADIATION

External beam radiation has been used for decades to direct high-energy radioactive rays at a cancer. Side effects have limited the dosage because the rays also hit the organs of the anatomical neighborhood. Therefore, the **radiation oncologist** must walk a tightrope between getting enough radiation to the tumor to kill it, while keeping the dosage to the adjacent organs low enough that he doesn't severely damage them.

Recent advances have greatly enhanced our ability to achieve this balance. We now use computers to target energy deep into the pelvis where the prostate lies. They allow dispersed beams to go through multiple paths in order to converge at the prostate, so it receives a lethal dose of energy while the rest of the pelvis receives smaller doses. **Conformal radiotherapy** and **intensity modulated radiation therapy** (**IMRT**) are the most advanced versions of such technology.

LOGISTICS

Before beginning therapy you will undergo simulation; this is basically a computerized programming based on a CT scan that will allow the radiation oncologist to create a dosage treatment plan. Within days you can begin daily treatments.

You arrive at the radiation oncology clinic (often located in a hospital) at approximately the same time each day. Treatments are administered Monday through Friday. Some feel this schedule is purposeful to allow time for healing on the weekend, but it is actually just a realistic approach to the work schedule. It appears that this is as good as daily treatment and is much easier to manage.

You may have a short wait, though the schedule usually runs on time. When your turn arrives, a technologist will bring you into the treatment room and ask you to lie on the table. When the machine is aimed properly at your prostate it is turned on, but the only way you will know it is on is by the sound—you cannot feel the beam. Within a few minutes you are done and ready to return to your usual activities for the remainder of the day. Most centers give around six weeks' worth of daily treatments.

MEASURING SUCCESS

Success is more difficult to measure following radiation than it is with surgery. The PSA should be zero—undetectable—following prostatectomy. The prostate is realistically the only source of PSA, so if PSA is detectable after its removal it is definite that prostate tissue remains. Cancerous prostate tissue that has escaped the gland (whether into the tissues nearby the prostate or through metastases) is the most likely explanation.

In contrast, radiation leaves prostate tissue in place that still produces PSA. Disagreement exists regarding how low PSA should go, but the goal is to get PSA below somewhere around 0.5 ng/dl. Because radiation does its damage slowly and on an ongoing basis, it may take two or three years to reach the bottom, or the *nadir*. If PSA never reaches this level or reaches bottom and begins to rise quickly, there is a real chance cancer will eventually recur.

However, there is no absolute level that determines how low PSA must go in order to be normal. In order to address that reality and to standardize the definition of success, the *American Society for Therapeutic Radiology and Oncology (ASTRO) Consensus Conference* created a new definition in the nineties.[1] The conference determined that it takes three consecutive PSA rises to indicate failure. This definition is fraught with hazard because PSA tends to jump around sometimes even in the absence of cancer, but it is the definition the most people can agree on for now.

SUCCESS EXPECTED WITH RADIATION

The likelihood of cure depends on how severe the disease is. The only way to truly define cure is to know that a man died (we hope of old age) without evidence of prostate cancer. Given that, a surrogate for cure often means that a person will remain disease free five years after treatment. This likelihood is broken down into three risk categories. The definition of these categories and the chance of being disease free in five years (according to the medical literature) are shown in table 1.

Table 1.
Historical Predicted Success Following Radiation Therapy[2]

Risk Group	PSA	Clinical Stage	Gleason Grade	Chance of Being Disease Free Five Years After Treatment
Low	<10	T1c–T2a	6 or less	85%
Intermediate	10–20	T2b	7	50%
High	>20	T2c	8 or more	33%

In order to understand this table you will need to review the **Clinical Staging** system and **Gleason scoring** system shown in chapter 13. Note that you are considered part of the category matching your highest finding by any of the three criteria (PSA, clinical stage, or Gleason score).

Keep in mind such tables cover widely divergent groups of patients. Therefore, I caution you to beware of prediction and statistical models. They give you some idea of what to expect, but are subject to significant limitations.

Another thing to understand about this table is that even if there is evidence of prostate cancer at five years (either using ASTRO criteria or findings of cancer on either rectal examination or radiographic studies), that is not always a serious finding. Because prostate cancer often is a slow-growing disease, an asymptomatic recurrence at five years might take several more years to become fatal. Therefore, if you are seventy at the time of radiation and experience a recurrence at seventy-five, it might take until you are eighty-five or ninety-five years old (or older) before serious problems will occur. In addition, the ASTRO criteria might define someone as having failure while the PSA is still below 1 ng/dl. This range is "normal" by traditional definitions. Therefore, failure "on paper" doesn't mean you are dying so beware of interpretations of success and failure.

Ultimately, success means living well and avoiding death by prostate cancer. This may be more likely than the above table and historical standards predict. I believe that success is markedly better now than it was when the historical numbers were generated a decade or more ago. For one thing, we have better technology. Far more important is that we currently treat a significantly different population of men. Prostate cancer is usually detected at much earlier stages than even a few short years ago. Therefore, we know that even when PSA, Gleason score, and other indicators appear the same, a later year of diagnosis is a favorable prognostic sign. In other words, *everything* else being equal, your prognosis is better now than it would have been even a few years ago.[3] As a result, at the Cleveland Clinic we have recently seen much better outcomes than shown in the above table. We believe it is because men treated today have a better prognosis than ever before. To demonstrate the more favorable findings, Dr. Jay Ciezki of the department of radiation oncology has provided the Cleveland Clinic's recent statistics in table 2.

Table 2.
Cleveland Clnic Outcomes with Radiation in the Current Era

Risk Group	PSA	Clinical Stage	Gleason Grade	Chance of Being Disease Free Five Years After Treatment
Low	<10	T1c–T2a	6 or less	90%
Intermediate	10–20	T2b	7	81%
High	>20	T2c	8 or more	69%

These same three risk groups continue to do better than patients in the past even beyond the five-year period. Low-risk patients have the same prognosis through eight years, and a majority of even high-risk patients continue to be disease free at that point. These newer numbers are cause for encouragement that your chance of doing well long term has never been better.

FOLLOW-UP

One frustrating thing for men who have undergone radiation is the fact it takes a while to know if it has been effective. Cancer cells continue to die for months. PSA may not reach its nadir for two or three years. Once it does, you will have a PSA and DRE every few months until you get so old it doesn't matter. After a few years this can safely be an annual checkup.

Few men need repeat biopsy following radiation. The only reason would be if there were suspicion of persistent cancer (because of rising PSA or abnormal DRE), *and* if knowing there was still cancer would change management. If a **metastatic workup** (as described in chapter 13) finds no cancer elsewhere, a prostate biopsy can be performed in that setting.

If cancer persists more than two years later, it is possible to consider either cryotherapy (as discussed in detail in the next chapter) or a **salvage prostatectomy**. The latter is an unreassuringly named operation that refers to removal of the prostate following radiation. Because of radiation-induced scarring, this operation is difficult and associated with significant complication rates.

Many urologists feel the complications do not justify the benefits of salvage prostatectomy, especially considering that there is no guarantee of cure. All the risks of radical prostatectomy are many times more likely to occur following radiation. In addition, there is a significant chance that radiation will scar the rectum to the prostate, which creates the possibility that a colostomy will be required. However, some men who chose radiation at the time of their original diagnosis will be young and healthy enough that they will be willing to accept such risks. Those who do should consider surgery only by a urologist with extensive experience in prostatectomy, and must understand up front the significant risks.

SIDE EFFECTS

The most common side effect of radiation therapy is the one usually talked about the least—fatigue. Most men barely notice anything is going on with their bodies for the first few weeks. However, toward the end of therapy, fatigue sets in.

It is not incapacitating; rather, it is like the fatigue of overwork. Although most of it comes from radiation, some may well be the cumulative effects of going to the doctor every day for six weeks. I often tell men that if I made them go to the grocery store each day for that duration—simply walking in the building and back out with groceries fifteen minutes later—they would become tired. Driving back and forth, parking in a location that is sometimes inaccessible, and walking into the building and back takes energy. Sitting in a medical environment waiting with other cancer patients who may be far more ill is further taxing. The treatment may then sap the last reserve you have. Fatigue is predictable.

However, fatigue is also manageable—and in an unexpected way. Exercise during treatment helps men cope better with fatigue.[4] Men who remain active during treatments actually maintain better energy levels than those who try to increase their rest. That is not to say that rest is bad—just that it should be used in moderation.

As much as any other treatment option, radiation side effects are based on the prostate's location in its anatomic neighborhood. The bladder, rectum, penile nerves, pelvic bones, and intestines surround the prostate. Each receives a tolerable dose of radiation in most cases. However, even with modern improvements such as **conformal radiotherapy** and **intensity modulated radiation therapy (IMRT)**, most patients will notice some effects on the neighboring organs.

The most common side effects are diarrhea and urinary **irritative symptoms**. Bleeding in the stool or urine is possible, but rarely is it severe. Most symptoms disappear within weeks. Finally, radiation reaching the small intestines occasionally leads to intestinal problems in the future.

Because these symptoms are usually minor, radiation is easier on most patients than major surgery *in the short term*. However, radiation damage occasionally continues to do its work over the years—and sometimes decades. Blood vessels may shrivel, leading to tissue injury. In the early years of radiation therapy, this escalation of symptoms sometimes made it the malevolent "gift that kept on giving."

Such long-term consequences of radiation have been greatly curtailed in recent years through contemporary techniques. However, one legacy we still see is the effect of radiation on erectile dysfunction. The penile nerves receive a full dose of radiation because the neurovascular bundles course along each side of the prostate. Since radiation does its damage over time, the immediate effect may be minimal. However, after three years the likelihood of impotence (approximately 50 percent if you start with completely normal erections, and higher if you already have erectile dysfunction prior to therapy) is about the same with either surgery or radiation, indicating things slowly improve after surgery but slowly worsen after radiation.[5]

Therefore, long-term effects may offset short-term ease, so the decision to have radiation in lieu of surgical removal of the prostate is complex. In addition, a prostate that has already shown the capacity to develop malignancy left in place risks a recurrence of the cancer or the development of a new cancer in the future. These risks must be weighed against the risks of surgery in order to make a fully informed decision.

SECONDARY MALIGNANCY

We know that radiation causes cellular damage—that's the idea. As a result, there appears to be a *very small* risk that radiation therapy can cause a secondary cancer in a nearby organ.

Don't be alarmed. First, the risk appears to be less than one-half of 1 percent.[6] In addition, it is unclear how much of this is a true risk and how much is simply a result of increased monitoring. In other words, patients who have had cancer are carefully followed, x-rayed, examined, and otherwise investigated. A second (unrelated) malignancy already present might be unable to escape detection for long with such careful investigation.

The primary site for such occurrence will be in the prostatic neighborhood. Rectal, bladder, and occasionally other cancers have been reported with sufficient rarity to allow you for the most part to escape worry. In addition, a secondary malignancy resulting from radiation should take years to develop. This minimizes the risk for most patients, but may concern young men. Obviously this low risk is not to be ignored, but pales in comparison to the other risks involved, including the potential risks of untreated prostate cancer.

RADIATION FOR SURGICAL FAILURES

Some people with continued cancer activity (as defined by a detectable PSA) following RRP will be candidates for radiation. There has also been a tendency on the part of physicians to recommend this for any person with high-risk disease, including those with positive surgical margins or high-grade cancer. In addition, men with a persistent or rising PSA following RRP have been treated similarly.

The problem with this concept is that most men in such circumstances do not actually require further therapy, since their cancers may not progress. Unfortunately, there is no way to tell which ones will, so a shotgun approach is tempting. However, the risk of postoperative side effects is much higher when this is done, especially **bladder neck contracture**, **stricture**, and **incontinence**.

In contrast to radiating everyone, most men should be treated only with *salvage radiotherapy*. This involves treating only those men whose cancer appears to be progressing in the prostatic bed (the site where the prostate once existed). Determining this is difficult. Therefore, an assumption is often made that the prostatic bed is likely the site of recurrence if the PSA is rising and no cancer shows up on a **metastatic workup**. Some physicians use the **ProstaScint scan** (as described in chapter 13) in this setting in order to try to identify a tumor recurrence. Its results are variable.[7]

TIMING OF SALVAGE RADIOTHERAPY

Success with salvage radiotherapy appears to be greater when radiation is started earlier, potentially when the PSA first becomes detectable. It should be *undetectable* following prostatectomy, so *any* detectable PSA suggests the possibility of cancer recurrence. However, this risks overtreatment since many men with a slightly elevated PSA may never experience clinical recurrence. Based on their review of available studies, ASTRO feels that the appropriate starting point is when the PSA reaches 1.5 ng/dl.

Side effects will be greater when radiation follows surgery, especially if it is in the first few months after the operation. The chance of all prostatectomy side effects will increase. This must be weighed against the risk of cancer progression.

PROTON AND NEUTRON BEAMS

Some centers advocate using *heavy particle beams* comprised of proton or neutron particles. The theoretical advantage of such machines is that their damage to cancer tissue may be more intense and effective to permanently damage cancer cells. They also dissipate more quickly so they have less penetration beyond the prostate.

To date these technologies are available at only a few centers. An advantage over regular radiation therapy remains to be demonstrated. Studies show they are as good, but have failed to convince the urological community they are better.[8]

SEEDS: BRACHYTHERAPY

Brachy (rhymes with "tacky") means "close." By placing radioactive pellets or "seeds" into the prostate, we can get the radiation source close to its target. The technique has been around in various forms for almost a century, but reached success only when we became able to place seeds accurately into the prostate under ultrasound guidance. A computer program determines the location and number of pellets required.

Many centers perform brachytherapy as a staged procedure. The first trip to the operating room allows the urologist and/or radiation oncologist to obtain ultrasound information that will be used for treatment planning. With this information in hand, they will order the seeds and bring you back to the operating room later for implantation. Needles deposit somewhere around one hundred seeds (varying by as much as 50 percent from that) into the prostate tissue. They remain, emitting their radiation over the coming months.

The *radioisotopes* chosen for seeds are based on their low-energy emissions. This allows them to cause extensive cell death nearby (in the prostate and its cancer), but this damage trails off quickly the farther that the rays travel. This limits damage to organs in the neighborhood. Naturally, they do not stop at the prostatic capsule so there is some damage to adjacent organs, usually at about the same rate as for external beam radiation. Therefore, seeds are not "better" than external beam radiation—they simply allow delivery of similar cancer killing doses of radiation in a one-time treatment instead of having to undergo daily treatments for several weeks. They emit their radiation over the coming months in order to accomplish the same goal, doing their work while you do yours.

One specific concern with brachytherapy involves the radiation risk to people around you. This is unlikely with minimal safeguards. Dr. Ciezki recommends that you hold babies or small children on your lap for no more than twenty minutes per hour—a minor limitation. Other radiation oncologists recommend more significant limitation, so you should discuss this with your doctor.

THE ISOTOPES

Radioisotopes are the energy source of the "seeds" or pellets that emit cancer-killing radiation. Iodine-125 is the most common. Its half-life is about sixty days, which means that half its energy dissipates every two months. Therefore, one-quarter remains at four months, one-eighth at six months, and so on. Palladium is a similar isotope, but its half-life is much shorter, at seventeen days. Its energy also drops off more quickly the farther that the rays travel from the source, so less radiation reaches the rectum and bladder.

It is unclear that there is a clear advantage to one isotope over the other, although it is possible palladium may have more short-term urinary effects and fewer long-term side effects. It may also be more effective than iodine-125 against high-grade cancer, but this is not universally accepted. In addition, its short half-life precludes its storage on site. It loses its energy by the day, so most centers have to order it for each individual case. If the treatment is cancelled for any reason, these expensive seeds would go to waste.[9]

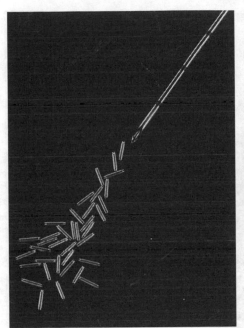

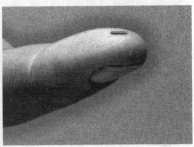

Figure 16-1. Radioactive brachytherapy "seeds" and needle used for their placement. (Courtesy Bard, Inc.)

Figure 16-2. Size of radioactive seed implant can be demonstrated by its size compared to the human finger. (Courtesy Bard, Inc.)

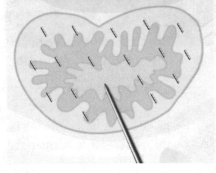

Figure 16-3. Schematic drawing showing how seeds are dispersed from the needle into the prostate (Courtesy Bard, Inc.)

PSA: ALL OVER THE MAP AFTER BRACHYTHERAPY

PSA levels actually *rise* after brachytherapy as a result of prostatic irritation. Recall that anything abnormal in the prostate can release PSA. After brachytherapy, much happens. First the seeds and needles disrupt the linings responsible for keeping PSA inside the gland. Then radiation causes diffuse changes that allow PSA to rise. Therefore, PSA will rise about 25 percent within the first three months,[10] and may take up to five years to decline all the way to its nadir.[11]

PSA also "bounces" in some men several months after brachytherapy.

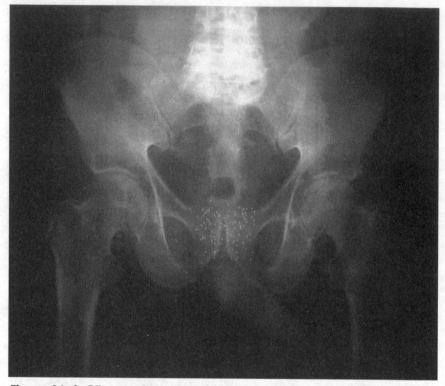

Figure 16-4. CT scan shows seed distribution (small white dots) in the pelvis of a man treated with brachytherapy. (Courtesy Bard, Inc.)

The reason this occurs remains a mystery, as is its effect on prognosis.[12] The main issue is to not panic when the PSA bounce occurs—it is normal and might even portend a better prognosis.

URINARY RETENTION

One specific concern with brachytherapy is the risk of urinary retention. About 4 percent of men will develop prostatic swelling and will be unable to urinate. If this occurs, we can perform a TURP on most men to restore normal voiding if they fail to respond to medications. However, men who have radioactive seeds in the prostate cannot undergo TURP for some time because of the radiation risk. Until the seeds "burn out," they must remain. This usually means waiting about ten months for men treated with I-125—a long time to wear a catheter. Because of the shorter half-life of palladium, its seeds burn out most of their activity within about three months—the time required to go through five "half-lives."

For this reason, men with **obstructive** voiding symptoms are not ideal candidates for brachytherapy. This is controversial and many physicians will treat these men with seeds, but I recommend men with significant obstruction to have external beam if they choose radiation.

COMBINATION RADIATION

Many centers perform both brachytherapy and external beam radiation in combination, but there is no clear advantage to doing so. We recommend using one or the other treatment, and regard their success and side effects as similar.

Again, they are simply *two ways of delivering the same treatment.* The energy can be delivered from outside radiating in (external beam) or from inside radiating out (brachytherapy). Doing both increases cost and provides no proven additional benefit.

IMPROVING (OR LESSENING) THE LIKELIHOOD OF SUCCESS

It is important to deliver an effective radiation dose in order to achieve cure. This is up to the physician, of course, but 70 to 72 CGy (the measure of radiation energy delivered during the complete treatment course) is needed for maximum success. For very low-risk cases (as defined earlier in this chapter), the doctor may drop this a little bit in order to lessen side effects.[13]

Hormonal ablation as a treatment is discussed in detail in chapter 22, but it is also used to enhance the effectiveness of radiation therapy. For one thing, it shrinks the cancer so more energy concentrates where needed. In addition, it seems to make the treatment more effective, perhaps rendering cancer cells more sensitive to radiation toxicity. The ideal timing and duration of such treatments remain unclear, but most start hormonal ablation before treatments begin and give one to three injections that last three to four months each.

Recovery is also affected by overall health. Smoking limits the effectiveness of radiation therapy. The mechanism for this is unclear, but potentially is related to limiting blood flow to tissues.[14] Anything that makes your own tissues healthier will hasten your recovery.

RADIATION FOR BONE METASTASES

When prostate cancer spreads to bones, it is usually treated with hormonal therapy. However, if there is a solitary lesion, it can be effectively treated for symptom relief by two weeks of radiation to the site. This can relieve pain and lessen the chance that a cancer-weakened bone will fracture spontaneously.

Cancer in the back can compress the spinal cord and create risk of paralysis. Radiation in this setting can prevent catastrophe. Fortunately, this situation is very rare and unlikely to occur in anything other than the very worst cases.

KEY POINTS

- Radiation energy kills cancer cells selectively but not exclusively.
- Two main options are available for radiation delivery. External beam radiation directs rays into the body from the outside, and brachytherapy emits radiation from the inside.

17.

CRYOTHERAPY:
FREEZING CANCER

It seems likely, given all the progress that has been made in the past decade, that cryosurgery will play an increased role in the future management of prostate cancer.

—Katsuto Shinohara, MD
University of California, San Francisco

N
o doubt ever existed that freezing cancer cells kills them. The problem has always been damage control. Until recently prostate cancer treatment with cryotherapy often caused unacceptable injury to organs of the neighborhood. This led to regular complications until technology finally caught up with cryobiology.

After years of frustration, we can now control freezing well enough to destroy prostate cancer while leaving vital organs nearby virtually unaffected. This technology has finally opened the door to the widespread—and safe—use of cryotherapy.

AN UNSAVORY HISTORY PRECEDES
A HOPEFUL FUTURE

Despite efforts by champions for its effectiveness, cryotherapy took decades to gain respectability. The procedure was pushed in an almost evangelical way by patients and physicians who refused to understand why the urological community regarded it with skepticism. This led to early results bordering on catastrophe.

To the credit of our profession, most urologists demanded scientific evidence before they were willing to seriously consider cryotherapy. Because of their foresight and scientific integrity, few patients suffered during an era when some reports showed over half of patients experienced major complications.[1] During the midnineties the technology was out of favor with all but the most ardent advocates. The pinnacle of criticism came when a speaker called it a "sham" at the annual meeting of the American Urological Association.

However, a dedicated few continued to work on improvements in it. Improvements in ultrasound monitoring allowed physicians to see the *freeze zone* better. Smaller *cryoprobes* (as described below) allow less traumatic probe placement. Temperature monitors warn when freezing approaches structures that should not be frozen. When this occurs, the machine can quickly be reversed so the tissue rewarms as quickly as it freezes. Finally, warming catheters protect the urethra. With the advent of these changes, urologists are again considering the possibilities of cryotherapy—and finally seeing success with acceptable side effects.

HOW CRYOTHERAPY WORKS

Any mountain climber knows the risk of damage to living tissues from freezing. Bringing prostate cancer to a hard freeze will do the same thing. Early cryosurgeons (remember we are referring to only a decade or two ago) used *cryoprobes* supercooled with liquid nitrogen. These probes were about the size of a #2 pencil (huge by today's standards) and were difficult to place precisely. In the late nineties markedly smaller probes were developed that use 3mm or smaller diameter probes. A recently developed system uses 1.5mm needle probes, not much bigger than the lead in a #2 pencil.

The freeze zone created by the 2.4 mm probe systems (manufactured by Endocare, Inc.) is approximately 4 cm in diameter and 4 to 5 cm in length. Its flame-shaped "iceball" correlates with the tapered shape of the prostate—larger near the base and conical at the apex. The "ice balls" created by 1.5 mm (17 gauge) probes (manufactured by Oncura Corp.) are smaller, approximately 2 cm in diameter. Cryosurgeons are still investigating whether it is better to have fewer probes and a tapered shape or more but smaller iceballs that can "sculpt" the prostate for a better fit to its normal shape; there is no consensus at this time.

Each uses an obscure law of physics called the *Joule-Thompson principle* to supercool its tip. Liquid argon is expanded rapidly in the outer of two

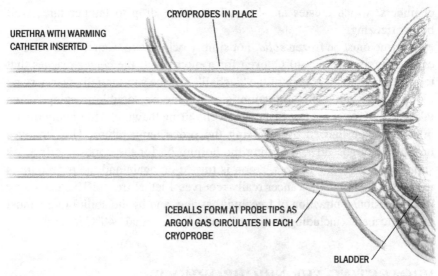

Figure 17-1. Cryoprobes placed into the prostate (upper part of illustration) are supercooled, creating "iceballs" around their tips (lower part of illustration) within minutes. (Courtesy Endocare)

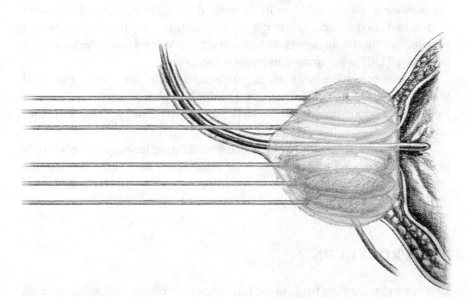

Figure 17-2. "Iceballs" have coalesced into one, freezing the prostate completely. (Courtesy Endocare)

chambers, which creates an almost immediate drop to temperatures well below freezing.

Tissue must be frozen *solid*, not simply below zero. Cancer cell death is essentially assured at −40°C, even for a moment. If the center reaches that temperature, the outer core of the "iceball" may be substantially warmer and barely below zero. This limitation is overcome by "double freezing." This takes advantage of the fact that cells swell during thawing. After being frozen once, they are thawed by reversing the probe temperature. This involves turning the argon off and turning the helium on for the opposite effect. As soon as the "iceball" freezes, argon is turned on again and the procedure is repeated. This time the cancer really receives a lethal freeze. This occurs by the expansion/contraction of freezing/thawing, and by the ability to get most of the "iceball" (including its outer layers) to the lethal −40°C level.

PROTECTING THE NEIGHBORHOOD

As with any prostate cancer therapy, cryotherapy can cause side effects or damage to adjacent organs. The **urethra** running right through the middle of the prostate is most vulnerable. In the early days of cryotherapy, it was often frozen and would literally slough or turn inside out. Its channel would remain, but the lining would at times melt away for a few weeks until it healed. A TURP was required to remove the tissue.

This complication has been largely eradicated by the use of a urethral warming catheter that circulates warm fluid through its chambers. Saline or salt water at approximately 40°C (104° Fahrenheit) usually protects the urethra.

Damage is also minimized by precise monitoring techniques currently in place. Probes placed near vital areas of interest tell us when to reverse the cooling process. Helium begins to warm the tissues within seconds so that the "iceball" doesn't grow beyond its intended borders.

THE PROCEDURE

Enemas and something to clean the intestines and rectum such as *magnesium citrate* will be administered the day before the operation. Antibiotics to prevent infection are given preoperatively.

After anesthesia is administered, the patient is positioned in a manner similar to a woman having a pelvic examination, and an ultrasound probe is placed into the rectum to guide placement of all probes.

Temperature-sensing probes are placed near the **urinary sphincter**, rectum, and prostatic apex. These probes will warn the physician if freezing is reaching somewhere it should not. Next, six or more (rarely, up to thirty with the smaller Oncura system) cryoprobes are placed into position. **Cystoscopy** confirms that none has entered the urinary tract and the urethral warming catheter is inserted.

Freezing begins slowly under ultrasound and computer monitoring. When the "iceball" reaches a lethal chill, the argon is turned off and helium is turned on to thaw the gland. The process is repeated as soon as it is thawed, and the entire procedure is completed within a couple of hours. The urethral warming catheter is sometimes left in place for an hour or so in the recovery room in order to minimize complications.

Following surgery most men are permitted to return home within twenty-four hours, often on the day of the procedure. A **catheter** or **suprapubic tube** will remain in place for a week or longer. The punctures heal spontaneously within days.

WHO IS A CANDIDATE FOR CRYOTHERAPY?

The most important factor to make you a candidate for cryotherapy is having cancer limited to the prostate or its immediate vicinity. Like other local therapies (prostatectomy and radiation), cryotherapy works only if cancer is contained in its targeted site.

Men with persistent cancer in the prostate following radiation therapy are obvious candidates. Because **salvage prostatectomy** is associated with such significant complications (as described in the previous chapter), cryotherapy is appealing as a method of treating localized recurrent cancer without major surgery. Complication rates for cryotherapy following radiation are indeed higher than they are with cryotherapy as an initial treatment, but appear to be lower than the rates with salvage prostatectomy.

Men with large prostates—measuring greater than 50 to 75 grams on ultrasound—are harder to treat. It is difficult to fully freeze all the tissue when the gland is bigger than that. Those within about 10 to 15 grams of that volume can reach it by taking hormonal ablation (as described in the chapter 22). Six months of hormone therapy will reduce the prostate volume by up to one-third, making some men candidates who would have not been otherwise.

In addition, it is possible that this improves the chance of cure since hormonal therapy is effective against prostate cancer. Some surgeons will treat larger glands, but it is more difficult.

Finally, cryotherapy at present is appropriate only for men who understand they will probably not have *spontaneous* erections following treatment. These men may still be sexually active if they use treatments such as those discussed in chapter 19, but very few will have normal erections without such assistance. Interestingly, because the nerves are frozen instead of severed, a very small number of men will recover natural erections even two years following treatment. However this is the exception and most men will not.

Some centers are now treating only the side of the prostate with known cancer (thereby sparing one of the two penile nerves). Such nerve-sparing cryotherapy is controversial, and it may be years before we can confirm that this will control prostate cancer. We currently perform such focal treatment extremely selectively, and only as part of an investigation protocol.

SUCCESS WITH CRYOTHERAPY

An undetectable PSA is our best indicator of absence of cancer in men who have undergone prostatectomy. However, cryotherapy and radiation leave some residual prostate tissue so PSA remains detectable in most men. Fortunately, tissue remaining after cryotherapy is typically near the urethra because of its preservation courtesy of the warming catheter. This minimizes serious complications but also leaves a source of detectable PSA. It also leaves a theoretical source of cancer recurrence in the uncommon situation where the tumor is near the urethra. Recall that most cancers are located peripherally, well away from the urethra, so the risk of residual cancer in that location is low.

There is no universal PSA level that confirms cure, but the PSA should reach a *nadir* of <0.5 ng/dl. A PSA nadir of <0.1 ng/dl is an even better indicator of long-term disease control. **ASTRO criteria**, as discussed in the previous chapter, are commonly used.

Cryotherapy seems to provide disease control and survival through five to seven-year follow-up that rivals surgery and radiation; nevertheless, this is short follow-up compared to experience with those options, so its durability will be watched closely.[2] Some have advocated that the ability to freeze beyond the prostate might give even better results than surgery or radiation for men with cancer extending outside the capsule, but this has yet to be shown.

COMPLICATIONS

Cryosurgical ablation of the prostate can cause any of the complications listed in the surgical prostatectomy chapter. Impotence is expected because the **neurovascular bundles** are intentionally frozen. Still, erections can occasionally return in a year or two because the nerve sheaths remain intact as a conduit for nerve regrowth.

In addition, a couple of specific issues with cryotherapy have limited its use in the past, but have been reduced substantially at this time. Penile or rectal pain occurs up to 10 percent of the time from freezing of the nerves in the area. This usually resolves, but can persist in some men. It is managed with medication, and sometimes using a nerve block or other options offered by a pain clinic specializing in pain relief, until it resolves.

Urethral sloughing occurs if the urethra becomes too cold. Nothing is required if tissue passes spontaneously, since complete healing will eventually occur. If not, a catheter must be placed to empty the bladder. Because the tissue heals poorly soon after cryotherapy, nothing more is done for a few months. In the worst-case scenario, a TURP can relieve the problem.

The worst specific complication is urethrorectal fistula. This occurs when both the rectum and urethra are damaged, leading to an opening between the two. Surgery to correct it, potentially involving a temporary colostomy, will be required. Fortunately, this occurs in modern cryotherapy series less than 1 percent of the time.[3]

KEY POINTS

- Intermediate results with cryotherapy rival those of surgery and radiation.
- Cryosurgical ablation of the prostate has been in use for decades, but only recently has the technology allowed its safe widespread use.
- Complications mirror those of radiation and surgery, but also include occasional cases of urethral sloughing and rectal injury. These usually heal spontaneously but sometimes require surgery.
- Most men will experience permanent impotence following cryotherapy.

18.

MAKING THE DECISION ON LOCALIZED PROSTATE CANCER

[Y]ou have to fight . . . arm yourself with all the available information. . . . Understand what has invaded your body."
—Lance Armstrong, world-class athlete, father, son, and conqueror
of urological cancer and the Tour de France more times than anyone in
history. (By the way, he did *all* these things after recovering from
metastatic urological cancer.)

N
ow you know the options and are nearly ready to make a decision. This is the hard part. Men struggle for weeks with the final call. They make up their minds just in time to change them. New information arrives—from a friend who had surgery, a cousin who had radiation, Internet ads for complementary treatments, and the latest celebrity to be diagnosed. It seems to never end.

I am a strong advocate of each patient making an *informed decision*—not giving *informed consent*. You should not give consent to allow the doctor to do something *to* you. Rather, you should be making a decision to request that the doctor do something *for* you. It is you that matters.

You must weigh the risks versus benefits of each option in consultation with your doctor. You should know the likelihood of success versus the likelihood of side effects. This may not be a specific number or percentage because such predictions cannot be accurately made for each individual. However, you should have a general idea and should be comfortable that you have the pertinent information before making a decision.

SECOND OPINIONS

A diagnosis of cancer can be bewildering. You may not think clearly as the doctor gives you a ton of information, then asks you to make a decision. For that reason, I usually suggest men go home, think it over, and come back in a week or two to move the process forward. I offer the option of a second opinion in the meantime.

If your urologist served you well, a second opinion may be a waste of time and money. He may have earned your trust by giving you the information you need, respecting your feelings on treatment options, and recognizing it is your decision while his responsibility is to help you make the right one. If this is the case, and if he is someone experienced in treating prostate cancer and has good recommendations from people you trust, you may need to look no further.

If that is not the case, then getting a second opinion is a good idea. It will allow you to get another perspective. If the approaches are similar, you gain assurance that you are in good hands and are getting good advice. If they differ, you must figure out which one is right for you and may have to enlist your primary care physician or another urologist to determine which way to go.

There are a couple of reasons that your doctor might object to a second opinion. First would be a lack of confidence in his diagnosis or recommendations. Strong physicians do not let this concern them. However, he might be concerned by a certain phenomenon in which the doctor giving the second opinion is at an advantage. As the most recent person to discuss the issues, he has the patient in front of him while he is trying to make decisions. Therefore, the patient may decide to go with the second doctor purely because that's who is there when he makes the decision. Therefore, you should be up front with your doctor. Let him know you will seek further advice, but also assure him you will let him know if for any reason you should decide to go with another physician.

SEEKING ADVICE

Your physicians are your best source of information. The urologist has extensive knowledge of prostate cancer. He has watched many men go through the process and you can benefit from his experience. A radiation oncologist can clarify concerns regarding radiation therapy. Finally, your primary care physician will have an unbiased perspective based on his own patients who have gone through the process. You trust him for other health issues, so feel free to rely on him for perspective on this as well.

The best source of information regarding whom to see for a second opinion is often your primary care physician. He may refer patients to more than one urologist, and will have knowledge of other experts whom he trusts. Another good source is the nursing staff (if you know any of them or know anyone who can introduce you), particularly those who work in the operating room of a major hospital. They know the surgeons better than anyone. They see the hands in action, and know the personalities under the pressure of the operating room lights. They're usually very honest about their thoughts on the subject.

WIVES, CHILDREN, AND OTHER INTERESTED PARTIES

An anonymous quote accurately notes that "patients don't get cancer—families do." You may be the one with the tumor, but your family will be intimately involved. Wives usually take one of three approaches. The first is to become the decision maker, inquisitor, and so on. Women are often more comfortable with health-care issues than men are, and may seek information while men sit passively by. This works for some couples, but overlooks the simple fact that it is *his* body, not hers.

The opposite occurs when wives sit passively through the discussion and then proclaim, "It's your body." In some ways this approach simply acknowledges the obvious, but also overlooks the reality that cancer has an impact on them both. Abdicating any role in decision making avoids having to take responsibility for the ultimate outcome, but also leaves the man without counsel from the one person who theoretically is his most trusted adviser.

A healthier approach is usually found in the middle. This is a decision in which both parties should participate. He is the one susceptible to side effects, although potential erectile dysfunction obviously affects them both. More importantly, his longevity has an impact on the rest of both their lives.

The most common comment from wives is, "I just want him around, whatever it takes." Once they fully explore the issues, they usually agree on management as long as they freely and openly communicate with each other.

HOW LONG DO I HAVE TO DECIDE?

Take a deep breath—there is no rush to make a decision. Prostate cancer usually develops very slowly and it progresses equally as slow. We believe it takes a decade or longer before any signs to arouse suspicion occur. It takes months for a prostate cancer cell to divide into two, and might take years before any of them escapes and spreads to other body areas. This provides you with time to make up your mind with the best solution for you. It also allows time to get your life—*not your affairs*—in order and to get ready to devote the necessary emotional energy to treatment.

We used to make men wait three months following diagnosis before we would consider surgery in order to allow swelling to subside after biopsy. Although we don't do this any longer, it should give you the perspective that a delay of three or four months doesn't alter your chance of cure. It is certainly more acceptable to wait this time period if it allows you to choose the right option for you instead of choosing the wrong option in haste.

Nevertheless, this doesn't give you license to avoid the decision altogether. Even if you choose **deferred therapy**, at least make the decision actively, not passively. Deciding to follow cancer closely is very different from failing to make a decision, which would risk serious consequences.

CHOICES, CHOICES

You are now at the first of three major forks in the road. *The first choice you must make is whether to treat the cancer at all.* Recall that most men with prostate cancer will die of something else, so the cancer becomes life threatening in a minority of cases. This means that watchful waiting is appropriate for many men, especially those with a less than ten- (or at most twenty-) year life expectancy. Many cases of prostate cancer will take longer than that to lead to death, so it is very possible you will live your normal life expectancy before cancer becomes an issue.

Obviously, if you actually do live longer than could be predicted, there is the chance that cancer could become serious; this might lead to reduced survival, but this is unlikely in appropriate candidates. In addition, if you truly watch carefully for signs of cancer progression, cure is still possible in many instances.

Although watchful waiting is appealing, we know from the Scandinavian experience that in large populations, men who choose watchful waiting are more likely to die of prostate cancer than those who proceed to surgery.[1] Their experience finds that prostatectomy prevents half of cancer deaths. Interestingly, this study was used in its early years to advocate that men not treat prostate cancer until the potential consequences became clear with time. Thus, once again this decision should not be made lightly. If so, active surveillance is mandatory.

HOW OLD IS TOO OLD?

Since prostate cancer usually takes years to progress, men with limited life expectancy may not require treatment. Cancer may take so long to grow that a man may live his normal life expectancy before it has time to cause much harm. The tricky part is that no one knows either how long each of us will live or how long each cancer will take before becoming serious or life threatening.

When I was training in the eighties, we were often taught that men over the age of seventy should be treated rarely, if at all. This was based on the flawed reasoning that most men that age will live less than ten years. If that reasoning were accurate, we would never see men in their eighties, nineties, and beyond—clearly not the case.

In order to define which older men will benefit from treatment, we must consider the fact that age is a poor predictor of potential longevity. I often meet sixty-year-old men who are in such poor health, they will likely never see seventy, but I also see octogenarians who may outlive their children. Age alone is not enough.

A recent study looked at predictive models of otherwise healthy men over the age of sixty-five who were treated for prostate cancer; it led to some interesting findings. The effect of treatment on life expectancy and quality of life were considered. Local therapy in men with *well-differentiated* (Gleason score 4 or less) tumors led to improved life expectancy up to age seventy-five, but didn't improve quality of life. Men with *moderately differentiated* tumors (Gleason score 5–7) received improved quality of life and additional life expectancy if treated up to age seventy-five. Men with *poorly differentiated* tumors (Gleason score 8–10) up to age eighty gained life expectancy and quality of life. Therefore, treatment must be individualized to the man and the cancer.[2]

THE SECOND FORK IN THE ROAD

If you decide to choose treatment, *the second fork is choosing radiation, surgery, or cryotherapy.* Consider each form of radiation to be similar to the other. The same can be said for surgery. (The third option, cryotherapy, is performed only one way, so it requires no further choices.) Therefore, you must decide if the advantages and disadvantages of one of these major categories meets your needs better than the others do. The table depicts the major issues involved in the decision.

Table 18-1. Advantages and Disadvantages of Options for Treatment of Localized Prostate Cancer

Treatment	Treatment and Recovery Time	Advantages	Disadvantages
Surgery		Cancer removed	Major surgery required; incontinence more common than non-surgical options in short term, but resolves in most men; impotence common in months after surgery and can be permanent
Retropubic (RRP)	6 weeks	Operation with longest track record; more surgeons skilled at this than other operations	Biggest operation; more blood loss than other operations
Lap/robotic	2–6 weeks	Less invasive than RRP; low blood loss	Lack of long-term data; few surgeons skilled in procedure
Perineal	2–6 weeks	Less invasive than RRP; low blood loss	More difficult than other operations to spare nerves; few surgeons skilled in procedure

Radiation		Avoids major surgery; less incontinence than surgery	Prostate remains; long-term side effects become almost as common as surgery, especially impotence
External Beam	6 weeks	Low risk of urinary retention; noninvasive	Time commitment
Brachy-therapy (seeds)	1–2 weeks	One-time treatment; you can continue to work while seeds release their energy	Requires anesthesia; if urinary retention occurs, cannot treat for months because of radiation
Cryotherapy	1–2 weeks	Minimally invasive freezes beyond capsule so may kill locally advanced cancer	Impotence almost definite; occasional risk of urethral or rectal injury

THIRD DECISION POINT: SURGERY

If you have chosen surgery, the next fork is which form of surgery to choose. The time-honored approach is the radical retropubic prostatectomy. Although the "biggest" operation, it is also the one that most urologists know they can perform safely and effectively. **Perineal prostatectomy** offers a smaller incision and potentially less blood loss, but makes it difficult to preserve potency. **Laparoscopic/robotic prostatectomy** is the newest version. In very skilled hands, it appears to be a realistic option, although there are limited studies to indicate its success rates and complication rates. Recovery may be quicker, and this may be the preferred option in the future when enough surgeons become facile with this technically challenging operation.

Regardless of choice, go into the operation with confidence that 95 percent of men who undergo prostatectomy survive prostate cancer at least ten years.[3] Such men whose cancer is confined to the prostate have a life expectancy that is essentially that of comparable men who have never had cancer at all!

To reiterate, my mentor and chairman of the Department of Urological Surgery at Vanderbilt University Medical Center, Dr. Joseph A. Smith, gives the best advice on the choice of surgical approach: "Choose your surgeon, not your operation." If you find a surgeon you trust, ask his advice. If he can assure you that his best results are with one of those three surgical options, that's all you need to know. Don't ask him to do it through an approach that he's still learning or not an expert in. Ask him which one he would do for a friend. If you are ready to choose surgery, ask him to perform that operation for you as well.

THIRD DECISION POINT: RADIATION

If you have chosen radiation, regard both forms as the same treatment through two different routes. External beam radiation directs radioactive beams into the prostate from the outside, whereas brachytherapy seeds emit radiation from within.

The advantage of brachytherapy is that it is a quick outpatient procedure. You can return to your routine quickly, while the seeds do their work. The advantage of external beam radiation is that it doesn't leave a permanent radioactive implant in place. In the uncommon event that **urinary retention** occurs, a **TURP** can open up the channel. If this occurs with brachytherapy, you have to wait ten or more months before the seeds can safely be removed.

PREVIOUS HERNIA SURGERY: AN UNANTICIPATED PROBLEM FOR SOME

The move to minimally invasive surgery led to the introduction of *laparoscopic hernia repair (LIHR)*. Instead of a large groin incision, a laparoscope is used to place a large sheet of surgical plastic mesh along the inside of the abdominal wall. It works well and sounds great.

However, an unforeseen downside became clear when urologists tried to perform retropubic prostatectomy in some of these men. The mesh obliterated all natural surgical planes used to safely remove the organ. Surgeons who encountered the problem were unable to remove the prostate and had to abort the procedure. Most surgeons will now decline to even attempt the operation if a man has had a bilateral LIHR because of this severe scarring and its attached mesh.

This should be taken into account, and if you have a large mesh (you may have to contact the surgeon who did the operation to find out) you may not be a surgical candidate. Other forms of hernia repair that do not involve the large sheet of mesh do not create the same concerns.

We now advocate aggressive prostate cancer screening *prior to* considering laparoscopic inguinal hernia repair in order to determine risk of future cancer, since it will preclude the ability to have prostate cancer removed in the future. Although the medical community at large has not yet fully recognized this risk, we also recommend men less than forty years old consider a traditional hernia repair instead of LIHR because if they develop prostate cancer in the future they may have forfeited their ability to have it removed.

My colleague Dr. Inderbir Gill has found, however, that prostatectomy on such men seems possible using laparoscopic/robotic prostatectomy because of its approach to the abdominal wall from the inside. If this experience is confirmed after thorough study, it may again allow men who have had laparoscopic inguinal hernia repair to undergo prostatectomy safely.[4]

NO FREE RIDES

I frequently meet patients who want treatment benefits without the risks. There is no such thing. I believe that all three curative options for localized prostate cancer—surgery, radiation, and cryotherapy—are viable options. Their differences are spelled out in this book, and you can tell there is no single right treatment for everyone.

That is sometimes misinterpreted as meaning that there is no difference in treatments. Some men will take the logical extension that brachytherapy is the way to go. It is

Men often tell me they have a friend or family member who chose a treatment option that is working great because they have gone two years with no signs of cancer. Occasionally this involves an alternative treatment.

The fallacy in this thought process is that prostate cancer—as emphasized throughout this book—usually progresses slowly. Of course they are doing well in two years. Many men with even the most serious cancer do well for that duration.

The slow progression times of most prostate cancers can make even a placebo look good, because few men will experience major problems in that short time period. Thus, beware of experiences you hear of that involves short time frames—less than five years' follow-up—they mean little as you make your decisions.

performed on an outpatient basis, is minimally invasive, and rarely causes impotence or incontinence in the short term. That sounds ideal, unless you recall that radiation toxicity can be more severe than surgical side effects on occasion (especially regarding bowel function and diarrhea).[5] Moreover, the cancer remains in place and success depends on the hope that radiation damage will kill it within the coming year or two with brachytherapy. Local tumor recurrence is possible.

Cryotherapy is similarly appealing as long as a man doesn't wish to be sexually active. Moreover, tissue surrounding the urethra may occasionally still harbor cancer in some men who choose cryotherapy, just as it has known side effects.

These are the reasons I say there are no free rides. Brachytherapy and cryotherapy are great minimally invasive options as long as you consider the whole picture. Similarly, some men choose surgical removal assuming it guarantees cure if they can tolerate postoperative recovery and side effects. They forget that there is no such thing as a guarantee in medicine. Cells that might have already escaped the prostate prior to the operation remain a concern, so cancer can sometimes recur despite a perfect operation.

Therefore, remember to take *all* issues—cure, side effects, personal feelings, time required, and other concepts covered in this book—into account and discuss them with your physician (and your wife) when making a decision. Doing so ensures your best chance of success, as well as the best chance you will be pleased with your decision.

NOMOGRAMS

There are more than forty different mathematical models called nomograms to predict the behavior of prostate cancer. Dr. Michael Kattan, now at the Cleveland Clinic Foundation, developed the most well known and easiest to use while at Memorial Sloan Kettering Cancer Center in New York. His nomograms allow you to enter some readily available data, including PSA, Gleason numbers, and stage in order to predict your likelihood of a good outcome. They are available at no charge at http://www.mskcc.org/mskcc /html/10088.cfm. Your urologist can readily give you the information needed to fill in the blanks. If you are considering external beam radiation, the radiation oncologist can tell you his plan for the prescribed radiation dose in order to fill in this information.

Another similar guide exists in the *Partin Tables*. Dr. Alan Partin assembled the data in the large Johns Hopkins University radical prostatectomy database. He wanted to give patients and physicians an idea of the likelihood that the cancer is limited to the prostate or if it has advanced. The *Partin Tables* are also available at no cost on the university's Web site at http://urology.jhu.edu/prostate/partintables.php.

The size of the database they are based on is the strength of the Partin Tables, but they have limitations. First is that they have large ranges in many categories, so that the table might show you having a chance of having **extracapsular extension** that is either likely or unlikely, depending on where you fit in the range given.

The second problem with the Partin Tables and other statistical predictions is that they apply only across large groups of people. Although we can predict that there is a 90 percent chance of something happening, for each individual there is either a 0 percent or 100 percent chance. It either happens or it doesn't. Therefore, you should remain aware that these numbers might show somewhat similar outcomes with the various options, while you may make a decision based on factors outside this mathematical prediction.

Finally, all prediction models are based on historical data. Information regarding patients from the past is fed into the models and their outcome is used to predict yours. However, recall that we now treat a very different group of patients than even a decade ago. Regardless of PSA, stage, or any other variable, men with prostate cancer today have a more favorable prognosis than ever before. Therefore, most men today can be expected to do better than the nomograms predict because these models have not yet incorporated data of the current group. This should not dissuade you from using prediction models in order to understand your disease, but you should realize that they may underestimate the chance of success.

OTHER WAYS TO KNOW HOW SERIOUS THE CANCER IS

The Gleason grade, stage, and PSA are universal pieces of data used to predict the behavior of prostate cancer and the need for aggressive intervention. A recent concept is that of **PSA doubling time (PSA-DT)**. This is exactly as it sounds—the time it takes for PSA to double. If this occurs in less than ten months, the cancer will almost inevitably lead to serious complications or death unless treated aggressively. Less than three months is even more concerning and is often associated with rapid disease progression, while doubling times measured in years often suggest an indolent tumor that may never require therapy.

Free PSA may also be useful prognostically. Men with a free PSA of less than 10 percent are more likely to have high-grade, potentially serious tumors. *PSA velocity* or rise in the year prior to diagnosis of greater than 2 ng/dl also suggests a cancer likely to progress rapidly unless treated successfully.

We discussed the concept of a staging or reassessment biopsy in chapter 10. Men choosing **watchful waiting** or **deferred therapy** can get a better idea of their prognosis a few months after diagnosis through a biopsy; the doctor may check to see if there is worsening of the Gleason score or an increase in cancer volume.

DOC, WHAT WOULD YOU DO IF YOU WERE ME?

This question is the most common one I hear. It may be the fairest one as well. However, it's also the one I'm least capable of answering. *I'm not you.*

I don't have your exact value system. I don't have your priorities. I don't have your history. Therefore, I don't answer the question with the answer most men want, which is for me to tell them what to do. Instead, I answer that if I were the patient, I would look in the proverbial mirror and ask myself what my priorities are. If my only priority were getting rid of the cancer, I would have a radical prostatectomy. If avoiding treatment side effects were my only priority, I would choose watchful waiting.

Not surprisingly, most men quickly realize they don't have a single priority, but rather a combination of priorities that will need to be individualized. Most men want a cure, but not at the risk of permanent side effects. Some want to avoid surgery because of biases they don't have to explain. Some have seen friends or family do very well from radiation, while others have seen men choose radiation only to experience cancer recurrence later.

I can't be these men, and I can't use the filters through which they view their options. However, once patients let me know how they feel about these issues, I can help them make a decision that most closely approaches their goals. For the young man wanting to live another forty years, this usually means a radical prostatectomy. For a man with a life expectancy of less than ten years, it usually means watchful waiting.

Predictably, most men are in the middle. They must weigh the desire to know the cancer is out (radical prostatectomy) versus avoiding major surgery (radiation or cryotherapy). They will have to choose concern regarding certain side effects versus concern regarding others. For example, a man whose greatest fear is incontinence might accept the greater chance of urinary and bowel urgency through radiation, whereas a man with chronic bowel problems might wish to minimize this risk by avoiding radiation.

A unique interaction occurs when the risk of impotence is considered. Although it has long been assumed that the risk is higher with surgery, we now know this is somewhat misleading. Indeed, immediately following surgery, the chance of impotence is very high. Over time, as tissues recover from the trauma of surgery, the risk of impotence continues to drop for the next year or two. On the other hand, the risk of impotence is very low immediately following radiation therapy, but climbs over the next few years. Adding this risk to the natural decrease in sexual function as a man ages over three to five years, we now know that a majority of men treated with either option will experience erectile dysfunction in that time frame.[6] This is contrary to popular belief, but demonstrates how biases should be based on facts or they will convince you to make a decision for the wrong reasons.

When we look at it dispassionately, we really can't say that one treatment is "best." Studies show it is difficult to prove any option as superior to the others.[7] The overall risk of most side effects (strictures, bleeding, etc.) overlaps among treatments. The likelihood of cure is similar, although it appears that higher-grade cancers may be less likely to respond to radiation. Therefore, each man must weigh his perspective on the risks and benefits to determine which alternative best meets his needs.

MAKING THE CALL

Once you make the three-forked decision described at the beginning of this chapter, let your urologist know you're ready to proceed with a plan. Review the information in the appropriate chapter regarding each treatment option, and find a good time to begin treatment. Any of the three curative options (surgery, radiation, or cryotherapy) will dominate your life for several weeks, so plan work accordingly.

If you want to delay treatment more than three to six months, it is still unlikely that cancer will progress rapidly. However, some men under these circumstances will consider temporary hormone deprivation therapy. Although needed infrequently, it does allow men to undergo treatment on a temporary basis while they defer definitive therapy. A good example might be one of my snowbird patients who was diagnosed in autumn but wanted to go south to Florida for the winter. He didn't have time to recover from surgery before the migration, but didn't want to go six to nine months untreated. Hormonal ablation allowed him to know that the cancer was being treated while he waited, and then he could undergo whichever treatment option he wanted upon return in the spring. There is always a small risk cancer could progress in that time frame, but this risk appears minimal. It should be noted that this deferment has not been well studied, so it is reserved for special situations.

NO LOOKING BACK

Buyer's remorse is bad enough with a house or a car, but has no role in cancer treatments. Once you make the decision, remain faithful to it with the confidence you made the best decision you could, using the best information you could get. Avoid second-guessing if the future brings new information or outcomes. It is easy to look back with the lamentation, "If I'd only known then what I know now." Well, you couldn't have known then what you know now, so dismiss that thought forever!

I liken this to a poker game. You make bets based on the likelihood of a good outcome. If you have a hand full of aces you bet accordingly. Occasionally you will lose and have an unexpected outcome, but that improbability wouldn't change the fact you'd still bet the farm the next time you have such a hand. Similarly, you will occasionally win with a bad hand, but you'd never choose the hand that is likely to lose on purpose.

Likewise with prostate cancer, make your decisions based on the cards in your hand and what you know today. If you choose an option likely to meet your needs and you end up with an unfavorable outcome, it doesn't change the fact that your decision was the right one at the time. Hold your head high—you made the decision the right way.

KEY POINTS

- There are several options to treat localized prostate cancer. None is clearly "better," but understanding the differences will allow you to make the right choice for you.
- Information is power. Find out all you can from credible sources and avoid information overload from well-intentioned friends and family or from the Internet.

- Choosing therapy for localized prostate cancer involves three major decisions:
    - (1) Do I treat the cancer or observe it closely?
    - (2) If treating, do I choose surgery, radiation, or cryotherapy?
    - (3) If choosing surgery, which route (retropubic, laparoscopic/robotic, or perineal) do I take? If radiation, which route (external beam or brachytherapy) do I take?
- Make a decision with the information available to you today. Make the best one you can and never look back.

19.

MAINTAINING SEXUAL FUNCTION

This is the monstruosity in love, lady—that the will is infinite and the execution confined; that the desire is boundless and the act a slave to limit.

—William Shakespeare

Victor had only one thing on his mind when I told him he had prostate cancer—sex. He was a young seventy-two. His wife was a younger forty-eight. He would not consider anything that would affect his ability to be sexually active at least once a week. "I'd rather be dead," he declared (boldly, I thought, since the potential widow was not there to hear his proclamation).

"I understand," I assured him (although I wasn't sure his wife would). Over the following half hour I presented the implications of his prostate cancer. We discussed all options for localized prostate cancer. A Gleason score of 3+3=6 wasn't too alarming. His PSA was less than 10. He was an excellent candidate for watchful waiting.

He concurred. "That way I can keep it up." I wasn't sure if he meant the activity or his anatomy, but didn't want to ask. I recommended careful surveillance with a PSA and DRE in six months, and a repeat biopsy within the year to be sure his cancer remained inactive. The most pointed advice I gave was a recommendation that his two sons approaching age fifty begin screening for prostate cancer immediately.

Three months later I was surprised to find Victor on my schedule earlier than expected. I wondered if he had changed his mind about treatment. Not uncommonly, men get home and begin to think, leading them to decide they were not comfortable with observation. "How do things stand?" I asked.

"Terrible . . . I'm in bad shape, Doc."

Medically he looked fine. A PSA drawn the previous week was actually a little bit lower than it had been at the time of diagnosis. "What do you mean?" He handed me a symptom score card designed to quantify erectile dysfunction. The low score made it clear why he was back so soon. This time his younger wife was at his side.

***

A majority of men with prostate problems—whether prostatitis, BPH, or cancer—will experience erectile dysfunction (ED) at some point. I make that seemingly alarming statement not because prostate trouble causes impotence, but because we know that a majority of *all* men will experience difficulties eventually. The good news is that these men—like nearly all men who experience sexual difficulties—can expect treatment success.

Victor was one such man. Cancer had not caused his problems, but perhaps the stress of the past few months had been a factor. He had chosen an appropriate option—watchful waiting. He made this decision less on my agreement with it than in his confidence that ED was possible only if he underwent treatment. He learned all too quickly, however, that impotence is simply a risk in men his age. He was about to learn of options to manage it successfully.

THE PROBLEM

Up to 30 million American men are affected by ED and the numbers are growing.[1] Almost two thousand American men roll over and say, "This never happened to me before," every night. The incidence goes up substantially with age, increasing significantly above the age of sixty-five. Note that this parallels the incidence of prostate cancer. Although both become more likely with advancing age, no age cutoff exists for a sexually fulfilling life. Some men enjoy sexual activity into their eighties and nineties.

Although impossible to document, almost every adult male experiences at least one occasion when he is not satisfied with the outcome. A vast majority of men will experience ongoing sexual difficulties at some point in life whether they have had prostate cancer or not.

SPECIFICS WITH PROSTATE CANCER PATIENTS

"Okay," you say. "That's fine and dandy that over half of men have at least some degree of impotence, but I don't care about those guys. I'm a cancer patient and my situation is different."

You are right. Your situation *is* different. Prostate cancer does not cause impotence, but the stress of having cancer combined with treatments for it definitely makes its victims prime candidates for sexual difficulties. Like Victor, even if you have not received treatment, you have the anxiety of being a "cancer patient." Most of those other guys don't have that stress. However, as noted throughout this book, most men with prostate cancer don't face life-and-death issues daily, so don't think of yourself as a "cancer patient." Think of yourself as someone living with prostate cancer, and we hope someone living successfully with it.

We know that prostate cancer treatments contribute to impotence, which is the real difference between you and the average ED patient. Surgery usually leads to at least temporary impotence, although half or more men with previously normal erections will regain them in the months after surgery. In contrast, radiation causes minimal impact initially, but a year later significant numbers of men experience some weakness in erections, and by three to five years after treatment, approximately the same percentage of radiation patients are as likely to have ED as those treated with surgery.[2] Most men who choose cryotherapy or are treated with hormonal therapy have already conceded the likelihood of permanent erectile dysfunction. For that matter, men treated for BPH may also experience problems. Therefore, men in all groups may need help with erections in the future.

The surprising statistic is that almost half of men managed through watchful waiting also experience erectile difficulties. Part of this may be due to the stress of their disease, but more likely is the result of the aging process. A number of men already have difficulties by the time their cancer is diagnosed. In my own practice, that is almost half of all men. After three to five more years of simple living and aging, 45 to 62 percent of men on watchful waiting will become impotent even without treatment.[3] Therefore, making decisions based on the long-term effects on erections may not be wise.

A SUCCESSFUL OUTCOME IS AT HAND

There has never been a better time to have erectile dysfunction. Not that this fate should be wished on anyone, but at least *we can now successfully treat virtually all cases no matter what the cause.*[4] Whereas men with erectile dysfunction were disregarded in years past because of medicine's inability to help them, we can now offer multiple effective treatment options. Most respond to oral medications, and those who don't can be treated through several other medical and surgical approaches. Indeed, it is a rare man who can't resume sexual activity if he and his partner are motivated.

Testing is rarely helpful for men with ED. Simply stated, if a man cannot achieve and maintain a satisfactory erection, he is a candidate for the *goal-oriented approach*. Instead of focusing on diagnostic tests to decide where the problem is, the focus is on achieving the real goal—*overcoming* the problem. It is based on the reality that treatment options are the same regardless of cause unless there is an obvious, readily reversible condition at the root of the problem. Treatment should be able to overcome ED regardless of the cause.

MEDICATIONS

Several treatments are available, but a trial of oral medication is usually initially considered. Medications such as Viagra, Cialis, and Levitra are well-known because of their ubiquitous advertising. There are relatively few downsides to a medication trial as the initial approach. They are very safe if you are healthy and as long as you are not taking nitroglycerin, since their most serious contraindication involves a potentially lethal drug interaction with nitroglycerin. Their side effects are otherwise temporary and not serious. In fact, most men who experience side effects still want to continue treatment because the medication worked. Some men report a mild headache, but conclude that it's worth it.

The most common reason men fail to respond to medications is that they haven't taken them properly. The most frequent error is in taking an inadequate dose. Many physicians are comfortable with prescribing fifty milligrams of Viagra since that is the dose in the free sample packs. However, this dose may not be enough for men with more significant problems such as those encountered following prostatectomy or radiation. Whichever medication you take, a full dose will probably be needed if ED is related to prostate cancer treatments. You will need to discuss this with your physician.

Some men don't realize that these drugs work only by allowing the erection cycle to function normally. Their real role isn't in creating an erection—it is actually in keeping the arteries open once the process starts. Without sexual stimulation, the penis may be unmoved. Only with stimulation—sometimes surprisingly little—will the medication exhibit activity.

Failure can also occur if the situation is rushed. It takes at least thirty minutes after ingestion for medication to reach the bloodstream—or the penis. Attempting intercourse before it has had time to take effect invites frustration.

Men following prostatectomy can also become frustrated by rushing into sex too soon after surgery. It takes several months for swelling and scarring around the penile nerves to resolve in many men. Medications may not be effective until this occurs. My experience is that medications usually have little effect until six months, and usually closer to ten months following surgery. I tell men that I don't mind writing them a prescription if they are in a rush, but caution them not to become discouraged if unsuccessful. Another attempt a few months later is likely to be satisfactory.

It is important to realize that performance anxiety usually complicates ED. Once men have difficulties, the stress of worrying about impotence becomes a contributor. This is an example of a vicious cycle. Avoiding this downward spiral is necessary to achieve treatment success.

People frequently ask which oral medication is better. Studies have failed to show that one is "better," but there are a few differences. Viagra has the longest record, so urologists know what to expect since it has been on the market since 1998. Levitra was released in 2003 with the suggestion that it takes effect a little faster, although this may or may not be clinically significant. Cialis came a few months later and has the potential advantage of being effective for about thirty-six hours. It will be in your system—not creating an erection—for that duration. I have patients who swear that each of the three is the only one that works for them. If your physician is comfortable with one I would recommend trying it first. You can try all three (one at a time, of course) and decide for yourself.

***

Victor was an ideal candidate for oral therapy. During his visit it became clear that stress was a big part of his sudden deterioration. In addition to his own cancer, both of his sons had elevated PSA levels and the younger one, living out of state, had been diagnosed with prostate cancer since his last visit. His older son, Anthony, was in the reception area of my office preparing for the appointment slot following Victor's. I reassured Victor that I would take good care of his son. We also discussed ED options. I wrote a prescription and recommended that he take the medication an hour before attempting intercourse, then sent him out to wait for Anthony.

A prostate biopsy was clearly indicated for the son. His PSA was 7.8 ng/dl, definitely high at his age. A few days later we discussed his pathology results—Gleason score 3+3=6 in several cores. Unlike his father, watchful waiting was not a wise choice for the forty-eight year old. After a complete discussion of the issues and the choices to be made, I scheduled a radical prostatectomy. Erections were also on Anthony's mind, but he was more concerned about being there for his teenage children. He had a several decades life expectancy ahead and was taking no chances. He wanted his cancer out.

CONSIDERING OTHER OPTIONS

Vacuum Devices

If still unsuccessful after four or five serious attempts at taking oral medications you may want to ask your urologist for more direct assistance. As with most things in life, there are tradeoffs with the more intricate options.

Vacuum constriction devices (VCD) are cylinders that fit over the penis which create a vacuum, causing the penis to fill with blood. A constriction ring (a thick, specially designed rubber band) holds blood inside the penis following its filling. The ring securely encircles the base of the penis (where it exits the body wall). It can hold blood inside the penis under pressure long enough for a man to have intercourse. Similar rings can also be used without a VCD to manage mild impotence.

Constriction rings and VCDs may be the safest treatments known to man—a death has never been reported from their use. Moreover, this affordable one-time expenditure enables use as frequently as desired. Unfortunately, they lack spontaneity and provide an erection that appears unnatural to some couples because of the presence of the constriction ring.

Because of the mechanical nature of VCDs and constriction rings, they are usually chosen by men in steady relationships. The ease of use, reliability of erection, and safety make them an effective option if you don't mind the "fidget factor" and lack of spontaneity of a mechanical device.

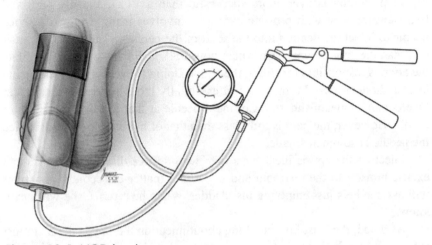

Figure 19-1. VCD in place.

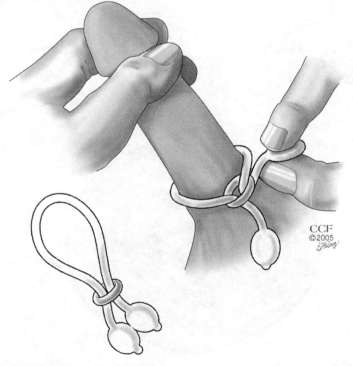

Figure 19-2. Constriction ring.

Injection Therapy

Injection therapy is even more successful than a VCD, and my preferred treatment for men with prostate cancer. It involves using a tiny "diabetic" needle to inject medication into the shaft of the penis—a site no more sensitive than the spot on your arm where your PSA is drawn—in order to dilate the arteries responsible for filling the penis. Doing so creates an erection that lasts an hour or two. Furthermore, it essentially looks natural to most men. Overcoming squeamishness regarding a needle at that location is the major hurdle. However, the pain is truly less than that of having blood drawn since the needle is so much smaller.

Injection therapy is ideal for a man who desires discretion. A man can excuse himself to the restroom and inject in a matter of seconds. A partner will assume he's just emptying his bladder. When he returns, she will never know.

As noted, the least favorite thing about injection therapy is the fact most men don't like the idea of putting a needle into their penis. This is more of a mental block than anything, so most motivated patients can overcome this concern.

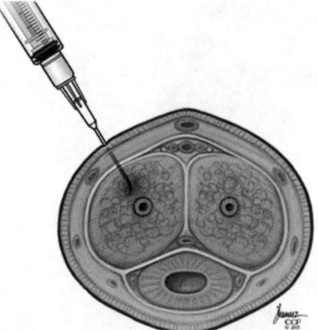

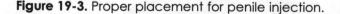

Figure 19-3. Proper placement for penile injection.

Penile Prosthesis

Most men will try at least one, if not all, of the above treatments before considering placement of a penile prosthesis, an inflatable device surgically implanted into the penis that can be triggered to cause an erection in seconds. Once the patient has recovered from implant surgery, the device will give a reliable erection on demand for years to come.

The advantage of a penile prosthesis is impressive in that almost anyone capable of withstanding an operation can regain erections. Some men assume prostatectomy makes treatment of ED more difficult, but penile prosthesis can overcome even the most severe case of erectile dysfunction. Don't let the permanence keep you from having a penile prosthesis if this is the right option for you. When men make the decision to have prosthesis surgery, their satisfaction scores outpace that of any other treatment, including oral medications.

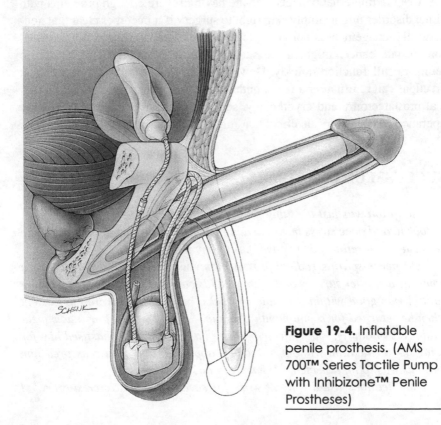

Figure 19-4. Inflatable penile prosthesis. (AMS 700™ Series Tactile Pump with Inhibizone™ Penile Prostheses)

MAKING THE CHOICE:
THE PROGRESSIVE TREATMENT MODEL

A logical description of the sequence that men might consider in treating erectile dysfunction involves the *Progressive Treatment Model*, which compares management of erectile dysfunction to management of *osteoarthritis*. Oral medications are usually the first line of treatment of either problem. Anti-inflammatory drugs such as ibuprofen or aspirin are used for arthritis, while erectile dysfunction patients usually try oral medications such as Viagra, Cialis, or Levitra.

Second- and third-line therapy for arthritis might involve physical therapy or steroid injection into the painful joint. Likewise, VCDs or injection of medications into the nonfunctioning penis might be second- or third-line therapy for erectile dysfunction. Finally, prosthetic joint replacement for arthritis that doesn't respond to simpler measures is comparable to prosthesis placement for erectile dysfunction.

Keep in mind that patients who are having severe enough problems with either disorder might simply skip right to surgery if it becomes clear that nonsurgical management is not going to meet their needs. Men who are treated for prostate cancer might make such a choice, especially if motivated to return to full function quickly. However, it is important to remember that erections can return after a few months (up to two years) following both radical prostatectomy and cryotherapy, so waiting may avoid an unnecessary operation to correct a side effect that might eventually abate on its own.

SUCCESSFUL OUTCOMES

A prescription was just the thing for Victor. He responded reliably each time he took it, and once stress began to diminish, he stopped needing it (although he requested a refill "just in case"). Anthony took a little more work.

The nerve-sparing radical prostatectomy went well. He was discharged home the day after surgery and I removed his catheter ten days later. Bladder control was good within a couple of weeks, but erections were nonexistent when he returned for a one-month checkup. "I tried some of my dad's medications . . . nothing," he lamented. "I need an implant." I chastised him for using the medication without a doctor's approval, and then reassured him that this was to be expected. "What can I do?" he asked.

"Medications usually won't work for several months after surgery," I

explained. "There is a lot of swelling and scarring around the penile nerves. Let's wait to see how things develop before considering an implant." I then offered to begin injection therapy if he truly was ready to resume intercourse. However, once I reminded him of the slow recovery period, he agreed to a patient approach. "Let's talk about it when you really feel ready."

Some partial erections in the coming weeks were only frustrating. He and his wife made several valiant attempts, and he had achieved orgasm twice through foreplay. This is common, as an erection is not necessary to do so. He was ready for more. I arranged an appointment with my impotence coordinator so he could receive a VCD or injection therapy.

Anthony learned to do injection therapy, but used it only six times over the next two months. By that time he began responding to oral medications enough for an erection capable of penetration. Things continued to improve and after six months he had reliable erections, although slightly less firm than he had preoperatively. His wife was satisfied, but Anthony wanted things to be the same as they had been initially, so he continued to take medications when they had intercourse in order to feel he hadn't lost a step.

Three years later, Victor is still being managed expectantly and takes ED medications occasionally. His son is disease free, takes medications primarily for confidence, and has two children heading to college soon.

KEY POINTS

- A majority of men will experience ED at some point. Those with prostate cancer are more likely than those without, but not by as much as many might think. Therefore, possible impact on erections may not be as important as some men believe when making treatment decisions.
- Erectile dysfunction should be managed with the seriousness of any other illness. With current medical and more intricate options, virtually all men can enjoy a fulfilling and satisfying sexual life with their partners.
- For more information, my previous book, *Overcoming Impotence*, provides a complete guide to successful management of erectile dysfunction. The facts in it enable men concerned about—or experiencing— erectile dysfunction to be sexually active for as long as they wish to be.

20.

DEALING WITH OTHER
SIDE EFFECTS

The misery is part of getting better.

—Lance Armstrong

Nick was a nervous man. He took almost three months to decide on treatment for Gleason score 4 + 4 = 8 prostate cancer. Mine was the second of five opinions he would receive. I worried he would put off the decision until it was too late, but he finally decided on surgery and asked me to do it. Concern for side effects made him crazy, but ultimately not as crazy as the idea of his high-grade cancer remaining untreated.

The operation was difficult because of his weight—283 pounds—but went well all things considered. He had been impotent for years and had no wish for sexual activity, so I performed a nonnerve-sparing prostatectomy. He was discharged two days after surgery and the postoperative period remained straightforward until leg swelling developed. I ordered a Doppler ultrasound because of concern for blood clots. It was negative, indicating that swelling was simply due to accumulation of extra fluid in an overweight man recovering from surgery.

Two days later his catheter was due for removal. While I removed it, he told me he had not eaten well since he left the operating room. He was concerned about an intestinal blockage because he had been constipated and belched a lot. I recommended a laxative and increased exercise, suspecting he was spending his time becoming one with the sofa. I also informed him that narcotics cause constipation, so he should minimize prescribed pain killers. "It's a beautiful Cleveland summer," I reminded him. "Get out. Walk in the metro parks—get some fresh air." I think he wanted to be hospitalized (assuming something was seriously wrong), but he heeded the advice anyway.

*We then discussed his pathology report. The final Gleason score was still 8, but there was **extracapsular extension**. The margins were negative so I felt we had gotten the entire tumor, but he was at high risk of recurrence because of the high grade and findings of extracapsular extension. Because of his obesity, I felt he was at higher than average risk of incontinence and didn't think the potential benefit of radiating his prostatic bed justified the likelihood of increased side effects. "Remember your bladder control will take a while to return," I cautioned and helped him put a pad in place in his shorts. The look of disgust was memorable.*

***

Many men faced with a diagnosis of prostate cancer fear the risk of complications as much as they fear dying of cancer. This is often reasonable because most of these men will not die of cancer.

Impotence, incontinence, and all the other issues covered in this book must be taken into consideration when choosing management. Side effects are possible with all options. They often take weeks or months to resolve, although most things eventually return to normal.

However, you should be reassured that we can manage essentially all side effects. In addition, BPH treatment also has some of the same potential side effects, so men who have such concerns will find answers to their problems in the coming pages.

INCONTINENCE

Incontinence is common in women; most handle it well and know to seek help. Men are the opposite. Many panic at the idea of a drop lost, but often will not ask for help. Loss of bladder control is the worst common side effect for most men.

Temporary incontinence is part of recovering from radical prostatectomy, and may also occur following radiation, cryotherapy, or BPH treatments. However, it resolves in most men in a matter of weeks or months as the external **sphincter** muscle becomes more efficient. Thereafter, incontinence severe enough to consider pad use should be expected in only about 5 percent of men if the operation is performed by a surgeon skilled in prosta-tectomy.[1] It is less common following radiation, although also possible as evidenced by reports in up to 6.6 percent of men in one study.[2]

Incontinence is possible because the prostate and bladder neck are responsible for a significant portion of bladder control. When they are removed during TURP or radical prostatectomy, your bladder control is dependent on the external urinary **sphincter** muscle. Fortunately, this muscle will strengthen and allow most men to recover good bladder control. If this muscle is not strong enough, however, incontinence is possible.

Until it resolves, most men will wear incontinence pads. Their use should drop off quickly. I usually observe a significant improvement around a month after the catheter is removed.

Many urologists recommend *Kegel exercises*—pelvic floor muscle–tight-ening workouts that logically should strengthen resistance to urine loss. This logic has not been proven true, however, so most men see no improvement with such efforts. Kegels are not harmful, but it is hard to see a major benefit.

An easily overlooked issue involves urinary "pooling" in the urethra. Recall that urine can become trapped in the urethra, especially if the penis is not directed straight down during urination. Elasticity lessens with aging—and even more following surgery or radiation—so the urethra may not squeeze its contents out until the penis has been replaced into the pants. If you have dribbling a few minutes after urination this is probably the cause. Reviewing the advice from chapter 3 can prevent an embarrassing spot that doesn't have to occur. Some men also benefit from taking the thumb and compressing the urethral area behind the scrotum, "stripping" it forward toward the penis in order to force the last few drops out *before* the penis returns to the pants.

IF INCONTINENCE PERSISTS

Several options exist for the uncommon man whose incontinence persists a year or more after surgery. Over-the-counter cold and allergy medications can boost a weak sphincter enough to make a difference if control is good but not perfect. Recall that urinary obstruction is relieved by blocking *alpha receptors* in the prostate and bladder neck. Doing the opposite—stimulating these receptors—resists urinary flow. These so-called *alpha agonists* (drugs that stimulate instead of block) constrict nasal passageways to help breathing in people with upper respiratory problems. Their constricting properties are problematic in men with underlying urinary obstruction, so they can cause urinary retention if taken by a man with BPH (thus, the warning labels on the package regarding that effect). In contrast, this constriction is actually helpful for men having difficulties holding urine back. Because these medications are not developed for this purpose, research involving this use is sparse; you should discuss it with your urologist. It is still unknown which ones will be most effective for urinary incontinence, but an attempt by using recommended doses of one is reasonable.

Some men develop **overactive bladder** following treatment. Uncontrolled bladder contractions capable of forcing urine through the sphincter can be blocked by **anticholinergic medications** (as described in chapter 8). Detrol LA, Ditropan XL, and a host of new medications being introduced can treat such symptoms.

A similar effect is possible with *imipramine*, an old antidepressant that seems to help people with incontinence through its effect on bladder contractions in addition to possibly constricting the bladder neck. Its potential side effects of sedation and mental status changes must be considered nonetheless.

Duloxetine is another antidepressant drug that seems to correct mild incontinence in women through its effect on the bladder and bladder neck. It is logical that it will have a similar effect in men, although no published studies have yet looked at this effect.

SURGERY FOR SEVERE INCONTINENCE

A year after surgery most men will have long since finished with pads, but about 5 percent will still have leakage. Thereafter things will probably not get a lot better, so consideration of a permanent solution is in order if you still have severe incontinence.

In contrast, radiation damage usually starts out inconsequential but increases over time. In most men it never becomes an issue, but those with significant radiation toxicity may develop progressive incontinence symptoms.

Temporary closure for men with severe incontinence can be obtained by an external cuff such as that shown below. The most reliable way to regain bladder control is through placement of an **artificial urinary sphincter** (**AUS**), an inflatable cuff that encircles the urethra in order to restrict flow. It entails an operation lasting an hour or so. The patient returns a few weeks later to learn how to activate it.

The AUS has a small button placed into the scrotum that can be squeezed in order to open the cuff each time you need to void. Urination ensues and the cuff autoinflates within minutes. It constricts around the urethra again before the bladder has time to fill.

A simpler option for men with mild incontinence is a **male sling**. This involves placement of an artificial material (usually medical-grade plastic) under the urethra. It is tacked to the pelvic bones in order to allow this plastic to compress the urethra just enough to help hold urine in until you intend to void. Thus, the artificial sphincter is stronger and more reliable for severe incontinence; the sling is simpler and a less involved operation for men with mild incontinence. The decision should be made with your doctor, and either one should be performed by a urologist skilled in such surgery.

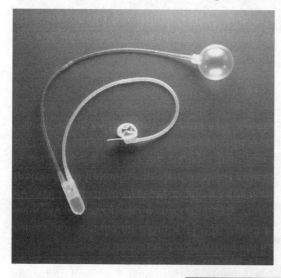

Figure 20-1. Artificial urinary sphincter. Fluid in the reservoir (bulb) fills the round cuff in order to compress the urethra in men with severe incontinence. (AMS 800™ Urinary Control System)

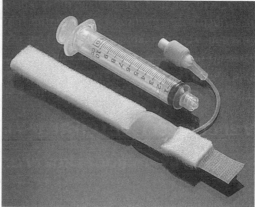

Figure 20-2. Temporary compression device for men with severe incontinence. (Courtesy Cook Urological)

BLADDER NECK CONTRACTURE AND STRICTURE

Bladder neck contracture and urethral stricture are scarring at their respective locations that narrow enough to constrict the urinary stream. Tissues heal together naturally through scarring, and their occurrence is based on the natural tendency of scar tissue to contract and shorten. If a linear scar shortens it goes unnoticed. However, if this line is brought end-to-end to create a circular scar, contraction can narrow the circle. Such is the case with the circular urethra and the bladder neck to which it is sewn.

Contractions occur around 5 to 10 percent of the time.[3] Treatment usually involves a relatively simple dilation procedure in the office. If a man can withstand a moderate level of temporary discomfort, a cystoscope may be inserted into the urethra to facilitate passage of a floppy-tipped wire through the narrowing. This serves as a guide for passage of a dilator; it is small on one end tapering up to a size large enough to dilate the narrowing to an adequate diameter. A single dilation will correct contractures in most men.

SIDE EFFECTS SPECIFIC TO RADIATION

Most of the side effects in this chapter are possible with all treatment options for localized prostate cancer. Radiation presents a couple of other issues. First is **radiation cystitis** and **proctitis**—that is, damage to the bladder and rectum, respectively. Their proximity in the anatomic neighborhood results in some radiation reaching these areas. With contemporary brachytherapy and external beam techniques, this is minimized. Mild symptoms occur in most men but can infrequently be severe. Your doctor can give advice on medications and dietary changes that may help. We recommend a bland diet, stool softeners to prevent straining, and Proctofoam (over the counter) for rectal problems.

Urinary retention occurs in up to 4 to 10 percent of brachytherapy patients.[4] This is minimized by carefully excluding men with preexisting urinary obstruction that may worsen with swelling from the implant. If you have obstructive symptoms, you should carefully discuss this with your doctor prior to implant. It is managed in the same way as it would be for any other man with this problem (as discussed in chapter 8)—with one big caveat. Radioactive seeds must not be manipulated for several months because of the risk to others by releasing radiation before they "burn out." No universal time frame is accepted, but we use ten months as the minimum. Until that time, brachytherapy patients with urinary retention must either use a **catheter** or do **clean intermittent catheterization** in order to empty the bladder.

UNUSUAL SIDE EFFECTS

Rectal injury occurs less than 1 percent of the time with any local therapy. If it occurs during surgery, it can usually be repaired with a few stitches. Such injury resulting from radiation or cryotherapy may rarely require surgical closure and temporary colostomy. These occur very rarely using current techniques.

About 15 percent of men who undergo radical prostatectomy will develop hernias within two years of surgery.[5] Some of these may occur due to normal aging, but the operation may contribute. Surgical repair is required only if bothersome.

Some men believe that their penis is shorter following surgery. We have traditionally attributed this to the effects of postoperative impotence. The theory was that the penis is essentially a blood-filled balloon. If not being filled with erections, the balloon will seem smaller. This may contribute to this perception. However, studies of actual measurements suggest the penis may be 5 to 15 percent shorter following prostatectomy.[6] The significance of this small change is up to the individual. This has not been studied in men undergoing radiation.

IMPACT OF DUAL THERAPY

Side effects increase when more than one treatment is used. The most common example of this is when radiation is administered following prostatectomy because of concern for positive surgical margins (as discussed in chapter 15). This makes all problems more likely, especially incontinence and bladder neck contracture. These risks must be considered and weighed against the potential increase in disease control. Prostatectomy and cryotherapy both entail higher risks of side effects following radiation failure as well.

***

It was no surprise when Nick called the Monday morning after his catheter was removed. "I can't stand it, Doc," he declared. "I'm totally incontinent."

I asked for clarification.

"I have no bladder control. I'm one of the bad ones."

After calming Nick down I discovered his *"total incontinence"* was less than it sounded. He indeed changed pads three times the first day, and used two pads a day thereafter. It was less than a week after catheter removal, so I was unalarmed. "Let's give it a little time," I urged. "It is too soon to tell." Nick wasn't happy, but realized there was nothing to be done in the short term. Once he took a laxative, it did away with constipation and his appetite was back, so at least he felt better.

At his one-month appointment Nick said he was still incontinent—losing a few drops of urine several times a day. One pad kept his pants dry, and he stayed dry all night long. Since he could see a trend toward improvement, he was the most relaxed I had seen him.

Three months later things were pretty much the same and Nick asked about placement of an artificial sphincter. However, on careful questioning it became clear his leakage always occurred within ten minutes of urination. We discussed the reasons why this occurs, and he acknowledged that he draped his penis across his pants instead of dropping them to allow the penis to be directed straight down, so it was likely he was trapping some urine in the urethra. The logic (as espoused in chapter 3) of measures to avoid dribbling made sense to him and he agreed to wait a little longer. When he returned six months later, his PSA was undetectable and he had not worn a pad since the week after his previous appointment. He was back to normal and clinically disease free.

KEY POINTS

- Temporary incontinence is common following surgery but usually resolves completely.

- Incontinence is uncommon (but possible) following radiation or cryotherapy.

- Medications or relatively minor surgery can usually correct incontinence that fails to improve spontaneously.

- Essentially all side effects can be managed. If you experience them, you should discuss your options with your doctor.

21.

LIVING WITH CANCER

*People die. That truth is so disheartening that at times I can't
bear to articulate it. Why should we go on, you might ask? Why
don't we all just stop and lie down where we are? But there is
another truth, too. People live . . . and in the most remarkable
ways.*
I still don't understand it.

—Lance Armstrong

Once a man is diagnosed with prostate cancer, he is changed forever.
He must immediately consider both the risk of death as well as the
risk of side effects from treatment—a double-edged sword.

It may be tempting to assume the role of "cancer patient." I strongly
encourage you not to. This makes you sound sick. It may make you think and
feel like you are sick. Avoid this trap. In most circumstances, *you are not
sick*.

FOLLOW-UP

Routine follow-up visits will become an intermittent part of your life. Initially these will occur every few weeks or months until your situation seems
stable. Your PSA level will be obtained around the time of most visits, and a
DRE may be needed as well.

Following radical prostatectomy, your PSA should be undetectable—

PSA anxiety can be unbearable for some men. Following apparently successful cancer treatment, some men continue to have excessive apprehension regarding the chance of cancer recurrence. Some men (and/or their wives) continue to fear the worst despite a final pathology reading showing organ-confined cancer with negative margins—suggesting that the cancer was completely removed.

Although they continue to do well—with a complete lack of cancer activity evidenced by an undetectable PSA—some men develop escalating stress levels as each follow-up visit approaches. From the time the PSA is drawn until they receive the results, they seem to be on a vigil awaiting word that cancer has returned.

I usually recognize these types early in their care. They may be the ones who ask questions about the chance of dying instead of the chance of living. They often want surgery as quickly as possible. Some would be willing to go straight from the clinic to the operating room in order to be liberated from their tumor without delay.

Once I recognize such men, I know to walk into the room and immediately tell them the PSA is undetectable (assuming that is true, which it usually is—then brace myself in case a bear hug or other expression of relief follows).

Some cannot believe the good news even when they hear it and need confirmation. "Zero, nada, nothing—perfect!" I sometimes must clarify.

zero. Since the prostate is the only significant source of PSA production, its removal should drive its level to undetectable within weeks.

Technically, machines cannot measure PSA below a certain level, usually 0.03 ng/dl, so most laboratories report an undetectable result as: "<0.03." This is often misinterpreted as being detectable by prostatectomy patients who know their PSA should be zero. It is easy to overlook the "less than (<)" sign in front of the number and conclude that the number implies that PSA persists. If you see your lab results and are unsure whether the PSA is undetectable, you should clarify this with your doctor.

Following radiation, PSA levels bounce around for several months. This can be unnerving to an anxious patient who wants to see the numbers approach zero. If I had my preference, I would not obtain a PSA on radiation patients for two years in order to avoid stressing them from such bounces. However, few patients have the patience to wait, so I inevitably concede. Those men whose PSA returns below 0.5 ng/dl are reassured and will usually do well. Those with PSA remaining above that level may still be fine, but are often stressed by the level until it reaches its nadir. Thereafter, the **ASTRO criteria** (as defined in chapter 16) are used to determine success. The **ASTRO criteria** are also used following cryotherapy, but PSA levels usually reach their nadir within just a few weeks since cancer cells die immediately.

Once you reach a steady state and cancer recurrence appears unlikely, your visits will usually become less frequent. My goal is to have a man who is likely to be cured reach a point whereby he requires only one checkup each year—just like any other man. This lessens his tendency to think of himself as a "cancer patient." For all but very high-risk individuals it usually allows time to intervene even if cancer ever does recur.

RISING PSA AFTER TREATMENT

An undetectable PSA suggests a successful outcome following prostatectomy, whereas the **ASTRO criteria** are used to gauge success following radiation (moreover, most urologists employ these criteria for cryotherapy success as well). Failure to meet these standards is defined as **biochemical failure**. In other words, biochemical (i.e., laboratory) evidence of cancer persistence exists.

Although PSA ideally will meet such criteria, a minimal elevation still might not be a serious finding. A study from the Cleveland Clinic found that men with a detectable PSA following surgery had a survival of at least ten years that was as good as those with a minimally detectable PSA.[1] This should reassure you to not panic if you receive such a report during your follow-up. Such men may need radiation to the surgical area or hormonal ablation, but they clearly are not usually in imminent danger.

One reason this is true is based on the use of *ultrasensitive PSA*. This assay can measure PSA levels that would have been undetectable by the machines of only a few short years ago. In that era, such men would have been reassured that their PSA was undetectable and most would have never developed cancer recurrence. The increased sensitivity of current machines allows detection of miniscule levels that might be produced by even a few benign glands.

The risk of cancer progression from an abnormal PSA following radiation or cryotherapy is not completely understood. However, we believe it is similar to the situation following prostatectomy—it suggests the need to consider further therapy, but doesn't mean cancer will inevitably progress. If the PSA level remains low (less than 0.4–0.6 ng/dl for men following prostatectomy; less than 2.0 ng/dl for men following radiation) nothing may be required. You should discuss the implications and options with your doctor.

If the recurrence is believed to be solely in the prostatic area, you may be a candidate for one of the local options that has not been used yet. For example, radiation to the prostatic bed might be used for men with biochemical failure following surgery. **Salvage prostatectomy** or cryotherapy might be used for radiation failure. Cryotherapy is unique, in that it can be repeated for local failure; radiation or salvage prostatectomy might also be considered.

As noted, a **PSA doubling time (PSA-DT)** of less than ten months suggests cancer progression is likely, so you should discuss options to manage this with your doctor. If biochemical failure is due to metastatic disease, hormonal therapy is first-line therapy. Chemotherapy remains an option even if this is unsuccessful (see chapter 23).

UROLOGICAL FOLLOW-UP

I advocate that all men treated for prostate cancer remain under the care of a urologist long term—at least through a ten-year period. The urologist will be most prepared to assist not only with cancer issues but with any concerns regarding urinary or sexual issues that might arise.

A man treated with radiation will usually be monitored by the radiation oncologist as well. A commonly employed schedule allows him to see both the urologist and radiation oncologist annually, with a six-month interval between visits. For example, he might see me in the summer and the radiation oncologist in the winter, so he is followed by both. This separates the visits in case anything comes up. Either one of the doctors involved could probably take over entirely, but I believe it is good practice to keep both involved.

Some men switch their care to their primary care physician after recovery from treatment. I find this problematic for three reasons. First, it is the responsibility of the treating specialist to assure that you continue to do well. A surrogate urologist in your hometown can suffice if you move or have been treated far from home. Second, a urologist will be attuned to your needs following treatment, especially those that pertain to urinary or sexual difficulties. Finally, some nonurologists will not understand that "normal" PSA is changed after treatment. As noted, a PSA of 3.5 ng/dl is not normal following radical prostatectomy. If a nonurologist checks the level and finds it "normal" by the traditional parameter of less than 4 ng/dl, he may overlook significant cancer recurrence before seeking a urological consultation.

DEALING EMOTIONALLY WITH CANCER

Cancer may arise in your prostate, but its effects are felt throughout your body. Your mind is one of the most susceptible areas to its influence. If the worry becomes overwhelming, it is not only harmful to you, but also may hinder your ability to make important decisions.

In order to maintain a clear head, you should exhibit significant self-awareness. Some men need to talk through such issues, while others think more clearly in solitude. You need to know which type you are.

You might seek counsel of your most trusted advisers, be they family, friends, clergy, or professional colleagues. Whichever you feel appropriate, you must be able to be completely open to them.

Faith plays a significant role in how some people deal with cancer. If you find it comforting you should utilize spirituality or philosophy to the fullest extent.

Support groups can be helpful if you are the type of man who is willing to interact in this setting. There are many such groups that can be accessed through your local cancer society, hospital, or county medical society. Man to Man and Us Too are the most well-known groups specifically for patients with prostate cancer. Their contact information is listed in the resources section at the end of the book.

Internet support groups can be helpful, but beware the anonymity of the Web. Some of these are designed for purposes other than supporting prostate cancer patients. They may be run by people trying to make money off other peoples' misery. Others may serve as a free platform for malcontents wanting to speak ill of something or someone. They may also be a gathering place for inaccurate information if the sponsors are not reputable or committed to factual rigor.

Any group counseling situation must be a supportive atmosphere. Stick with it if you find it comforting, or if it helps you sort through the information needed to make decisions. However, such groups can occasionally degenerate into a scene of woe if certain personalities dominate. This may make you feel worse. If so, you will be better off avoiding the situation.

VITAMINS, DIET, AND ACTIVITIES

Remember that the prostate is only one small part of you. Take care of your entire self in order to enjoy a productive life. Your diet should entail foods that you enjoy, but also that you know are good for you. Fast foods, sugars, and soft drinks may taste good at the moment, but have little nutritional value and might interfere with your digestion as well as your intake of healthier options. The body uses protein to repair damage (such as that done by surgery or radiation) and to fight diseases such as cancer. You should get an adequate amount in your diet. If you are nauseated (uncommon, but occurs occasionally with prostate cancer treatments) or have difficulty eating adequate amounts of food, drug stores stock a number of protein supplements that may allow you to tolerate adequate intake in a small volume. Your doctor can recommend a registered dietician for assistance with this or any dietary concerns. A multivitamin a day makes sense, but there is no evidence that cancer can be cured by any vitamins or nutritional supplements.

Unless you are severely ill or are in the first six weeks following surgery, you should maintain an active lifestyle. Exercising at least thirty minutes a day at least three times a week increases strength, helps maintain appetite, and can help you have the energy to overcome cancer and any side effects that may occur.

Avoid the temptation to bury your stress with alcohol or nicotine. This is a time you need to think clearly, and neither will help accomplish that goal. Inevitably, they only add more stress, so avoid their trap.

WHEN CAN I RELAX?

You know that most men with prostate cancer live their lives out and die of something other than cancer. Since the odds are in your favor, try to think positively. Unless your doctor has told you that you have a very serious situation, assume you have an excellent chance of surviving—and thriving—long term.

Five-year survival is used to judge cure with most cancers. The logic is that if cancer is going to recur, it will do so during that time frame or probably never will. You are thus believed cured if you are disease free at that point. Because prostate cancer is typically slower growing than most, five years is not long enough to know whether it will progress. However, biochemical success (as defined above) at five years is very encouraging. If there is no evidence of disease ten years following treatment, you are probably cured, although you and your doctor will need to discuss this.

Very rarely, patients develop cancer recurrence more than ten years later. Exceptions are uncommon enough that you should quit worrying if you haven't already. Continue to follow-up with your physician and feel confident that you are probably going to be fine.

WHAT ABOUT MIRACLE CURES?

Religious miracles are beyond the scope of this book, but miracles definitely don't come from people selling things on the Internet or late-night television. They aren't found in a small village in a third-world country selling laetrile, coffee enemas, or other spectacular but unsound promises of a cure. They also aren't concealed by the government in a way to keep the masses from receiving necessary relief.

The logic of the naivety required to take such treatments is obviously flawed if you take even a moment to consider the reality. First, the government may frustrate us, but it is not in the business of hiding cures for major diseases. The first politician or bureaucrat who released such a finding would be destined for coronation. Second, if such treatments really worked, some pharmaceutical conglomerate would find a way to get them approved and then to charge you far more than it cost to produce them. Finally (and don't be shocked), the guys who sell shark cartilage or other miracles out of shacks in third-world countries or through irresponsible Internet sites aren't as attuned to the finer nuances of prostate cancer as your physician and his team are.

Miracles are achieved one step at a time by doctors, nurses, and patients working together to defeat cancer through proven treatments. These miracles make our days.

KEY POINTS

- Most men live with—not die from—prostate cancer.

- Men with prostate cancer will be monitored by their PSA levels and sometimes DRE for the remainder of their lives.

- PSA should remain undetectable following prostatectomy. The ASTRO criteria indicate that success is likely unless you have three consecutive rises in PSA after it reaches its nadir.

- No one ever died from a rising PSA. An abnormal level following treatment is concerning, but may not indicate a serious situation. Your doctor will probably investigate it and tell you if further intervention is needed.

- Everyone needs to achieve a healthy lifestyle, but it is especially important for men with prostate cancer. This includes diet, exercise, and attention to maintaining mental wellness in this challenging time.

22.
HORMONAL THERAPY: A NOBEL EFFORT FOR ADVANCED PROSTATE CANCER

We wanted to see if hormone therapy would do for elderly gentlemen what it would do for their best friends, elderly male dogs.
—Dr. Charles Brenton Huggins, Nobel laureate who
discovered the effect of hormonal ablation on prostate cancer

Pain in his left hip and lower back was the first sign that Roger had a problem. He took several over-the-counter medications for presumed arthritis, but the pain worsened. He finally went to his family physician. An examination of the seventy-four-year-old man was unremarkable until the DRE. "What's taking so long, Doc?" he asked. There was no tenderness, but the physician noted a rock hard prostate that seemed to be growing into the adjacent tissues.

"I'm sending some blood work," the physician said without answering the question. "And I want you to see a urologist." He knew there was only one possible explanation—prostate cancer.

My receptionist scheduled him to have a biopsy the day of his first appointment because we know Roger's family physician well enough to know that his impression is usually right. After a brief history and physical examination, the one advantage I had over the family physician was that I had the PSA results—more than 5,000 ng/dl. With that knowledge the only thing left to do was to get tissue confirmation of the diagnosis. (Some urologists will assume the diagnosis when it is this obvious, but classically we will treat cancer only after a biopsy confirms it.)

A few days later I sat down with Roger and his family to discuss the pos-

itive biopsy. He had a huge cancer, and I suspected that it had caused his worsening bone pains. No local therapy would cure his cancer if it were as widespread as I believed, so I recommended we begin hormonal therapy as a means of controlling cancer no matter where it had spread.

***

The first (and so far, only) urologists to earn the Nobel Prize were Dr. Charles B. Huggins and Dr. Clarence Hodges, who showed in 1941 that protecting prostate cancer cells from the male hormone **testosterone** would slow their growth. After finding that removing their testicles caused the prostate to shrink in dogs in their laboratory, they tried similar treatments in men with prostate cancer. It sounds a little strange to remove the testicles instead of the cancerous gland, but it makes sense when you realize that testosterone is the engine that drives the growth of prostate cancer.

Their discovery made two major contributions. The first was to show the world that the young specialty of urology was on track to become a major branch of medicine. The second and most important was to completely change our management of this previously untreatable disease.

Prior to that time, patients whose cancers had spread had no treatment option. This was also the first time anyone demonstrated that cancer could be dependent on hormonal control.

ADVANCED PROSTATE CANCER

In contrast to the term *localized prostate cancer*, the term *advanced prostate cancer* is nebulous. It can be taken to imply cancer has moved beyond the prostatic capsule, but most urologists do not consider a small amount of cancer limited to the periprostatic area as advanced. However, local invasion of the *seminal vesicles, bladder,* or *pelvic muscles* is considered a serious finding and qualifies for the designation.

Cancer that has advanced to lymph nodes or bones, the two most common sites, is called **metastatic**. Although we can contain such cancers sometimes for years—and sometimes through a normal life expectancy—we cannot reliably cure them (although some encouraging results have been noted with extensive pelvic **lymphadenectomy** if cancer is limited only to the pelvic lymph nodes).

Because prostate cancer usually progresses slowly, most men with metastatic disease are not in imminent danger. Unlike most cancers, prostate cancer is usually treatable even when advanced. In fact, some men with advanced prostate cancer may be observed until symptoms develop, avoiding the cost and side effects of treatment until necessary. The implications are addressed below.

The best measure of severity appears to be **PSA doubling time (PSA-DT)**. If PSA levels double rapidly, it is likely that cancer will progress similarly as fast. The time that seems to be critical is about ten months. PSA-DT shorter than that portends a serious situation, and should be addressed accordingly. This can be misleading at very low levels, however, because a PSA rising from 0.2 to 0.4 ng/dl may not be significant. At these low (and technically normal) levels a little natural variation might be responsible. In contrast, a PSA rising from 20 to 40 rg/dl in less than ten months clearly suggests a serious situation.

EFFECT OF HORMONAL BLOCKADE

Prostate tissue—benign or malignant—is deprived of normal growth stimulation when testosterone reaches castration levels (below 50 ng/dl). Eunuchs (from birth, which is very rare these days in the absence of major birth defects) won't grow an appreciable prostate or develop clinical prostate cancer. As a result, most prostate cancer cells regress from hormonal blockade whether this is achieved through surgery or medications. Tumors thus shrink whether they are located in the prostate or have spread, and the gland becomes almost one-third smaller over a six-month period.

This slows cancer growth,

AN AMERICAN IN PARIS

When prostate cancer spreads elsewhere it is still prostate cancer. Many people are confused by this, calling it "bone cancer" or "lymphatic cancer" or cancer of whatever site it has reached. None of these labels is correct. In fact, they are misleading because prostate cancer acts like prostate cancer no matter its location. Treatment for "bone cancer" is very different because that type of cancer is very different.

My analogy is that of a traveler. An American who travels abroad is still an American no matter where he is. His presence in Paris doesn't make him French, no matter how long he is there. Likewise, a deposit of prostate cancer in bones or lymph nodes is still prostate cancer and will behave similarly and respond to treatments designed for prostate cancer—not other cancers.

causes it to regress, and sometimes relieves urinary obstruction. Tumors throughout the body will respond, and pain will often disappear within days.

Rendering a man without significant levels of testosterone is called *castration*. However, this term should be distinguished from **orchiectomy**, which means the removal of a testicle. In contrast, castration means that the hormones of *both* testicles are blocked. This can be accomplished either medically or by removal of both testicles, called bilateral **orchiectomy**.

SURGICAL ORCHIECTOMY

The gold standard option for removal of testosterone is surgical castration. Testicles are conveniently in a superficial location amenable to removal under local anesthesia. Testosterone levels drop in minutes. Though veterinarians and ranchers have known for years how to take advantage of this, men are less tempted by this approach. The reason for a reticence to have the testicles removed is obvious, which has led to the development of the alternatives described below. However, surgical orchiectomy remains the definitive and fastest form of hormonal ablation.

The operation is performed through a single incision in the middle of the scrotum just large enough to deliver the testicle through. The cord to each is cut and tied in minutes. Most orchiectomies are performed under anesthesia in the operating room, but we have had good success in the office simply with a local anesthetic. Recovery takes a couple weeks and hormonal ablation is permanent.

Despite the convenience and minimal cost, it is not surprising that most men reject the suggestion of orchiectomy. The psychological implications of castration are difficult to underestimate. They may be partially overcome by placement of a testicular *prosthesis*—a soft plastic device that looks like a normal testicle. Some men will request these be placed to minimize the impact of orchiectomy on their *body image*.

A study in the *Journal of Urology*[6] reported that men were willing to pay almost four hundred dollars a month to take medications for the rest of their lives in order to avoid orchiectomy—four hundred dollars a month for the ability to have nonfunctioning testicles in place. This attests to men's desire to maintain normal body image even in the face of cancer. Only one or two people ever see them (the man and his partner), but, as one patient said, "They sure do dress a man up."

MEDICAL CASTRATION

We can now perform *medical castration* by injecting medications that block testosterone. The testicles are effectively turned off so that they can remain in place, albeit for cosmetic purposes only. These agents are very expensive, but are generally covered by insurance. Most men on hormonal therapy choose medications over surgery.

There are several options, but the most common are variations of two drugs called *LHRH agonists* (agonists stimulate chemical reactions in the body). The abbreviation is for their effect of acting like *leutinizing hormone (LH) releasing hormone* in order to cause LH to rise and release testosterone.

This sounds counterintuitive to *increase* testosterone. It works by essentially burning out testosterone receptors by overloading them. After about two weeks they are unable to handle the load and no longer allow LH to stimulate testosterone production. Testosterone concentration in the body then goes to "*castrate levels*" or the same as they would be following surgical castration.

The first LHRH agonist was **leuprolide**, currently found in slow-release depot formulations labeled **Lupron**, **Eligard**, and **Viadur**. The second drug is **goserelin**, branded **Zoladex**. They are considered medically equivalent drugs. The differences come in their methods of administration since their effectiveness and side effects are identical.

Goserelin is given as a tiny pellet injected into the fat under the skin of the lower abdomen. The needle is a little larger than a standard injection needle, but still well tolerated and only takes a matter of seconds to inject. It releases its active ingredient over the next one to three months. Some men are concerned that the inert pellet remains, but it is no different than a stitch or surgical staple that remains unnoticed forever.

Leuprolide can be injected intramuscularly (as in the Lupron or Eligard brands) as depot preparations. A simple shot in the backside releases a constant dosage for one, three, four, or six months. Another way to give leuprolide is by a titanium encased implant (Viadur) with leuprolide on one end and "osmotic tablets" on the other. As the implant absorbs normal body fluids, the tablets expand ever so slowly and push leuprolide out at a constant rate for a year. It is placed through a small incision between the muscle bellies of the *triceps* and *biceps*. The groove between them running down the inner part of the upper arm is easy to access under a tiny local anesthetic injection. The implant is placed into the fat just below the skin so it can be felt if you press hard enough. It is four by forty-five millimeters, or about the size of a matchstick. Once a year it runs out of medication and must be replaced in a similar fashion in the doctor's office. A similar option, *Vantas*, contains a twelve-month dosing of *histrelin*, a similar drug, while Trelstan (triptorelin) is another three-month drug.

The FDA, Medicare, urologists, and medical oncologists agree there is no therapeutic advantage of one of the above options over the other. There may be differences in cost (which change frequently) or convenience, which is the real deciding factor on my part. I have patients on all the above options. Zoladex comes in a three-month release that seems an appropriate timetable for many patients with prostate cancer. Leuprolide comes in three- and four-month versions, so the latter is nice for someone who needs a little less frequent follow-up. Viadur works for the man with stable disease that comes in only once a year. In Cleveland this is often an advantage for the large numbers of retirees who live here in the summer but go south for the winter.

I rarely use the one-month versions since most of my patients neither need monthly follow-up nor like a shot that often. They are helpful, however, as a way to see how a patient responds before committing him to a yearlong Viadur.

TESTOSTERONE "FLARE"

Recall that for the first couple of weeks testosterone actually goes up. This is called a *surge*, or *flare*, and theoretically might cause cancer growth to speed up for that short time. In order to block this, an **antiandrogen** is sometimes given for two to four weeks. These drugs, which are discussed in greater detail below, can block this surge to prevent a temporary increase in cancer growth.

The clinical implications of the surge are unclear for most men, but those with cancer encroaching upon their spinal cord from advanced disease could have enough enlargement to cause paralysis. This situation is very rare (see below), but anyone thought to be at risk should receive either an antiandrogen or hormonal blockade using something other than an LHRH agonist, usually meaning an orchiectomy or medications capable of temporary blockade such as *ketoconazole*.

Another option to prevent the flare is a new drug called **abarelix (Plenaxis)**. In contrast to LHRH agonists, it is an LHRH *antagonist*. In other words, instead of revving up LHRH in order to burn out receptors, it actually blocks LHRH, so it cannot release testosterone. According to the manufacturer, side effects and uncommon allergic reactions mean that patients should be observed in the office for thirty minutes following each monthly dose.[1]

SIDE EFFECTS

Blocking testosterone essentially puts a man through menopause or its male version, sometimes called *andropause*. This sometimes leads to menopausal symptoms such as fatigue, anemia, muscle loss, and osteoporosis. The latter becomes serious only after several years of hormonal ablation. A *DXA scan* can detect decreased bone density caused by osteoporosis in time to begin medications to prevent this complication.

Hot flashes occur in a majority of men. (Wives often express a degree of empathy since they have experienced the same.) Medications such as *megesterol* (*Megace*) can relieve hot flashes if they are bothersome enough to justify a daily pill.

The effect of hormonal ablation on sexuality is complex. Despite assumptions that testosterone is required for erections, we know that some men continue to be sexually active following this treatment. The same experience dates to the use of eunuchs in ancient times, when harems required men to protect them, among other duties. The one duty forbidden by these men was prevented by castration—or so it was thought. As it turns out, many of these men could (and did) still have intercourse. Since testosterone is key to *libido*, these men may not have sought or enjoyed intercourse as much as they would have if their testosterone were normal—but that didn't keep them from serving such duties. Similarly, although most men have reduced desire for intercourse following hormonal ablation, some maintain an active sex life.

Breast swelling (called *gynecomastia*) occasionally develops. This can be prevented by a few days of therapy applying radiation to the breasts, but it is rarely needed.

Finally, cognitive impairment can occur with prolonged LHRH therapy. These side effects must be considered with your physician before deciding on hormonal ablation.[2]

A KINDER, GENTLER HORMONAL ABLATION?

Antiandrogens such as bicalutamide, flutamide, and nilutamide are drugs that actually prevent testosterone (the body's primary *androgen*, or male hormone) effects. They prevent its entry into cancer cells by blocking its receptors. Their use is based on the fact that a small amount of testosterone is produced in the adrenal glands, so even castration doesn't completely shield cancer from testosterone exposure. Antiandrogens can block the remainder and theoretically increase effectiveness of hormonal ablation.

Because less than 5 percent of total androgens are produced in the adrenal glands, their contribution to cancer growth appears to be limited. Antiandrogens have failed so far to lead to major improvements in survival.[3] Controversy exists in the urology community regarding whether to prescribe them for most patients. Prevention of *flares*, as described above, is the exception.

These agents in combination with hormonal ablation have been described as providing **maximal androgen blockade**. However, this has not been proven beneficial in all clinical trials to date. The three that showed benefit to antiandrogens found a survival advantage of three to six months. These medications can cause a number of side effects, including nausea, liver problems, and diarrhea. For this reason, a large review concluded that "the extensive body of data does not support routine use of antiandrogens in combination with medical or surgical castration as first line hormonal therapy in patients with metastatic prostate cancer."[4] Some advocates use antiandrogens *in place of* hormonal ablation in order to minimize side effects. This remains investigational at this time.

THE HIDDEN SIDE EFFECT: COST

LHRH therapy is very expensive. Depending on which drug you take and how often you get it, costs can be hundreds of dollars per month. A majority of the men taking them are of Medicare age, so it covers 80 percent of the cost. A Medicare supplement will cover the additional 20 percent, so there is no out-of-pocket expense if you have both. Men without full coverage might spend a fortune on these medications, potentially influencing them to have a surgical orchiectomy instead.

TIMING OF HORMONAL THERAPY

The Veterans Administration Cooperative Urological Research Group (VACURG) showed that early initiation of hormonal therapy delays disease progression, and that the earlier it is started, the more likely it is to prevent progression.[5] However, the risks of doing so, as outlined in this chapter, must be considered when deciding if it is appropriate.

Some urologists advocate intermittent hormonal therapy in order to decrease cost and side effects. They wait until PSA begins to rise before giving the next dose. Another option involves measuring blood concentration of testosterone and giving the next dose when levels begin to rise. The Southwest Oncology Group (SWOG) is currently following a group that will eventually number more than three thousand men in order to determine the role of this approach.

HORMONAL ABLATION AS AN ADJUVANT TO LOCAL THERAPY

Radiation effectiveness appears to be greater when a "boost" of hormonal therapy is started before radiation and continued for a few months. The impact is most significant for high-risk patients (as defined in chapter 16).

There are several possibilities of why hormonal therapy for men with **metastatic** disease improves radiation success. First is that hormone therapy has direct activity against cancer. Second, it shrinks the tumor by about one-third, so there is less cancer left for radiation to kill. Finally, it may actually sensitize cancer cells to toxic effects of radiation, improving its effectiveness. However, side effects and cost must still be considered. Hormonal therapy is thus usually added to local therapy mainly for men with high-risk disease.

Hormonal therapy is useful for reducing prostate size for men undergoing cryotherapy. If the gland is outside the size range considered appropriate for cryotherapy (less than fifty, or at most seventy-five grams), a reduction of one-third can make a man a candidate who would not have been otherwise.

In contrast to radiation and cryotherapy, there is little role for hormonal ablation in men who choose radical prostatectomy. Although early reports using hormonal therapy in order to "downstage" cancer looked promising, we now know outcomes are no better when hormonal therapy is given pre-operatively.[6]

HORMONAL ABLATION AS PRIMARY THERAPY

Although hormonal therapy was developed to treat metastatic prostate cancer, many men with organ-confined prostate cancer are currently treated with hormonal ablation. This is based on the presumption that it will prevent cancer progression, and is usually reserved for older men or those with limited life expectancy. It allows them to be treated without undergoing what they perceive as more aggressive curative options such as surgery, radiation, or cryotherapy. The role of hormonal therapy in this setting has not been defined as well as it has for metastatic or recurrent prostate cancer.

HORMONE RESISTANCE

Some cancer cells will inevitably become independent of hormonal influence and unaffected by hormonal ablation. These **hormone-resistant** cells are a minority population compared to **hormone-sensitive** cells in most tumors. However, when hormone-sensitive cells are blocked, the resistant cells have a competitive advantage. They will continue to grow, and will eventually be responsible for cancer progression.

Higher-grade cancers are less likely to be sensitive to hormonal ablation. In combination with their rapid growth rate, their invulnerability explains why they become more dangerous and are more likely eventually to become life threatening.

Some patients have very high-grade tumors that are composed almost entirely of hormone-resistant cells. These very dangerous cancers are indeed very rare. When they advance and take over as the major part of the tumors, the cancer is said to be hormone refractory. At this point most urologists will continue with hormonal ablation to control the hormone-sensitive cells, but may recommend additional therapy for the hormone-resistant component. Antiandrogens are sometimes considered, although evidence of their effectiveness is lacking as noted above.

Occasionally a patient seems to have hormone-refractory prostate cancer but the problem is actually that treatment is not achieving castrate levels of testosterone. Therefore, when that the treatment seems no longer to be effective, the first thing to do is to check a serum testosterone level. If above castration levels (each lab will have its own level determined as normal), then a change in therapy to achieve adequate hormonal blockade is in order. This is usually not the case, but should be confirmed. When cancer fails to respond to hormonal therapy the only remaining option is chemotherapy (as discussed in the next chapter).

***

A bone scan confirmed cancer had spread to multiple sites in Roger's bones. A CT scan also showed a large number of pelvic lymph nodes to be involved. He had already been given a three-month injection and had taken two weeks of an antiandrogen in order to prevent flare, so I reassured him that there was a good chance he would feel better soon. I reiterated what I had told him when we started the injections, that erectile dysfunction would probably occur soon. "Not yet," he proudly noted.

Indeed, when Roger was due for his next shot, all pain was gone. He hadn't realized it but he had been losing weight because of a poor appetite, but it had now finally returned. His PSA had dropped from over 5,000 to about 90 ng/dl—still very high but showing a clear trend downward. It was 9 ng/dl three months later, and was 1.8 ng/dl the next time.

"Am I cured?" he asked at that time. The look on his face betrayed his foreknowledge of the truth.

"No," I truthfully admitted. "Cure is not possible with metastatic cancer—at least not yet." His expression remained unchanged. "But," I added, "right now your cancer is under control."

We proceeded to discuss his side effects. Hot flashes were an occasional nuisance, but not enough to accept my offer for a prescription. He was gaining a little puffiness and extra weight. He also answered in the affirmative when I asked about erectile dysfunction.

"We have a lot of options to allow you to be sexually active," I reassured. "But your libido—interest in having sex—will still be low as a natural result of your cancer treatment." I was making that statement as much for his wife as I was for him, since sometimes wives erroneously think that the change is related to them. "Would you like to consider treatment to allow you to gain an erection?"

"I thought I would miss it, but I have to admit I don't."

His wife jumped in. "No, we're both fine just the way things are. I'm not interested and he's lost interest, so we're just happy he's doing well."

KEY POINTS

- Advanced prostate cancer is usually treated with hormonal ablation, preventing the tumor-stimulating effects brought on by the male hormone testosterone.

- Bones and lymph nodes are the most common sites that prostate cancer will spread to. It remains prostate cancer, however, even if now located elsewhere.

- Unlike most cancers, advanced prostate cancer is usually treatable. Long-term survival is possible in many men.

- Options include surgical orchiectomy or injection of agents that block testosterone production. Effects are the same, but cost is substantially higher with medications.

- Side effects of hormonal therapy are common and must be weighed against benefits.

23.
ADVANCED PROSTATE CANCER: CHEMOTHERAPY AND OTHER OPTIONS FOR HOPE

You play through it. That's what you do. You just play through it.
—Heather Farr, professional golfer and cancer patient (1965–1993)

A few months after beginning treatment with hormonal ablation, Roger's PSA began to rise rapidly. It had bottomed-out at less than 2 ng/dl but had doubled a year later. He still felt well but the reversal was concerning. Six months later it had reached double digits. "What do we do now?" he asked with alarm.

"First, remember that PSA is not the disease," I reassured him. "Cancer is the disease. PSA is just a chemical released into the bloodstream." I acknowledged my concern and ordered an evaluation. A testosterone level confirmed that the LHRH agonist continued to keep testosterone at castrate levels. A bone scan and CT scan were scheduled.

When Roger returned a week later the studies confirmed that cancer had returned to many of the same places it had been prior to beginning hormonal therapy. "What now?" he asked.

***

When I was in medical school and residency we were taught that half of all men with prostate cancer had incurable disease at the time of diagnosis. How times have changed! It is uncommon at this time to find men with widespread prostate cancer.

Despite that good news, some patients still develop **metastatic disease**.

373

Some have cancer in bones or lymph nodes at the time of diagnosis, but most men with advanced cancer currently have been treated for years when cancer finally reaches a **hormone-resistant** state. In years past, hormone resistance meant a man had no more options. Although we are still a long way from curing such men, chemotherapy now promises hope where a decade ago there was none.

WHAT IS ADVANCED DISEASE?

Advanced disease is sometimes in the eyes of the beholder. Some men with a PSA creeping up following therapy will believe the worst and become convinced they are dying. This can be more traumatic than it should be.

For example, men who develop a detectable PSA following prostatectomy may never develop clinical signs of disease. From the time PSA begins to rise, it takes an average of eight years before most men develop symptoms, and another five years *on average* to die.[1] Many of these men *never* develop evidence of disease beyond an elevated PSA, and live a normal life expectancy. This may be due to a few rogue prostate cells that remain in the bladder neck. Therefore, if PSA only begins to rise at age seventy, most men will live their normal life expectancy anyway. If treatment is administered, the prognosis might even be better.

Urologists cannot agree on a PSA level that requires treatment. Following prostatectomy, you should usually not become alarmed unless PSA rises above 0.4 to 0.6 ng/dl. Many men with PSA under that range may never develop disease progression, whereas men whose PSA rises above that range often will eventually develop metastatic disease.[2]

It is probably more appropriate to consider advanced disease the situation where a **metastatic workup** reveals cancer outside the prostate. If this is the case, treatment is usually in order. First-line therapy involves hormonal ablation. Only if this fails are the options in this chapter commonly considered.

WHAT ABOUT MARGIN POSITIVE STATUS?

When men have cancer at the margins (or cut edges) of the prostate following prostatectomy they often worry that cancer was left behind. This is usually not the case. In the past we gave radiation therapy to the prostate "bed" in this circumstance, but this appears to have been overtreatment. Now we recommend careful observation. If PSA becomes undetectable and then begins to rise a few months later, it raises suspicion that cancer might be present locally outside the prostate's original home. Radiation will sometimes kill any wandering cells in the neighborhood.

In contrast, if the PSA remains detectable after surgery, cancer is usually present somewhere unknown. Recall that a metastatic workup cannot detect microscopic cells, so even if negative it is reasonable to begin hormonal therapy. If it has already failed, systemic chemotherapy is potentially beneficial. Studies have suggested men with high-risk prostate cancer may benefit from chemotherapy prior to surgery, but long term results are needed before this becomes standard.

WHAT HAPPENS IN HORMONE REFRACTORY DISEASE?

Simply put, cancer cells duplicate faster than they die in hormone-refractory disease, creating a situation where the tumor grows through accumulation. Hormonal ablation causes **hormone-sensitive** cells to regress, but eventually the **hormone-refractory** cells grow out of control. This may take longer than a man's life expectancy in most patients, explaining why most men with prostate cancer do not die of the disease. However, hormone-refractory cells in some men begin growing faster and overwhelm his ability to fight their growth.

Prostate cancer has a clear affinity for bone. This can cause pain, anemia (from taking over the blood-producing marrow), and/or weakness that can lead to fractures. Spinal column involvement can cause paralysis in very rare cases. Lymph nodes are involved about 20 percent of the time in advanced disease, while metastases to "soft tissue" organs such as lung or liver occur in fewer than 10 percent of such cases.[3]

When cancer advances locally outside the prostate it can obstruct the **ureters** because of their neighborhood location at the base of the bladder. Involvement of one may go unnoticed, but if both are obstructed, kidney failure will ensue. This can be relieved with soft rubber tubes called *stents* placed through the blockage, but this is usually a temporary measure.

SHOULD I PARTICIPATE IN RESEARCH?

It was not until around the arrival of the twenty-first century that we finally saw successful treatment of prostate cancer with chemotherapy. Effective agents were all identified as a result of research protocols. Thus, during the time before their release, the only way to access such medications was to participate in research.

Some people are threatened by the idea of "experimental" medicine. This is understandable, since no one wants to think of himself—as some patients phrase it—"as a guinea pig." However, there are significant benefits to participation, beyond the positive feelings you get as part of the process to improve treatment and to help mankind.

Newer agents and various dosing schedules and combinations are the focus of a number of studies. Participation in one might allow you access to options that are otherwise out of reach. Moreover, research protocols are cutting edge, and usually involve the most up-to-date physicians. Their expertise contributes to your care, and the expertise of a team of top-notch physicians around the country or world may play a role in your care as well.

The final specific issue with prostate cancer research hits home when you recall that it is often a heritable disease. Whether the research protocol helps you or not, it might provide the key to a successful outcome one day for your sons or grandsons if they ever face the same disease.

TREATMENT OPTIONS

Although a majority of cancer cells are hormone resistant at this point in the disease process, hormonal ablation is usually continued in order to prevent the hormone sensitive cells from proliferating uncontrolled. In contrast, men who have been on **antiandrogens** (as discussed in the last chapter) should discontinue their use as there seems to be a paradoxical effect created by doing so. This so-called *antiandrogen withdrawal syndrome* is not well understood, but can ironically slow tumor growth for a few months in men who had been on these medications.

Chemotherapy has not shown much promise for metastatic prostate cancer until the past decade. Several agents have shown significant activity, but only three options are approved at present for metastatic prostate cancer. The first is an old drug rarely used today called estramustine, which has both hormonal and chemotherapeutic effects.

Two newer chemotherapy options are *docetaxel* (*Taxotere*) and *mitoxantrone* (*Novantrone*). Both are injected every few weeks in the doctor's office and are used in combination with prednisone. Although they will not cure men with advanced disease, they offer hope where previously there was none and both have been shown to increase life expectancy by a few months.[4] They *palliate* or relieve symptoms in many men with even the most advanced tumors.

ASSISTANCE TO CHEMOTHERAPY

Zoledronic acid (*Zometa*) is a new option that takes advantage of prostate cancer's affinity to bone. It is the first of a group of drugs called *bisphosphonates* that block cancer growth in bone, help prevent osteoporosis caused by LHRH therapy, and help prevent fractures. Its use is usually reserved for advanced disease.

    Strontium 89 is a radioisotope that accumulates in bone in a manner similar to calcium. This leads it to attach to sites where bone turnover is in high gear, such as where cancer occurs. It releases its radiation over about a week, killing the cancer. The main side effect is bone marrow suppression, leading to anemia. In addition, it is removed from the body in urine; if a patient has urinary retention (not too rare in severe cases of prostate cancer), it can cause damage to the bladder from dwelling too long in contact with the bladder lining.[5]

IS THERAPY ALWAYS APPROPRIATE?

Men with hormone-refractory prostate cancer are faced with difficult decisions. Knowing cure is currently impossible, many will still choose to fight the disease using chemotherapy. Some will resort to alternative therapy despite the paucity of data to support its use.

    However, some will choose to end their resistance. They may choose quality of life over continued acceptance of side effects of treatments they know may help keep their disease in check for a time, but will eventually fail to contain it.

    If or when such a decision is made, everyone involved—doctors, family, and friends—must respect it. A number of books are available on dealing with end-of-life issues. In addition, I would highly recommend counseling for the men and their partners who reach this stage if they are having difficulty dealing with their situation.

Sometimes advanced prostate cancer will grow upward into the bladder, which can obstruct the **ureters** as they pass through its wall above the prostate. If this occurs on one side only, there may be little effect and kidney function may remain normal because one kidney can do enough work to compensate for loss of the other one. However, kidney failure will rapidly ensue if both ureters become obstructed, and death can follow (variably, depending on the individual) within days or weeks.

This may be successfully overcome by a stent—a hollow rubber tube the width of a matchstick and long enough to reach from the kidney, through the obstruction, and into the bladder. It is either placed surgically through a **cystoscope**, or by a radiologist via a needle placed through the skin and into the kidney.

The decision to place a stent can be very difficult. Failure to relieve obstruction can lead to death within days, so the stent can literally be lifesaving. However, often the cancer has advanced to a near-terminal stage by the time complete kidney failure occurs. Moreover, kidney failure is regarded as one of the most peaceful ways that life might end; most patients simply become sleepy and die peacefully within a few days if kidney failure is total. Thus, stent placement might involve invasive procedures and external tubes that provide only temporary relief, while circumventing one of nature's gentler ways to end life.

Whether this is worth it is a personal decision. Even a short-term extension of life is important to some men, especially if there is an important date or life event coming up. For instance, a daughter's wedding, an anniversary, or a grandson's graduation might be important to bring closure to a man or his family. Reaching that goal might be worth any amount of effort. In contrast, some men will conclude that nature—or their maker—has signaled that their days are over. Such men should be granted the dignity of their choice.

HOSPICE

If a man reaches the point that cancer can no longer be contained, care is usually best provided by a hospice—an organization dedicated to end-of-life support services. Hospice can provide emotional sustenance in its assistance with the final phase of life, while providing palliation of symptoms, including pain and nausea. As we make progress toward prevention of prostate cancer death, we can hope hospice services will become needed rarely. Until we reach that goal, men with cancer no longer responding to therapy should ask their physicians to help them take advantage of this invaluable resource.

KEY POINTS

- Three chemotherapy options currently exist: estramustine, docetaxel, and mitoxantrone. The latter two are often used in conjunction with prednisone.

- Current chemotherapy options are not curative, but can delay disease progression and may be used for effective symptom relief in men with hormone refractory cancer.

- Trials are in place that may show benefit from new chemotherapy options in men with high-risk disease who undergo chemotherapy.

24.

HOPE FOR THE FUTURE

Cancer was the best thing that ever happened to me—but I wouldn't want to do it again.

—Lance Armstrong

Recall that half of men with prostate cancer had advanced, incurable disease at the time of diagnosis until recently. In a short two decades, we now detect most cases while it is still *organ confined* and usually curable. Furthermore, men treated with what appears to be the same disease do better than their counterparts from a decade or two ago. Stage for stage, grade for grade, and regardless of PSA levels, men treated today are more likely to be cured than men treated at any point in the past.

Despite the wonderful news in the above paragraph, however, we still have much work to do. Researchers from around the world are working to improve cure rates and minimize side effects. Others hope to achieve an even greater goal: To find the key to prevention that could obviate the need for either.

FUTURE DIRECTIONS FOR DIAGNOSIS

The identification of PSA created a revolution in prostate cancer diagnosis. We were suddenly able to detect most cancers while still curable—an advance of tectonic proportions that ended an era when half of prostate cancer cases went unrecognized until it was too late. However, as noted, we still cannot tell whether an elevated PSA is from cancer or from some benign condition (such as BPH). Thus, many men without cancer must undergo biopsy. Work to find a better marker is underway, and it is feasible we may identify a blood or urine test specific to cancer that will allow men with a benign PSA elevation to avoid biopsy.

Several agents are under investigation for identification of prostate cancer from urinary testing. One such test, an assay for the *uPM3* molecule, is one of the most promising. Others use the *DD3* gene and the *uPM3* molecule in combination with PSA. Drs. Thomas Weimbs and Ryan Hedgepeth at the Cleveland Clinic are investigating urinary markers called *matrix metalloproteinases* (enzymes found in the urine). Bringing such tools to clinical use could change our screening paradigm if we can be confident that they are as accurate as they appear during initial investigations.

Although MRI has not yet proven widely useful for staging prostate cancer, it may have a role in diagnosis.[1] Using improved techniques, possibly involving injection of agents designed to elucidate a tumor, the biopsy may be directed into suspicious lesions through MRI guidance. Laser imaging may one day improve the accuracy of a prostate biopsy, although its benefit compared to standard procedures is still being defined.

Serum proteomics (analysis of serum proteins) may someday in the very distant future replace prostate biopsy. Simply drawing blood for analysis through laser *desorption/ionization* in an instrument called a *flight mass spectrometer* may one day determine who has prostate cancer and who does not.[2]

The issue of a *false negative* biopsy continues to be a problem because biopsy is simply a sampling technique and can miss small cancers. Therefore, repeat biopsy is required if suspicion of cancer persists. At the Cleveland Clinic we are currently involved in a multicenter investigation in cooperation with study leaders at Johns Hopkins University to see whether a new tissue marker (abbreviated GSTP1) can be used on the biopsy tissue to determine which patients with a negative biopsy actually have cancer that the biopsy missed. If successful, this would allow us to avoid repeat biopsy in men who truly have no malignancy and to treat those whose biopsy missed the tumor.

Another area of exploration involves risk analysis. We know that men with a positive family history of prostate cancer are at increased risk. Dr. Una Lee, Dr. Julian Kim, and I are currently evaluating additional genetic risk factors at the Cleveland Clinic Foundation that may lend insight into cancer development. We are looking into the relationship of prostate cancer in families with the hereditary breast cancer gene, BRCA-2, in order to understand this or other genes and factors that determine prostate cancer risk.

FUTURE DIRECTIONS FOR STAGING

In my opinion, the greatest need in prostate cancer care is an indicator to tell us which cancers are **clinically significant** and which are **clinically insignificant**. We are now very good (but by no means perfect) at detecting prostate cancer, but we are nowhere near as good at knowing which ones we can safely leave alone. The Gleason score is the best indicator we currently have, but it is limited by sampling error. Moreover, some men with Gleason scores in the intermediate range (say, 6 and 7) will develop rapidly progressive cancer, while the majority will not. Knowing at the time of diagnosis which will progress would allow us to treat only those at risk.

The greatest hope for this goal probably lies in molecular medicine. A number of researchers are looking at thousands of genes and other proteins using *microarrays*—tests that can investigate in a short time what researchers in the past might have spent a career attempting. If these efforts are successful, men with minimal risk cancer will be able to avoid the "burden of cure." Moreover, those at significant risk will usually be cured and confident that their tumor needed to be aggressively dealt with.

One possible prognosticator to determine whose cancer is destined to progress has been identified and nicknamed Hedgehog. It refers to a chemical pathway in prostate cancer cells that sends a signal to cancer cells telling them to reproduce and spread if it is turned on. This may someday serve as a way to know which cancers are **clinically significant** and which ones are not. It also may serve as a target for therapy if researchers can find a way to turn this signal off.[3]

FUTURE DIRECTIONS FOR PREVENTION

The outcome of several ongoing trials will have an impact on prostate cancer prevention strategies. The Prostate Cancer Prevention Trial (discussed in chapter 5) proved that we could reduce the risk of prostate cancer by one-fourth by administering **finasteride**. However, it is still unclear whether some of those who do develop cancer might be actually at *increased* risk of dying because of their higher-grade cancers. This will be elucidated as these data mature, but some study insiders believe that further evaluation will confirm their bias that this will not be the case. A similar nationwide trial (REDUCE) is currently underway to investigate the possibility that the similar drug, *dutasteride*, could have a similar or even greater preventive effect.

The SELECT trial is now closed to new enrollees. Approximately thirty-two thousand men are taking either a placebo or combinations of vitamin E and selenium. If early reports of the effect of these two agents are confirmed, we may all need to take one or both of them daily. However, as noted earlier, vitamin E carries some potential risks as well. Finally, a host of other agents that have perhaps not even been considered yet might prove to be the "magic bullet" that prevents prostate cancer in most men.

FUTURE DIRECTIONS FOR INFORMATION TRANSFER

Most medical information traditionally is transferred directly from physician to patient and back again. This model will persist, but the information age offers opportunities to improve patient care and wellness through innovative approaches.

One example involves Internet-based patient interactions. Some large hospital systems now allow patients who are seeing physicians in certain specialties to view parts of their medical records online by using password-protected access. This enables them to review laboratory, radiology, or pathology reports in a more leisurely and in-depth manner than is possible in an office visit.

Online consultation is now possible using sites such as eCleveland-Clinic.org or Partners Telemedicine. By entering your information into a series of fields, you can receive a second opinion for many conditions, including prostate cancer, within a few days. If your biopsy results or radiology findings need to be reviewed, they can be sent by mail or courier and confirmed quickly. This is especially valuable for people living a great distance from a major cancer center, saving them the time and cost of travel. If you need to be physically present, a follow-up visit in person can be arranged after it is determined that this is necessary. The most significant limitation involves current licensing laws that determine when doctors can render advice or care to persons in other states. This may require rethinking such laws to keep up with emerging technology.

Telepathology and teleradiology will probably play a role in the future as well. One example was developed by Olympus, which makes a microscope system that allows the pathologist to read a biopsy on a high-definition computer screen instead of straining to see through the little eyepieces we traditionally think of for microscopy. Moreover, an Internet link enables the pathologist to share the image with a colleague miles away. This can allow a pathologist in a small town to receive immediate collaboration if the diagnosis is in doubt instead of waiting to forward slides to an expert in another location. Its potential for patients in areas without pathologists (such as third-world countries) is obvious.

We have recently found great success using the Group Shared Medical Appointment for urology patients, including those with prostate cancer or elevated PSA. Instead of the one-on-one interaction of the traditional office visit, we have a simultaneous appointment involving up to fifteen patients with similar diagnoses. This allows a more relaxed visit where the doctor, nurse, physician's assistant, impotence coordinator, and other providers see the patients together in a group setting. It is not a lecture—rather, it is an appointment involving person-to-person interactions in the presence of others. Patients who need an examination are taken into a private area for the necessary check, and then return to the group for the remainder of the scheduled time. Satisfaction scores are high from patients and providers, as both parties feel the longer appointment (typically ninety minutes) allows everyone to get all issues covered better than during the rushed atmosphere of the traditional model. This concept is in the early stages, and we foresee exploring its value in multiple areas.

FUTURE DIRECTIONS FOR TREATMENT

The progress made in treatment during the past two or three decades has been amazing. Prior to that time, radical prostatectomy was an operation fraught with hazard—and almost assured of complications. Vast numbers of urologists are now comfortable with the operation and achieve excellent results—and usually cures. Significant numbers now also are mastering laparoscopic/robotic prostatectomy. If early results fulfill their promise and confirm success and complication rates matching those of the retropubic version, this could become the preferred approach.

Impotence is no longer a fact of life following prostatectomy. Most men can remain sexually active following surgery, although assistance may be required. Long-standing incontinence is uncommon now, but men still don't like wearing pads even for a few weeks or months. We have shown that we can decrease the time it takes for continence to return by placing a *sling* of absorbable material such as animal *small intestine submucosa* or absorbable suture mesh under the urethra at the time of prostatectomy. This remains investigational at this time, but is another step towards minimizing postoperative urinary problems.[4]

Radiation therapy has seen similar improvements. New technologies have led to further reductions in side effects, while allowing increased tumor-killing doses to be delivered where needed. It is probably inevitable that such technological advances in radiation physics will continue.

Cryotherapy has gone from pariah to an accepted option only in the past decade. Serious side effects have been reduced purely through improved technology to a rare occurrence. An especially promising concept is the possibility of nerve-sparing cryotherapy. Since we now detect most cancers at their initial stage, the paradigm requiring treatment of the entire prostate is being challenged. Some surgeons already treat the side of the known cancer only, thereby sparing the contralateral penile nerves. Early reports suggest this may lead to maintenance of erections in such men.[5] The success of this approach may depend on the assurance that there is not a second *satellite tumor* on the opposite side of the gland. Improved biopsy accuracy, perhaps using GSTP1 or similar molecular markers (as described above), may allow focal treatment with the confidence that all of the cancer has been addressed. If cancer recurs on the opposite side following such treatment, it is possible that curative cryotherapy may then be applied only when required instead of prophylactically at the time of the initial treatment.

Chemotherapy has only recently developed a significant role in prostate cancer care. Now that oncologists have identified viable cellular and molecular targets for drugs, it is likely that a number of new agents will be introduced for men with **hormone-resistant** prostate cancer.

Perhaps the most exciting thing on the horizon is gene therapy. By vaccination of modified tumor cells or specific proteins, it is possible that we will be able to treat both localized and advanced prostate cancer through alterations of its genetic structure. Researchers around the globe continue to work on this enticing—but so far confounding—technology.

FUTURE DIRECTIONS FOR BPH

A drug in clinical trials appears to treat both BPH and the irritative symptoms of **overactive bladder**. Naftopidil may be able to manage both obstructive and irritative symptoms in men with BPH, obviating the need for two drugs as is currently sometimes required. In addition, it might allow easier treatment, since there would be no need to determine which type of symptom is the problem—both would be covered.

Injection of ethanol gel or other agents directly into the prostate has

PAYING FOR THE FUTURE: NO FREE RIDES

The efforts underway to improve the care of men with prostatic diseases described here are only the tip of the iceberg that will continue to offer men hope in the future. There is no doubt that similar projects are going on in university and medical center laboratories, pharmaceutical companies, and governmental research facilities throughout the world that haven't yet been publicized. This all offers great hope to you—and to your sons or grandsons, who may be at risk of similar problems.

Such efforts come at great expense—and someone must pay the bill. For each discovery that "hits a home run," many more well-designed investigations fail to yield major advancements. Fewer than one in five thousand compounds screened for a new drug makes it to market; it takes twelve to fifteen years for the few that succeed.[7] The final cost for the winner averages over $800 million—before a single prescription is written.[8]

University and major medical center research budgets limit how rapidly projects can proceed. Many worthy projects fall by the wayside because there is no money to get them off the ground. Government spending on healthcare research is subject to the political winds, and there are more projects and researchers vying for support than there are dollars available. Private foundations provide vital financing, but could never cover the unmet needs. Insurers essentially decline any support of research activities, deeming such projects "experimental."

It is tempting to feel that such research must go on despite the costs. However, there will always be a balance between the cost of research and what patients, companies, the federal government, and insurers will be willing to pay. I hope you will keep this balance in mind as you form opinions on healthcare and research financing. It is never easy when you are the one footing the bill—but is also not easy when it is you, your son, or your grandson who needs the advances that never got financed.

shown promise as a treatment for BPH that would theoretically create an adequate channel matching that of TURP without the need for surgery. Researchers, including my friend and colleague Dr. Raymond Rackley, have been able to relieve BPH symptoms by injection of botulinum toxin (Botox).[6]

Developments in laser technology have become the mainstay of BPH treatment advancements lately. With engineers diligently working on newer generations of such technology, lasers will continue to be faster, more specific in their targeting, and potentially more affordable.

Finally, it is feasible that the next generation of drugs such as dutasteride and finasteride may be able to prevent or permanently arrest the development of BPH.

FUTURE DIRECTIONS FOR HOPE

You now know that most men with prostate problems can be managed successfully. Our results will only become more reliable as we detect such problems early and treatments continue to improve.

You also know that men diagnosed with prostate cancer today have a better prognosis than those at any time in history. Regardless of stage, grade, PSA level, or any other factor, you are more likely to survive prostate cancer and reach your life expectancy than you would have ever before. Most men who have prostate cancer will never develop serious symptoms, nor will they die of their disease.

Thus, I encourage you face the problem head-on. Get the best information you can, choose a doctor that earns your confidence, and make a plan for management that best meets your individual needs. Doing so will likely lead to a long, healthy future for you.

The 10 Biggest Prostate Myths

Myth 1: Prostate enlargement is the be all and end all.

Size is not the important issue with benign prostate problems. Obstruction is. Recall the metaphor of Dr. Ulchaker: "I don't care how big your doughnut is; I care how big your doughnut hole is."

Myth 2: Prostate cancer usually causes symptoms.

Symptoms in men with prostate cancer are usually due to something other than the cancer—often BPH. Cancer only causes symptoms when very advanced, so do not allow the absence of symptoms to influence your thinking.

Myth 3: A normal PSA is 4 or less.

The number of 4 ng/dl as a "normal" value for PSA was determined before we knew as much as we do now regarding prostate cancer diagnosis. Each man probably has a level that is "normal" for him, depending on his age, size of his prostate, and some other issues. In the absence of a better definition, normal for most healthy men should be considered 2.5 ng/dl or lower.

Myth 4: You only need a DRE *or* a PSA to detect prostate cancer.

Either PSA or DRE can be normal in men with prostate cancer. Their combination is the best way to detect prostate cancer while curable.

Myth 5: There are symptoms that are exclusive to the prostate.

No symptoms are automatically attributable to the prostate. Unfortunately, it gets a bad rap for many pelvic, urinary, and sexual symptoms because of its anatomic neighbors.

Myth 6: Prostatitis is usually the source of urinary, sexual, or painful symptoms in the lower abdomen and pelvis.

A majority of men with such symptoms have a diagnosis other than prostatitis. Identifying the real cause, whether urological or musculoskeletal, can lead to a solution instead of floundering with prostatic treatments for nonprostatic problems.

Myth 7: PSA is dangerous.

Nobody ever died of PSA. It is a serum marker for prostate problems—sometimes malignant, sometimes not.

Myth 8: All men need a PSA.

The American Urological Association and the American Cancer Society recommend that men above the ages of forty and forty-five (respectively) have a DRE and a PSA annually until they reach the age that prostate cancer diagnosis would not yield benefit. This is usually when they have a life expectancy of less than ten to fifteen years. Nonetheless, some men may choose to forgo this recommendation as long as they accept the reality below.

Myth 9: If you live long enough, you get prostate cancer.

This is the one myth that has *some* (misleading) truth to it. **Clinically insignificant** prostate cancer may arise eventually in most men if they reach very old age. These tumors typically remain unknown throughout a man's lifetime, as evidenced by one of their nicknames, *autopsy prostate cancer*. In contrast, **clinically significant** prostate cancer will arise in approximately 17 percent of men, and is usually suspected and diagnosed through PSA and DRE. This will result in the death of approximately 3.4 percent of American men.

Myth 10: The prostate is involved in erections.

Because of its proximity to the penile nerves, anything done to the prostate risks injury to these delicate structures. This, along with the correlation in age of men with prostate problems (including cancer), makes erectile dysfunction appear to have more of a relationship to the prostate than it really does.

GLOSSARY

Abarelix (Plenaxis): Drug that blocks the release of testosterone by blocking its releasing hormone.

Alpha blockers: Drugs used to treat urinary obstruction by blocking chemical *alpha receptors* in the prostate and bladder neck.

Anastomosis: The site where the bladder neck is sewn to the urethra to complete reconstruction during **radical prostatectomy**.

Antiandrogen: A medication that actually blocks the effect of testosterone at the cellular level.

Anticholinergic medications: Drugs that block bladder contractions in order to treat **overactive bladder** or bladder spasms.

Apex: The conical portion of the prostate located where the urethra exits the gland.

Artificial urinary sphincter (AUS): An inflatable cuff that can be surgically placed to encircle the urethra in order to restrict flow in men who experience severe urinary incontinence.

ASTRO criteria: Used to determine whether radiation therapy is successful or not. Following the point at which the PSA reaches its lowest level after treatment (called the nadir), three consecutive rises are thought to indicate a likelihood of cancer progression.

Atypical small acinar proliferation (ASAP): A pathological finding during biopsy that is often found to be malignant if a repeat biopsy is performed.

AUA symptom score: A scoring system used to quantify urinary obstructive symptoms. A level below 9 or 10 is considered mild. A score between 10 and 20 is moderate, and higher scores are considered to indicate severe obstruction.

Autologous blood donation: The process of storing your own blood for use for transfusion during surgery.

Avodart. *See* **dutasteride.**

Bedside bag: A plastic container that attaches to the bedrails to collect urine from a **catheter**.

Benign: The opposite of malignant; implies that a tumor or other condition is noncancerous.

Benign prostatic hyperplasia or **hypertrophy (BPH)**: Noncancerous prostatic growth that can obstruct urinary flow.

Biochemical failure: A situation in which PSA levels indicate that cancer persists despite treatment. For surgical patients, this will include anyone with a detectable PSA, whereas the **ASTRO criteria** are used to gauge success following radiation.

Biopsy: The act of obtaining tissue to check for cancer. Sometimes used to describe the actual tissue sample.

Bladder neck: The portion of the bladder that funnels inside the prostate. It and the prostate in combination comprise a significant part of urinary continence.

Bladder neck contracture: A narrowing of the urethra caused by a fibrous waistband at the bladder neck, usually because of scarring following prostate surgery.

Bladder scan: A portable ultrasound machine that rapidly determines the amount of urine remaining in the bladder after a person voids.

Bone scan: Imaging study that uses injection of **radioisotopes** to detect prostate cancer activity in the bones.

Brachytherapy: Surgically placing radioactive "seeds" or pellets into the prostate. These seeds emit their radioactivity into the prostate slowly over the coming weeks.

Cardura. *See* **doxazocin**.

Castration: Removal of all testicular-produced **testosterone** in order to treat prostate cancer by depriving it of its main growth factor. May be achieved by medications to block its production, or by surgical removal of the testicles.

Catheter: A hollow tube—usually with an inflatable balloon on the end to hold it in place—used to drain the bladder.

Central zone (also called transition zone): The inner portion of the prostate. Its growth is usually due to BPH instead of cancer, which can cause urinary **obstruction**.

Clean intermittent catheterization (CIC): Instead of leaving a catheter through the urethra to constantly drain the bladder, the patient puts one in just long enough to empty the bladder and then removes it.

Clinical stage: Used to describe how far advanced a cancer is based on clinical information—that obtainable prior to surgical removal.

Clinically insignificant prostate cancer: Low-grade cancer with a low potential for spreading or causing harm.

Clinically significant prostate cancer: The type of cancer that can become dangerous—or deadly.

Complexed PSA: PSA that is bound or complexed to protein in the bloodstream. Its elevation suggests a higher likelihood of prostate cancer.

Computerized tomography (CT): A computerized x-ray image that pictures the body in slices, as if each slice were a playing card to examine one by one as you go through the deck.

Conformal radiotherapy: An advanced form of external beam radiation that allows dispersed beams to go through multiple paths in order to converge at the prostate, so it receives a lethal dose of energy while the rest of the pelvis receives smaller doses.

Cryotherapy: Freezing cancer cells to a lethal temperature using small probes placed through the **perineal skin**.

Cystoscopy: Placement of a small scope through the urethra into the urinary bladder. Performed using an instrument called a **cystoscope**.

Deferred therapy with curative intent: Similar to traditional **watchful**

waiting, deferred therapy involves an intentional strategy of observation until signs of danger arise.

Digital rectal examination (DRE): Palpation of the prostate and adjacent tissues with a gloved finger through the rectum.

Doubling time: The amount of time it takes for PSA to double, or for prostate cancer cells to divide throughout the tumor so that its size doubles.

Dorsal vein complex: A group of veins carrying blood primarily from the penis. Their presence is responsible for most blood loss during **radical prostatectomy**.

Doxazocin (Cardura): An **alpha blocker** medication that relaxes the prostate and bladder neck in order to improve urinary flow.

Dutasteride (Avodart): A **5-alpha reductase inhibitor** medication that shrinks the prostate.

Eligard. *See* **Leuprolide.**

Epidural anesthesia: A catheter is used to anesthetize the patient below the middle of the abdomen for prostate or other surgery.

External beam radiation: Administers lethal doses to radiation to a cancer while the patient lies on a machine that focuses several radiation beams toward the prostate.

Extracapsular extension: Cancer reaching beyond the prostatic capsule.

Finasteride (Proscar): A **5-alpha reductase inhibitor** medication that shrinks the prostate.

5-alpha reductase inhibitors: Medications that shrink the prostate by blocking the enzyme that converts **testosterone** into its active form, dihydrotestosterone.

Flomax. *See* **tamsulosin.**

Foley catheter. *See* **catheter**.

Frequency: Simply implies that you void frequently.

Free PSA: The portion of PSA that is floating free in the bloodstream, instead of complexed or bound to proteins. A low percentage of free PSA increases the likelihood that an elevation in PSA is due to cancer.

Gleason score (*easily confused with the* **Gleason grade**): A system designed to denote how aggressive a cancer is. The difference is that the two most common *grades* of cancer identified in the biopsy specimen are added together to give a Gleason *score*.

Goserelin (Zoladex): One of a group of medications called LHRH antagonists. They slow the progression of prostate cancer by blocking the release of its primary growth factor, testosterone.

Grade: Determines the aggressiveness of a cancer. High-grade cancers are more likely to grow uncontrollably than are low-grade ones.

Hematospermia: Blood in the semen; usually not significant.

Hematuria: Blood in the urine. Its presence requires urological investigation, as it sometimes indicates a serious problem.

Hereditary prostate cancer: Cancer caused by genes that run in the family.

Hesitancy: Delay prior to beginning the stream.

Hormone resistant (*also*, **hormone refractory**): The state when cancer cells overcome their dependence on **testosterone**.

Hormone sensitive: The state when cancer cell growth is dependent on **testosterone**.

Hytrin. *See* **Terazosin**.

Incontinence: Involuntary loss of urine.

Initiation: First step in triggering the development of prostate cancer.

Intensity modulated radiation therapy (IMRT): The most advanced version of external beam radiation technology.

Intermittency: The classic spurt-spurt as a man tries to completely empty his bladder despite a partially obstructing prostate.

Irritative symptoms: Urinary symptoms suggesting bladder irritation, including **urgency, frequency**, and **nocturia**.

Laparoscopic radical prostatectomy: Removal of the prostate using a laparoscopic approach.

Leg bag: A plastic container that attaches to the patient's leg to collect urine from a **catheter**.

Leuprolide: One of a group of medications called LHRH antagonists. They slow the progression of prostate cancer by blocking the release of its primary growth factor, testosterone.

Lupron. *See* **Leuprolide.**

Lymphadenectomy: Surgical removal of lymph nodes.

Lymph nodes: Glands of the body's immune system designed to protect from harmful things such as infection or cancer. If cancer cells overwhelm their protective abilities, a satellite tumor can begin.

Malignant: A tissue area that has the potential to grow out of control. Synonymous with *cancer*.

Margin positive: Describes cancer cells present at the margin of removed tissue. suggesting the possibility that some cells remain inside the patient.

Maximal androgen blockade: The use of **antiandrogens** in combination with hormonal ablation.

Metastatic: Cancer that has spread to an area other than where it began.

Metastatic workup: An evaluation utilizing imaging techniques such as **bone scan**, **CT scan**, or other studies used to determine if cancer has spread.

Mount Everest Sign: The white appearance that looks like the famous snowy peak that is used by the urologist as a landmark to determine where to inject the **periprostatic nerve block** for prostate biopsy.

Nerve-sparing prostatectomy: Removing the prostate while leaving the nerves responsible for erections intact.

Neurovascular bundles: The nerves and associated blood vessels responsible for erections that run alongside the prostate.

Nocturia: Frequent urination during hours normally reserved for sleep.

Obstructive symptoms: Slow stream, **hesitancy**, **intermittency**, or other signs of urinary obstruction.

Orchiectomy: The removal of one or both testicles usually performed to block **testosterone** in order to treat prostate cancer.

Organ-confined (localized) prostate cancer: Cancer limited to the prostate.

Overactive bladder (OAB): Sensation of urgency or other **irritative** symptoms often caused by mild bladder contractions.

Oxidative DNA damage: Damage caused by *oxygen free radicals* or other harmful agents that disrupt DNA, leading to a change in the cell's genetic makeup. Unless the body repairs the damage, malignancy may result.

Pathological (staging): Most accurate staging, based on actually examining the removed prostate.

Pelvic lymphadenectomy: Surgical removal of pelvic lymph nodes in order to **stage** (determine the extent of) a cancer.

Perineal body: A small fibrous tendon where all the muscles come together in the middle of the pelvic floor.

Perineal prostatectomy: Removing the prostate through the **perineum**.

Perineum: The area between the scrotum and the rectum.

Periprostatic block: A nerve block performed at the beginning of a transrectal ultrasound guided prostate biopsy that allows the doctor to remove small cores of prostate tissue painlessly.

Postvoid residual volume: The amount of urine remaining in the urinary bladder after completing urination.

Primary bladder neck obstruction: Contraction of muscle fibers in the bladder neck causing urinary obstruction.

Proctitis: Radiation damage to the rectum.

Progression: The second step in prostate cancer development, which involves triggering of significant growth. Must follow **initiation**.

Proscar. *See* **Finasteride**.

Prostadynia: Term used to describe a painful prostate.

ProstaScint Scan: Imaging study that takes advantage of an *antibody* bound to a *radioisotope* (111-indium) which allows a scanner to identify abnormal areas of accumulation.

Prostate specific antigen (PSA): Protein produced by the prostate to turn semen into its more liquefied form several minutes after ejaculation. It use clinically is in the diagnosis and monitoring of prostate cancer.

Prostatic intraepithelial neoplasia (PIN): A potentially precancerous abnormality in the prostate found in approximately one out of five men who undergo prostate biopsy.

Prostatitis: Inflammation of the prostate. It is occasionally caused by infection, but most men who are under the impression they have prostate infection actually have symptoms caused by something other than bacterial infection.

PSA density (PSAD): A concept based on the ratio of PSA to the size of the prostate.

PSA doubling time (PSA-DT): The time it takes for PSA to double. If PSA is elevated and this occurs in less than ten months, the cancer is likely to lead to serious complications or death unless treated aggressively.

PSA velocity: Rate of rise in PSA over time (also called PSA slope).

Radiation cystitis: Radiation damage to the bladder.

Radiation oncologist: A physician who uses radiation to treat prostate and other cancers.

Radical prostatectomy: Surgery to remove the cancerous prostate. Options include retropubic, laparoscopic/robotic, and perineal.

Radioisotope: Radioactive material. One type is injected into the bloodstream through an intravenous (IV) puncture that is used to detect **metastases** during **bone scan**. Another type is embedded in radioactive seeds that are placed into the prostate during **brachytherapy**.

Residual volume: The amount of urine remaining in the bladder *after* voiding.

Robotic prostatectomy: Removal of the prostate using the assistance of a robotic instrument that facilitates the surgeon's movements inside the body.

Salvage prostatectomy: A complex operation involving removal of the prostate following radiation.

Saturation biopsy: Prostate biopsy involving twenty or more cores or samples. Required hospitalization prior to the development of **periprostatic block**, but it can now easily and safely be performed in the office setting.

Saw palmetto: Made from the bark of the small palm tree, genus *Serenoa repens*, it is used by many men to treat BPH and occasionally cancer. Its effectiveness and safety have not been established.

Screening and **early detection**: Efforts to detect prostate cancer at an earlier and potentially curable stage.

Sextant biopsy: Outdated biopsy scheme obtaining six cores of prostate tissue to check for cancer.

Sphincter: A muscle encircling an orifice. The **external urinary sphincter** is especially important because it is responsible for urinary continence following treatment of BPH or prostate cancer.

Systematic biopsy: Biopsy technique taking samples from throughout the prostate in an attempt to optimize cancer detection.

Tamsulosin (Flomax): An **alpha blocker** medication that relaxes the prostate and bladder neck in order to improve urinary flow.

Terazosin (Hytrin): An **alpha blocker** medication that relaxes the prostate and bladder neck in order to improve urinary flow.

Testosterone: The primary male hormone. Serves as both a growth factor for prostate tissue, including cancer, and as stimulus for libido.

Transition zone. *See* **central zone**.

Transurethral microwave therapy (TUMT): Heat treatment using directional microwaves the heat the prostate for thirty to sixty minutes in order to block BPH symptoms.

Transurethral resection of the prostate (TURP): Operation to enlarge the opening through the prostate for men with **obstruction**.

Ultrasound residual volume. *See* **Bladder scan**.

Ureter: Tube that carries urine from the kidneys to the bladder.

Urethra: Urinary tube running from the bladder, through the prostate, and out the penis.

Urethral stricture: Cause of obstructive symptoms by a fibrous waistband in the urethra.

Urgency: An abnormal—usually sudden—urge to void.

Urge incontinence: When **urgency** is so severe that an accident occurs.

Urinary retention: The complete inability to void.

Urodynamics: Involved testing to determine the cause of urinary symptoms if simple tests fail to do so.

Uroflowmetry: Measurement of urine flow rate by voiding into a funnel-shaped flow meter that quantifies the volume released per second.

Viadur: One of a group of medications called LHRH antagonists. They slow the progression of prostate cancer by blocking the release of its primary growth factor, testosterone.

Watchful waiting: Management of a condition through careful monitoring instead of actually taking treatments.

Zoladex (*see also* **goserelin**): One of a group of medications called LHRH antagonists. They slow the progression of prostate cancer by blocking the release of its primary growth factor, testosterone.

RESOURCES

American Cancer Society
1599 Clifton Road NE
Atlanta, GA 30329-4251
1-800-227-2345
http://www.cancer.org/index_4up.html
Comprehensive cancer resources Web site.

American Foundation for Urologic Disease (AFUD)
300 W. Pratt St.
Suite 401
Baltimore, MD 21201
1-800-242-2383
http://www.afud.org
Dedicated to research and education regarding urological diseases, including
    prostate cancer, impotence, incontinence, etc.

American Board of Medical Specialties
1-800-776-2378 (United States)
1-613-730-8177 (Canada)
http://www.certifieddoctor.org
Enables you to determine if your doctor has been certified by the American
    Urological Association or other specialty boards.

American Urological Association
1120 North Charles Street
Baltimore, MD 21201
410-223-4310
Largest organized body of urologists in the world. Patient information on
    many urological conditions, including prostate cancer and BPH.

Canadian Cancer Society
10 Alcorn Avenue
Suite 200
Toronto, Ontario
Canada M4V 3BJ
416-961-7223
Dedicated to cancer education and research.

Cancer Care, Inc.
1180 Avenue of the Americas
New York, NY 10036
800-813-HOPE (800-813-4673)
Dedicated to cancer education and research.

Cancer Hotline
R.A. Bloch Cancer Foundation, Inc.
4410 Main Street
Kansas City, MO 64111
816-WE-BUILD (816-932-8453)
Prostate cancer information.

CancerNet (National Cancer Institute)
http://wwwicic.nci.nih.gov/clinpdq/screening/Screening_for_prostate_cancer
    .htm
Cancer information from the National Cancer Institute.

Cancer Support Network
5895 Devereau Lane
Pittsburgh, PA 15232
412-661-8949
Cancer patient support.

Chronic Prostatitis Clinic
http://www.dshoskes.com/cpclinic.html
For help dealing with prostatitis, urinary complaints, and pelvic pain.

Home and Health Solutions
21475 Lorain Rd., Suite #2
Fairview Park, OH 44126
440-333-7050
Support and access to incontinence information and assistance.

Impotence Institute of America
10400 Little Patuxent Parkway
Suite 485
Columbia, MD 21044
1-800-669-1603
Information regarding erectile dysfunction.

Man to Man
c/o American Cancer Society
1599 Clifton Road, NE
Atlanta, GA 30329
1-800-ACS-2345 (1-800-227-2345)
Support group for men with prostate cancer and their wives.

The Mathews Foundation for Prostate Cancer Research
1010 Hurley Way
Suite 195
Sacramento, CA 95825
1-800-234-6284
Prostate cancer information and research.

National Association for Continence
PO Box 8310
Spartanburg, SC 29305
1-800-BLADDER (1-800-252-3337)
Information regarding continence issues for both men and women.

National Coalition for Cancer Survivorship
1010 Wayne Avenue
5th Floor
Silver Spring, MD 20910
301-650-8868
Cancer information resource.

OncoLink
http://cancer.med.upenn.edu/disease/prostate/index.html
Oncology Web site.

Prostate Cancer InfoLink
http://www.comed.com/Prostate/
Prostate cancer information Web site.

Patient Advocates for Advanced Cancer Treatments, Inc.
1143 Parmelee, NW
Grand Rapids, MI 49504
616-453-1477
http://www.paactusa.org.
Oncology Web site.

Prostate Cancer Foundation (*formerly* **CaP CURE**)
1250 Fourth Street
Santa Monica, CA 90401
310-570-4705
http://www.prostatecancerfoundation.org
Foundation dedicated to prostate cancer education and research.

Theragenics Corporation
5325 Oak Brook Parkway
Norcross, GA 30093
1-800-458-4372
Information regarding brachytherapy.

Us Too International, Inc.
5003 Fairview Avenue
Downer's Grove, IL 60515
1-800-80-US-TOO (1-800-808-7866)
Support group for men with prostate cancer and their wives, dedicated to research and education.

NOTES

CHAPTER FOUR

1. S. J. Jacobsen, E. J. Bergstralh, S. K. Katusic, H. A. Guess, C. H. Darby, M. D. Silverstein, J. E. Oesterling, and M. M. Lieber, "Screening Digital Rectal Examination and Prostate Cancer Mortality: A Population-Based Case-Control Study," *Urology* 2, no. 52 (August 1998): 173–79.

CHAPTER FIVE

1. F. C. Lowe and E. Fagelman, "Phytotherapy in the Treatment of Benign Prostatic Hyperplasia: An Update," *Urology*, no. 53 (1999): 671–78.

2. J. R. Hebert et al., "Nutritional and Socioeconomic Factors in Relation to Prostate Cancer Mortality: A Cross-National Study," *Journal of the National Cancer Institute* 21, no. 90 (November 1998): 1637–47.

3. E. Giovannucci, "A Review of Epidemiologic Studies of Tomatoes, Lycopene, and Prostate Cancer," *Exp Biol Med (Maywood)* 10, no. 227 (November 2002): 852–59.

4. E. Giovannucci, "Tomatoes, Tomato-Based Products, Lycopene, and Cancer: Review of the Epidemiologic Literature," *Journal of the National Cancer Institute*, no. 91 (1999): 317.

5. Hebert et al., "Nutritional and Socioeconomic Factors."

6. "Men and Black South African Men," *Cancer Res*, no. 39 (1979): 5101; E. Giovannucci et al., "A Prospective Study of Dietary Fat and Risk of Prostate Cancer," *Journal of the National Cancer Institute*, no. 85 (1993a): 1571.

7. L. N. Kolonel, A. M. Nomura, and R. V. Cooney, "Dietary Fat and Prostate Cancer: Current Status," *Journal of the National Cancer Institute*, no. 91 (1999): 414.

8. J. Garrard, S. Harms, L. E. Eberly, and A. Matiak, "Variations in Product Choices of Frequently Purchased Herbs: Caveat Emptor," *Arch Intern Med* 19, no. 163 (October 2003): 2290–95.

9. *Urology Times*, (June 2004): 1.

10. J. C. Carraro et al., "Comparison of Phytotherapy (Permixon) with Finasteride in the Treatment of Benign Prostate Hyperplasia: A Randomized International Study of 1098 Patients," *Prostate*, no. 29 (1996): 231–40.

11. L. C. Clark et al., "Effects of Selenium Supplementation for Cancer Prevention in Patients with Carcinoma of the Skin: A Randomized Controlled Trial," *JA.M.A.*, no. 276 (1996): 1957.

12. K. Yoshizawa et al., "Study of Prediagnostic Selenium Level in Toenails and the Risk of Advanced Prostate Cancer," *Journal of the National Cancer Institute*, no. 90 (1998): 1219.

13. N. M. Corcoran, M. Najdovska, and A. J. Costello, "Inorganic Selenium Retards Progression of Experimental Hormone Refractory Prostate Cancer," *J Urol*, no. 171 (2004): 907–10.

14. O. P. Heinonen et al., "Prostate Cancer and Supplementation with Alpha-tocopherol and Beta-carotene: Incidence and Mortality in a Controlled Trial," *Journal of the National Cancer Institute*, no. 90 (1998): 440.

15. E. L. Miller III, R. Pastor-Barnuso, D. Dalal, et al., "Meta-Analysis: High-Dosage Vitamin E Supplementation May Increase All-Cause Mortality," *Annals of Internal Medicine* 142, no. 1 (2005), http://www.annals.org/cgi/content/full/0000605-200501040-00110v1 (accessed November 11, 2004).

16. A. Morales, D. Eidinger, and A.W. Bruce, "Intracavitary Bacillus Calmette-Guerin in the Treatment of Superficial Bladder Tumors," *J Urol*, no. 116 (1976): 180–83.

17. I. M. Thompson et al., "The Influence of Finasteride on the Development of Prostate Cancer," *New England Journal of Medicine* 3, no. 349 (July 2003): 215–24. Epub June 24, 2003.

18. R. O. Roberts et al., "A Population-Based Study of Daily Nonsteroidal Anti-inflammatory Drug Use and Prostate Cancer," *Mayo Clin Proc.* 3, no. 77 (March 2002): 219–25.

19. A. F. Badawi et al., "Age-Associated Changes in the Expression Pattern of Cyclooxygenase-2 and Related Apoptotic Markers in the Cancer Susceptible Region of Rat Prostate," *Carcinogenesis* 9, no. 25 (September 2004): 1681–88. Epub April 29, 2004.

20. J. S. Jones, *Overcoming Impotence* (Amherst, NY: Prometheus Books, 2003).

21. M. F. Leitzmann "Ejaculation Frequency and Subsequent Risk of Prostate Cancer," *JA. M.A.* 13, no. 291 (April 2004):1578–86; G. G. Giles et. al., "Sexual Factors and Prostate Cancer," *BJU Int* 3, no. 92 (August 2003): 211–16.

CHAPTER SIX

1. J. C. Nickel et. al., "Treatment of Chronic Prostatitis/Chronic Pelvic Pain Syndrome with Tamsulosin: A Randomized Double Blind Trial," *J Urol* 4, no. 171 (April 2004): 1594–97.

2. E. A. Calhoun et al., "The Economic Impact of Chronic Prostatitis," *Arch Intern Med* 11, no. 164 (June 2004): 1231–36.

CHAPTER SEVEN

1. C. G. Chute et al., "The Prevalence of Prostatism: A Population-Based Survey of Urinary Symptoms," *J Urol*, no. 150 (1993): 85–89.

CHAPTER EIGHT

1. C. G. Roehrborn, "Effectiveness and Safety of Terazosin versus Placebo in the Treatment of Men with Symptomatic Benign Prostatic Hyperplasia in the HYCAT Study," *Urology*, no. 47 (1996): 169–78.

2. G. M. Clifford, and R. D. Farmer, "Medical Therapy for Benign Prostatic Hyperplasia: A Review of the Literature," *Eur Urol* 1, no. 38 (July 2000): 2–19.

3. R. S. Kirby, "Terazosin in Benign Prostatic Hyperplasia: Effects on Blood Pressure in Normotensive and Hypertensive Men," *Br J Urol*, no. 82 (1998a): 373–79.

4. Clifford and Farmer, "Medical Therapy for Benign Prostatic Hyperplasia."

5. H. A. Guess, J. F. Heyse, and G. J. Gormley, "The Effect of Finasteride on Prostate-Specific Antigens in Men with Benign Prostatic Hyperplasia," *Prostate*, no. 22 (1993): 31–37.

6. G. J. Gormley et al., "The Effect of Finasteride in Men with Benign Prostatic Hyperplasia," *N Engl J Med*, no. 327 (1992): 1185–91.

7. C. L. Foley and R. S. Kirby, "5 Alpha-Reductase Inhibitors: What's New?" *Curr Opin Urol* 1, no. 13 (January 2003): 31–37.

8. "The Long-Term Effect of Doxazosin, Finasteride, and Combination Therapy on the Clinical Progression of Benign Prostatic Hyperplasia," *N Engl J Med* 25, no. 349 (December 2003): 2387–98.

9. H. Boon et al., "Use of Complementary/Alternative Medicine by Men Diagnosed with Prostate Cancer: Prevalence and Characteristics," *Urology* 5, no. 62 (November 2003): 849–53.

10. H. Lepor and F. C. Lowe, "Evaluation and Nonsurgical Management of Benign Prostatic Hyperplasia," in *Campbell's Urology*, 7th ed., ed. M. P. Walsh, Alan B. Retnik, and E. Darracott Vaughan Jr. (Philadelphia: Saunders, 1998), p. 1388.

11. Ibid., p. 1393.

12. R. M. Hoffman, R. MacDonald, and T. J. Wilt, "Laser Prostatectomy for Benign Prostatic Obstruction," *Cochrane Database Syst Rev* 1, (2004): CD001987.

13. Ibid.

14. Ibid.

15. R. Bruskewitz, "Medical Management of BPH in the US," *Eur Urol* suppl 3, no. 36 (1999): 7–13.

16. Health Care Financing Administration: B.E.S.S. Data, Washington, DC, 1997.

17. C. D. Holman et al., "Mortality and Prostate Cancer Risk in 19,598 Men after Surgery for Benign Prostatic Hyperplasia," *BJU Int* 1, no. 84 (July 1999): 37–42.

18. J. D. McConnell et al., "Benign Prostatic Hyperplasia: Diagnosis and Treatment Clinical Practice Guideline," *Agency for Health Care Policy and Research Publication*, no. 94–0582 (1994).

19. Ibid.

20. J. Lapides et al., "Clean, Intermittent Self-Catheterization in the Treatment of Urinary Tract Disease," *Trans Am Assoc Genitourin Surg*, no. 63 (1971): 92–96.

21. S. A. McNeill et al., "Sustained-Release Alfuzosin and Trial without Catheter after Acute Urinary Retention: A Prospective, Placebo-controlled Trial," *BJU Int*, no. 84 (1999):622–27.

22. S. Khoury et al., "International Consultation on Urological Diseases: A Decade of Progress," *Prostate* 2, no. 45 (October 2000): 194–99.

CHAPTER NINE

1. American Cancer Society, "Cancer Facts & Figures 2004," *American Cancer Society, Inc.* (2003): 4.

2. B. F. Hankey et al., "Cancer Surveillance Series: Interpreting Trends in Prostate Cancer—Part I: Evidence of the Effects of Screening in Recent Prostate Cancer Incidence, Mortality, and Survival Rates," *Journal of the National Cancer Institute*, no. 91 (1999): 1017.

3. I. H. Derweesh et al., "Continuing Trends in Pathological Stage Migration in Radical Prostatectomy Specimens," *Urol Oncol* 4, no. 22 (July–Aug 2004): 300–306.

4. http://www-dep.iarc.fr/globocan/globocan.html (accessed March 23, 2004).

5. American Cancer Society, "Cancer Facts & Figures 2004," *American Cancer Society, Inc.* (2003): 4.

6. http://www.ahrq.gov/clinic/gcpspu.htm (accessed October 12, 2004).

7. A.V. D'Amico, K. Cote, A. A. Loffredo et al., "Advanced Age at Diagnosis Is an Independent Predictor of Time to Death from Prostate Carcinoma for Patients Undergoing External Beam Radiation Therapy for Clinically Localized Prostate Cancer," *Cancer*, no. 97 (2003): 56–62.

8. W. A. Sakr et al., *European Urology*, no. 30 (1996): 138–44.

CHAPTER TEN

1. W. A. Sakr et al., *European Urology*, no. 30 (1996): 138–44.

2. G. D. Steinberg et al., "Family History and the Risk of Prostate Cancer," *Prostate*, no. 17 (1990): 337.

3. B. S. Carter et al., "Hereditary Prostate Cancer: Epidemiologic and Clinical Features," *J Urol*, no. 150 (1993): 797.

4. P. A. Kupelian et al., "Familial Prostate Cancer: A Different Disease?" *J Urol*, no. 158 (1997): 2197.

5. Carter et al., "Hereditary Prostate Cancer."

6. P. A. Wingo et al., "Racial and Ethnic Differences in Advanced-stage Prostate Cancer: The Prostate Cancer Outcomes Study," *Journal of the National Cancer Institute*, no. 93 (2001): 388–95.

7. A. Jemal et al., "Cancer Statistics, 2002," *CA Cancer J Clin* 1, no. 52 (2002): 23–47.

8. G. G. Schwartz, and B. S. Hulka, "Is Vitamin D Deficiency a Risk Factor for Prostate Cancer? (Hypothesis)," *Anticancer Res*, no. 10 (1990): 1307.

9. American Cancer Society, "Cancer Facts & Figures 2003," *American Cancer Society, Inc.* (2003).

10. P. Hill et al., "Diet and Urinary Steroids in Black and White North American Men and Black South African Men," *Cancer Res*, no. 39 (1979): 5101.

11. E. Giovannucci et al., "A Prospective Study of Dietary Fat and Risk of Prostate Cancer," *Journal of the National Cancer Institute*, no. 85 (1993a): 1571.

12. L. N. Kolonel, A. M. Nomura, and R. V. Cooney, "Dietary Fat and Prostate Cancer: Current Status," *Journal of the National Cancer Institute*, no. 91 (1999): 414.

13. G. G. Schwartz, and B. S. Hulka, "Is Vitamin D Deficiency a Risk Factor for Prostate Cancer? (Hypothesis)," *Anticancer Res*, no. 10 (1990): 1307.

14. R. T. Prehn, "On the Prevention and Therapy of Prostate Cancer by Androgen Administration," *Cancer Res*, no. 59 (1999): 4161.

15. E. E. Calle et al., "Overweight, Obesity, and Mortality from Cancer in a Prospectively Studied Cohort of U.S. Adults," *N Engl J Med*, no. 348 (2003): 1625–38.

16. S. J. Freedland et al., "Obesity and Biochemical Outcome Following Radical Prostatectomy for Organ Confined Disease with Negative Surgical Margins," *J Urol* 2, no. 172 (August 2004): 520–24.

17. E. Giovannucci, "Medical History and Etiology of Prostate Cancer," *Epidemiol Rev* 1, no. 23 (2001):159–62.

18. R. J. MacInnis et al., "Body Size and Composition and Prostate Cancer Risk," *Cancer Epidemiology and Biomarkers* 12, no. 12 (December 2003): 1417–21.

19. A. W. Hsing et al., "Insulin Resistance and Prostate Cancer Risk," *Journal of the National Cancer Institute*, no. 95 (2003): 67–71.

20. M. F. Leitzmann et al., "Ejaculation Frequency and Subsequent Risk of Prostate Cancer," *JA. M.A.* 13, no. 291 (April 2004): 1578–86.

21. R. K. Ross et al., "A Cohort Study of Mortality from Cancer of the Prostate in Catholic Priests," *Br J Cancer*, no. 43 (1981): 233–35.

22. D. Smith, S. Frankel, and J. Yarnell, "Sex and Death: Are They Related? Findings from the Caerphilly Cohort Study," *British Medical Journal*, no. 315 (1997): 1641–44.

CHAPTER ELEVEN

1. J. A. Eastham et al., "Variation of Serum PSA Levels: An Evaluation of Year-to-Year Fluctuations," *JA. M.A.*, no. 289 (2003): 2695-2700.

2. S. D. Cramer et al., "Association Between Genetic Polymorphisms in the Prostate-Specific Antigen Gene Promoter and Serum Prostate Specific Antigen Levels," *J NCI*, no. 95: 1044–53.

3. M. B. Tchetgen et al., "Ejaculation Increases the Serum Prostate-specific Antigen Concentration,"*Urology* 4, no. 47 (April 1996): 511–16.

4. W. J. Catalona et al., "Measurement of Prostate-specific Antigen in Serum as a Screening Test for Prostate Cancer," *N Engl J Med*, no. 324 (1991): 1156–61.

5. G. Tibblin et al., "The Value of Prostate Specific Antigen in Early Diagnosis of Prostate Cancer: The Study of Men Born in 1913," *J Urol* 4, no. 154 (October 1995): 1386–89.

6. J. A. Antenor et al., "Relationship between Initial Prostate Specific Antigen Level and Subsequent Prostate Cancer Detection in a Longitudinal Screening Study," *J Urol* 1, no. 172 (July 2004): 90–93.

7. P. H. Gann, G. H. Hennekens, and M. J. Stampfer, *JA. M.A.* 4, no. 273 (January 1995): 289–94.

8. J. E. Oesterling et al., "Serum Prostate-Specific Antigen in a Community-based Population of Healthy Men: Establishment of Age-Specific Reference Ranges," *JA. M.A.*, no. 270 (1993): 860.

9. J. C. Presti Jr. et al., "Extended Peripheral Zone Biopsy Schemes Increase Cancer Detection Rates and Minimize Variance in Prostate Specific Antigen and Age Related Cancer Rates: Results of a Community Multi-practice Study," *Journal of Urology* 1, no. 169 (January 2003): 125–29.

10. J. C. Presti Jr. and P. R. Carroll, "Use of Prostate Specific Antigen (PSA) and PSA Density in the Detection of State T1 Carcinoma of the Prostate," *Semin Urol Oncol* 3, no. 14 (1996): 134–38; D. W. Keetch et al., "Prostate Specific Antigen Density versus Prostate Specific Antigen Slope as Predictors of Prostate Cancer in Men with Initially Negative Prostatic Biopsies," *J Urol*, no. 156 (1996): 428–31.

11. B. Djavan et al., "Optimal Predictors of Prostate Cancer in Repeat Prostate Biopsy: A Prospective Study in 1,051 Men," *J Urol*, no. 163 (2000): 1144–48.

12. I. M. Thompson et al., "Prevalence of Prostate Cancer among Men with a Prostate-specific Antigen Level < or = 4.0ng per Milliliter," *N Engl J Med* 22, no. 350 (May 2004): 2239–46.

13. L. A. G. Ries et al., eds., *National Cancer Institute, SEER Cancer Statistics Review, 1975–2001*, http://seer.cancer.gov/csr/1975_2001/.

14. G. W. Horninger et al., "Prostate Cancer Mortality after Introduction of Prostate-Specific Antigen Mass Screening in the Federal State of Tyrol, Austria," *Urology* 3, no. 58 (2001): 417–24.

15. F. Labrie et al., "Screening Decreases Prostate Cancer Death: First Analysis of the 1988 Quebec Prospective Randomized Controlled Trial," *Prostate* 2, no. 38 (1999): 83–91.

16. R. O. Roberts et al., "Decline in Prostate Cancer Mortality from 1980 to 1997, and an Update on Incidence Trends in Olmsted County, Minnesota," *J Urol*, no. 161 (1999): 529–33.

17. S. L. Yao and G. Lu-Yao, "Interval after Prostate-Specific Antigen Testing and Subsequent Risk of Incurable Prostate Cancer," *J Urol* 3, no. 166 (2001): 861–65.

18. K. S. Ross et al., "Comparative Efficiency of Prostate-specific Antigen Screening Strategies for Prostate Cancer Detection," *JA. M.A.* 11, no. 284 (2000): 1399–1405.

19. P. H. Gann, G. H. Hennekens, and M. J. Stampfer, *JA. M.A.* 4, no. 273 (1995): 289–94.

CHAPTER TWELVE

1. M. Nadji et al., "Prostatic-Specific Antigen: An Immunohistologic Marker for Prostatic Neoplasms," *Cancer*, no. 48 (1981): 1229–32.

2. H. Ragde, H. C. Aldape, and C. M. Bagley Jr., "Ultrasound-Guided Prostate Biopsy: Biopsy Gun Superior to Aspiration," *Urology*, no. 32 (1988): 503–506.

3. K. K. Hodge et al., "Random Systematic versus Directed Ultrasound-guided Core Biopsies of the Prostate," *J Urol*, no. 142 (1989): 71–75.

4. J. M. Carey and J. H. Korman, "Transrectal Ultrasound Guided Biopsy of the Prostate: Do Enemas Decrease Clinically Significant Complications?" *J Urol*, no. 166 (2001): 82–85; G. Vallancien et al., "Systematic Prostatic Biopsies in 100 Men with No Suspicion of Cancer on Digital Rectal Examination," *J Urol*, no. 146 (1991): 1308–12.

5. M. Davis et al., "The Procedure of Transrectal Ultrasound Guided Biopsy of the Prostate: A Survey of Patient Preparation and Biopsy Technique," *J Urol*, no. 167 (2002): 566–70.

6. Hodge et al., "Random Systematic versus Directed Ultrasound-Guided Core Biopsies."

7. T.A. Stamey, "Making the Most out of Sex Systematic Sextant Biopsies," *Urology*, no. 45 (1995): 2–12.

8. T. A. Stamey et al., "The Prostate Specific Antigen Era in the United States

Is Over for Prostate Cancer: What Happened in the Last 20 Years?" *J Urol* 4, no. 172 (October 2004): 1297–1301.

9. J. Rabets et al., "Prostate Cancer Detection with Office-based Saturation Biopsy in a Repeat Biopsy Population," *J Urol*, no. 172 (July 2004).

10. Ibid.

11. Ibid.

12. P. Nash et al., "Transrectal Ultrasound Guided Prostatic Nerve Blockade Eases Systemic Needle Biopsy of the Prostate," *J Urol*, no. 155 (1996): 607.

13. M. S. Soloway and C. Obek, "Periprostatic Local Anesthesia before Ultrasound Guided Prostate Biopsy," *J Urol* 1, no. 163 (January 2000): 172–73.

14. A. Zisman et al., "The Impact of Prostate Biopsy on Patient Well-being: A Prospective Study of Pain, Anxiety, and Erectile Dysfunction," *J Urol*, no. 165 (2001): 445–54.

15. K. A. Roehl, J. A. V. Atenor, and W. J. Catalona, "Serial Biopsy Results in Prostate Cancer Screening Study," *J Urol* 6, no. 67 (2002): 2435–39.

16. J. C. Rabets et al., "Marcaine Provides Rapid, Effective Periprostatic Anesthesia for Transrectal Prostate Biopsy," *BJU Int* (2004).

17. A. S. Alavi et al., "Local Anesthesia for Ultrasound Guided Prostate Biopsy: A Prospective Randomized Trial Comparing Two Methods," *J Urol*, no. 166 (2001): 1343–45.

18. J. S. Jones et al., "Periprostatic Local Anesthesia Eliminates Pain of Office-Based Transrectal Prostate Biopsy," *Prostate Cancer and Prostatic Diseases*, no. 6 (2003): 53–55.

19. C. Obek et al., "Is Periprostatic Local Anesthesia for Transrectal Ultrasound Guided Prostate Biopsy Associated with Increased Infectious or Hemorrhagic Complications? A Prospective Randomized Controlled Trial," *J Urol*, no. 168 (2002): 558–61.

20. Lou Liou abstract.

21. C. Magi-Galluzzi et al., "Prostate Cancer and Prostatic Intraepithelial Neoplasia Detection Rate by Saturation Needle Biopsy," USCAP Annual Meeting, San Antonio, TX February 2005.

22. G. K. Lefkowitz et al., "Is Repeat Prostate Biopsy for High-grade Prostatic Intraepithelial Neoplasia Necessary after Routine 12-Core Sampling?" *Urology* 6, no. 58 (December 2001): 999–1003.

23. G. K. Lefkowitz et al., "Follow-up Interval Prostate Biopsy 3 Years after Diagnosis of High Grade Prostatic Intraepithelial Neoplasia Is Associated with High Likelihood of Prostate Cancer, Independent of Change in Prostate Specific Antigen Levels," *Urol* 4, no. 168 (October 2002): 1415–18.

24. D. W. Keetch, W. J. Catalona, and D. S. Smith, "Serial Prostatic Biopsies in Men with Persistently Elevated Serum Prostate Specific Antigen Values," *Journal of Urology*, no. 151 (1994): 1571–74.

25. A. P. Berger et al., "Complication Rate of Transrectal Ultrasound Guided Prostate Biopsy: A Comparison among 3 Protocols with 6, 10, and 15 Cores," *J Urol*, no. 171 (2004): 1478–81.

26. F. W. Cheney, "The American Society of Anesthesiologists Closed Claims Project: What Have We Learned, How Has It Affected Practice, and How Will It Affect Practice in the Future?" *Anesthesiology* 2, no. 91 (1999): 552–56.

27. J. S. Jones, M. Oder, and C. D. Zippe, "Saturation Biopsy with Periprostatic Block Can Be Performed in Office," *J Urol*, no. 168 (2002): 2108–10.

28. A. Patel et al., "Parasaggital Biopsies Add Minimal Information in Repeat Saturation Prostate Biopsy," *Urology* 1, no. 63 (2004): 87–89.

29. J. Rabets et al., "Prostate Cancer Detection with Office-Based Saturation Biopsy in a Repeat Biopsy Population," *J Urol*, no. 172 (July 2004).

CHAPTER THIRTEEN

1. E. Kübler-Ross, *On Death and Dying* (New York: Macmillan, 1969).

2. J. S. Jones and H. W. Follis, "The Decreasing Incidence of Stage T1a and T1b Prostatic Adenocarcinoma in the Era of PSA Screening," North Central Section American Urological Association Annual Meeting, Chicago, IL, January 18, 2002.

3. S. F. Shariat et al., "Lymphovascular Invasion Is a Pathological Feature of Biologically Aggressive Disease in Patients Treated with Radical Prostatectomy," *J Urol*, no. 171 (2004): 1122–27.

4. J. E. Oesterling et al., "The Use of Prostate Specific Antigen in Staging Patients with Newly Diagnosed Prostate Cancer," *JA. M.A.*, no. 269 (1993): 57–60.

5. Ibid.

6. M. Skacel et al., "Multitarget Fluorescence In Situ Hybridization Assay Detects Transitional Cell Carcinoma in the Majority of Patients with Bladder Cancer and Atypical or Negative Urine Cytology," *J Urol*, no. 169 (2003): 2101-2105.

7. "Post-RP Imaging Modality Yields Disappointing Results," *Urology Times*, September 1, 2002, http://ut.adv100.com/urologytimes/article/articleDetail.jsp?id=34513 (accessed November 11, 2004).

8. L. E. Ponsky et al., "Evaluation of Preoperative Prostascint Scans in the Prediction of Nodal Disease," *Prostate Cancer and Prostatic Dis* 2, no. 5 (2002): 132–35.

9. Personal communication, 2004.

CHAPTER FOURTEEN

1. E. M. Messing and I. Thompson Jr., "Follow-up of Conservatively Managed Prostate Cancer: Watchful Waiting and Primary Hormonal Therapy," *Urol Clin North Am* 4, no. 30 (November 2003): 687–702.

2. L. Holmberg et al., "Scandinavian Prostatic Cancer Group Study Number 4:

A Randomized Trial Comparing Radical Prostatectomy with Watchful Waiting in Early Prostate Cancer," *New Engl J Med* 11, no. 347 (2002): 781–89.

3. M. I. Patel et al., "An Analysis of Men with Clinically Localized Prostate Cancer Who Deferred Definitive Therapy," *J Urol* 4, no. 171 (April 2004): 1520–24.

4. H. B. Carter et al., "Expectant Management of Nonpalpable Prostate Cancer with Curative Intent: Preliminary Results," *J Urol* 3, no. 167 (March 2002): 1231–34.

5. F. R. William and W. Whitmore Jr., "Lecture: Back to the Future—The Role of Complementary Medicine in Urology," *J Urol*, no. 162 (1999): 411.

6. E. J. Small et al., "Prospective Trial of the Herbal Supplement PC-SPES in Patients with Progressive Prostate Cancer," *J Clin Oncol* 21, no. 18 (November 2000): 3595–03.

7. US Food and Drug Administration, "State Health Director Warns Consumers About Prescription Drugs in Herbal Products," MedWatch, February 7, 2002, http://www.fda.gov/medwatch/SAFETY/2002/spes_press1.htm (accessed November 11, 2004).

CHAPTER FIFTEEN

1. D. M. Quinlan, J. I. Epstein, B. S. Carter, and P. C. Walsh, "Sexual Function Following Radical Prostatectomy: Influence of Preservation of Neurovascular Bundles," *J Urol*, no. 145 (1991): 998–1002.

2. F. Van der Aa et al., "Potency after Unilateral Nerve Sparing Surgery: A Report on Functional and Oncological Results of Unilateral Nerve Sparing Surgery," *Prostate Cancer and Prostatic Dis* 1, no. 6 (2003): 61–65.

3. A. Fergany et al., "No Difference in Biochemical Failure Rates with or without Pelvic Lymph Node Dissection during Radical Prostatectomy in Low-Risk Patients," *Urology* 1, no. 56 (July 2000): 92–95.

4. T. Clarke et al., "Randomized Prospective Evaluation of Extended versus Limited Lymph Node Dissection in Patients with Clinically Localized Prostate Cancer," *J Urol* 1, no. 169 (January 2003): 145–47.

5. H. J. Korman et al., "Radical Prostatectomy: Is Complete Resection of the Seminal Vesicles Really Necessary?" *J Urol* 3, no. 156 (September 1996): 1081–83.

6. H. John and D. Hauri, "Seminal Vesicle–Sparing Radical Prostatectomy: A Novel Concept to Restore Early Urinary Continence," *Urology* 6, no. 55 (June 2000): 820–24.

7. M. Menon, A. Shrivastava et al., "Vattikuti Institute Prostatectomy: A Single-Team Experience of 100 Cases," *J Endourol* 9, no. 17 (November 2003): 785–90.

8. J. C. Hu et al., "The Effect of Clustering of Outcomes on the Association of Procedure Volume and Surgical Outcomes," *Ann Intern Med* 8, no. 139 (October 2003): 658–65.

9. W. J. Catalona et al., "Potency, Continence and Complication Rates in 1870 Consecutive Radical Retropubic Prostatectomies," *J Urol*, no. 162 (1999): 433–38.

10. B. R. Straatsma et al., "Posterior Chamber Intraocular Lens Implantation by Ophthalmology Residents: A Prospective Study of Cataract Surgery," *Ophthalmology*, no. 90 (1983): 327–35

11. J. L. Epstein, "Pathologic Assessment of the Surgical Specimen," *Urol Clin North Am*, no. 28 (2001): 567–94.

12. M. O. Koch and J. A. Smith Jr., "Blood Loss During Radical Retropubic Prostatectomy: Is Preoperative Autologous Blood Donation Indicated?" *J Urol* 3, no. 156 (September 1996): 1077–79; Discussion, 1079–80.

13. http://www.redcross.org/faq/0,1096,0_315_,00.html#379 (accessed July 19, 2004).

14. M. Davis et al., "The Use of Cell Salvage During Radical Retropubic Prostatectomy: Does It Influence Cancer Recurrence?" *BJU Int* 6, no. 91 (April 2003): 474–76.

15. A. J. Stephenson et al., "Salvage Radiotherapy for Recurrent Prostate Cancer after Radical Prostatectomy," *JA. M.A.* 11, no. 291 (March 2004): 1325–32.

16. N. S. Goldstein et al., "Minimal or No Cancer in Radical Prostatectomy Specimens: Report of 13 Cases of the 'Vanishing Cancer Phenomenon,'" *Am J Surg Pathol* 9, no. 19 (1995): 1002–1009.

CHAPTER SIXTEEN

1. P. F. Schellhammer et al., "Prostate-Specific Antigen after Radiation Therapy: Prognosis by Pretreatment Level and Post-Treatment Nadir," *Urol Clin North Am* 2, no. 24 (May 1997): 407–14.

2. A. V. D'Amico et al., *Campbell's Urology*, 8th ed., ed. M. P. Walsh, Alan B. Retik, and E. Darracott Vaughan (Philadelphia: Saunders, 2002), p. 3148.

3. I. H. Derweesh et al., "Continuing Trends in Pathological Stage Migration in Radical Prostatectomy Specimens," *Urol Oncol* 4, no. 22 (July–August 2004): 300–306.

4. P. M. Windsor, K. F. Nicol, and J. Potter, "A Randomized, Controlled Trial of Aerobic Exercise for Treatment-Related Fatigue in Men Receiving Radical External Beam Radiotherapy for Localized Prostate Carcinoma," *Cancer* 3, no. 101 (August 2004): 550–57.

5. L. R. Schover et al., "Defining Sexual Outcomes after Treatment for Localized Prostate Carcinoma," *Cancer* 8, no. 95 (October 2002): 1773–85; A. L. Potosky et al., "Five-Year Outcomes after Prostatectomy or Radiotherapy for Prostate Cancer: The Prostate Cancer Outcomes Study," *Journal of the National Cancer Institute* 18, no. 96 (September 2004): 1358–67.

6. P. A. Johnstone et al., "Second Primary Malignancies in T1-3N0 Prostate

Cancer Patients Treated with Radiation Therapy with 10-Year Follow-up," *J Urol* 3, no. 159 (March 1998): 946–49.

7. "Post-RP Imaging Modality Yields Disappointing Results," *Urology Times*, September 1, 2002, http://ut.adv100.com/urologytimes/article/articleDetail.jsp?id=34513 (accessed November 11, 2004).

8. J. D. Slater et al., "Proton Therapy for Prostate Cancer: The Initial Loma Linda University Experience," *Int J Radiat Oncol Biol Phys* 2, no. 59 (June 2004): 348–52.

9. R. Peschel et al., "Long-Term Complications with Prostate Implants: Iodine-125 vs. Palladium-103," *Radiat Oncol Investig*, no. 7 (1999): 278–288.

10. C. Ianuzzi, R. Stock, and N. Stone, "PSA Kinetics Following I-125 Radioactive Seed Implantation in the Treatment of T1-T2 Prostate Cancer," *Radiat Oncol Invest*, no. 7 (1999): 30–35.

11. H. Ragde et al., "Ten-Year Disease Free Survival after Transperineal Sonography-Guided Iodine-125 Brachytherapy with or without 45-Gray External Beam Irradiation in the Treatment of Patients with Clinically Localized Low to High Grade Prostate Carcinoma," *Cancer*, no. 83 (1998): 989–1001.

12. C. Patel et al., "PSA Bounce Predicts Early Success in Patients with Permanent Iodine-125 Prostate Implant," *Urology* 1, no. 63 (January 2004): 110–13.

13. L. Potters et al., "Monotherapy for Stage T1–T2 Prostate Cancer: Radical Prostatectomy, External Beam Radiotherapy, or Permanent Seed Implantation," *Radiother Oncol* 1, no. 71 (April 2004): 29–33.

14. T. Pickles et al., "The Effect of Smoking on Outcome Following External Radiation for Localized Prostate Cancer," *J Urol* 4, no. 171 (April 2004): 1543–46.

CHAPTER SEVENTEEN

1. R. L. Cox and E. D. Crawford, "Complications of Cryosurgical Ablation of the Prostate to Treat Localized Adenocarcinoma of the Prostate," *Urology* 6, no. 45 (June 1995): 932–35.

2. A. E. Katz and J. C. Rewcastle, "The Current and Potential Role of Cryoablation as a Primary Therapy for Localized Prostate Cancer," *Curr Oncol Rep* 3, no. 5 (May 2003): 231–38.

3. K. Shinohara, "Prostate Cancer: Cryotherapy," *Urol Clin North Am* 4, no. 30 (November 2003): 725–36.

CHAPTER EIGHTEEN

1. L. Holmberg et al., "A Randomized Trial Comparing Radical Prostatectomy with Watchful Waiting in Early Prostate Cancer," *N Engl J Med*, no. 347 (2002): 781.

2. S. M. H. Alibhai , "Do Older Men Benefit from Curative Therapy of Localized Prostate Cancer?" *J Clin Oncol* 17, no. 21 (2003): 3318–27.

3. G. W. Hull et al., "Cancer Control with Radical Prostatectomy Alone in 1000 Consecutive Patients," *J Urol*, no. 167 (2002): 528–34.

4. Personal communication, October 12, 2004.

5. J. T. Wei et al., "Comprehensive Comparison of Health-Related Quality of Life after Contemporary Therapies for Localized Prostate Cancer," *J Clin Oncol* 2, no. 20 (January 2002): 557–66.

6. A. L. Potosky et al., "Five-Year Outcomes after Prostatectomy or Radiotherapy for Prostate Cancer: The Prostate Cancer Outcomes Study," *Journal of the National Cancer Institute* 18, no. 96 (September 2004): 1358–67.

7. L. Potters, E. A. Klein, M. W. Kattan, C. A. Reddy, J. P. Ciezki, A. M. Reuther, and P. A. Kupelian, "Monotherapy for Stage T1–T2 Prostate Cancer: Radical Prostatectomy, External Beam Radiotherapy, or Permanent Seed Implantation," *Radiother Oncol* 1, no. 71 (April 2004): 29–33.

CHAPTER NINETEEN

1. H. A. Feldman et al., "Impotence and Its Medical and Psychological Correlates: Results of the Massachusetts Male Aging Study," *J Urol*, no. 151 (1994): 54.

2. L. R. Schover et al., "Defining Sexual Outcomes after Treatment for Localized Prostate Carcinoma," *Cancer* 8, no. 95 (October 2002): 1773–85.

3. T. Siegel et al., "The Development of Erectile Dysfunction in Men Treated for Prostate Cancer," *J Urol* 2, no. 165 (February 2001): 430–35; G. Steineck, et al., "Scandinavian Prostatic Cancer Group Study Number 4: Quality of Life after Radical Prostatectomy or Watchful Waiting," *N Engl J Med* 11, no. 347 (September 2002): 790–96.

4. J. S. Jones, *Overcoming Impotence* (Amherst, NY: Prometheus Books, 2003).

CHAPTER TWENTY

1. J. A. Eastham and P. T. Scardino, *Campbell's Urology*, 8th ed., ed. M. P. Walsh, Alan B. Retik, and E. Darracott Vaughan (Philadelphia: Saunders, 2002), p. 3089.

2. R. M. Benoit, M. J. Naslund, and J. K. Cohen, "Complications after Prostate Brachytherapy in the Medicare Population," *Urology*, no. 55 (2000): 91–96.

3. E. S. Geary et al., "Incontinence and Vesical Neck Strictures Following Radical Retropubic Prostatectomy," *Urology*, no. 45 (1995a): 1000–1006.

4. G. S. Merrick et al., "The Dosimetry of Prostate Brachytherapy-induced Urethral Strictures," *Int J Radiat Oncol Biol Phys*, no. 52 (2002): 461–68.

5. P. C. Walsh, "Anatomical Radical Retropubic Prostatectomy: Detailed Description of the Surgical Technique," *J Urol*, no. 171 (2004): 2114.

6. M. Savoie et al., "A Prospective Study Measuring Penile Length in Men Treated with Radical Prostatectomy for Prostate Cancer," *J Urol* 4, no. 169 (April 2003): 1462–64.

CHAPTER TWENTY-ONE

1. F. M. Jhaveri et al., "Biochemical Failure Does Not Predict Overall Survival after Radical Prostatectomy for Localized Prostate Cancer: 10-Year Results," *Urology* 5, no. 54 (November 1999): 884–90.

CHAPTER TWENTY-TWO

1. D. Weckermann and R. Harzmann, "Hormone Therapy in Prostate Cancer: LHRH Antagonists versus LHRH Analogues," *Eur Urol* 3, no. 46 (September 2004): 279–88.

2. A. Koupparis, A. Ramsden, and R. Persad, "Cognitive Effects of Hormonal Treatment for Prostate Cancer," *BJU Int* 7, no. 93 (May 2004): 915–16.

3. M. Laufer et al., "Complete Androgen Blockade for Prostate Cancer: What Went Wrong?" *J Urol* 1, no. 164 (July 2000):3–9.

4. Ibid.

5. D. P. Byar and D. K. Corle, "Hormone Therapy for Prostate Cancer: Results of the Veterans Administration Cooperative Urological Research Group Studies," *NCI Monogr*, no. 7 (1988): 165–70.

6. M. S. Solowayet al., "Lupron Depot Neoadjuvant Prostate Cancer Study Group: Neoadjuvant Androgen Ablation before Radical Prostatectomy in Ct2bnxmo Prostate Cancer: 5-Year Results," *J Urol* 1, no. 167 (January 2002): 112–16.

CHAPTER TWENTY-THREE

1. C. R. Pound et al., "Natural History of Progression after PSA Elevation Following Radical Prostatectomy," *JA. M.A.*, no. 282 (1999): 1591.

2. C. L. Amling et al., "Defining Prostate Specific Antigen Progression after Radical Prostatectomy: What Is the Most Appropriate Cut Point?" *J Urol* 4, no. 165 (April 2001): 1146–51.

3. M. A. Eisenberger and M. A. Carducci, *Campbell's Urology*, 8th ed., ed. M. P. Walsh, Alan B. Retik, and E. Darracott Vaughan (Philadelphia: Saunders, 2002), p. 3210.

4. D. P. Petrylak et al., "Docetaxel and Estramustine Compared with Mitox-

antrone and Prednisone for Advanced Refractory Prostate Cancer," *N Engl J Med* 15, no. 351 (October 2004): 1513–20.

5. P. L. Jager, A. Kooistra, and D. A. Piers, "Treatment with Radioactive (89)Strontium for Patients with Bone Metastases from Prostate Cancer," *BJU Int* 8, no. 86 (November 2000): 929–34.

CHAPTER TWENTY-FOUR:

1. J. S. P. Yuen et al., "Endorectal Magnetic Resonance Imaging and Spectroscopy for the Detection of Tumor Foci in Men with Prior Negative Transrectal Ultrasound Biopsy," *J Urol*, no. 171 (2004): 1482–86.

2. J. Li et al., "Detection of Prostate Cancer Using Serum Proteomics Pattern in a Histologically Confirmed Population," *J Urol* 5, no. 171 (May 2004): 1782–87.

3. T. Sheng et al., "Activation of the Hedgehog Pathway in Advanced Prostate Cancer," *Mol Cancer* 1, no. 3 (October 2004): 29.

4. J. S. Jones et al., "Sling May Enhance Return of Continence Following Radical Prostatectomy," *Urology* 6, no. 65 (2005): 1163–67.

5. G. Onik et al., "Focal 'Nerve-Sparing' Cryotherapy for Treatment of Primary Prostate Cancer: A New Approach to Preserving Potency," *Urology* 1, no. 60 (July 2002): 109–14.

6. R. Rackley and J. Abdelmalak, "Urologic Applications of Botulinum Toxin Therapy for Voiding Dysfunction," *Curr Urol Rep* 5, no. 5 (October 2004): 381–88; M. K. Plante, J. B. Folsom, and P. Zvara, "Prostatic Tissue Ablation by Injection: A Literature Review," *J Urol* 1, no. 172 (July 2004): 20–26.

7. http://www.pharma.org/publications/quickfacts/01.03.2001.34.cfm (accessed January 8, 2004).

8. Department of Health and Human Services, National Institutes of Health, *Medicines by Design—ABCs of Pharmacology.*

INDEX